"The COVID-19 pandemic has been in most ways disastrous, but it has fostered a wave of interesting social science studies about how individuals and societies have responded. This book is one of the more interesting and useful of the comparative accounts of governments facing the pandemic. With a wide array of cases, and a framework based on trust, this book provides numerous insights into the ways in which governments can respond to crisis."

B. Guy Peters, *University of Pittsburgh, USA.*

"*Policy Styles and Trust in the Age of Pandemics* provides forensic investigations of how ten governments responded to the COVID-19 crisis in the year 2020. Highly informative, the individual chapters are ideal for case study analysis in class. But their comparison is also leveraged to test hypotheses on policy styles during a crisis. It sheds novel light on the crucial role of trustworthy bureaucracies. The volume is a milestone in our understanding of governance, what to expect from policy responses to a fast-burning crisis and why we must build trust in bureaucracies."

Claudio M. Radaelli, *School of Transnational Governance (EUI) and University College London, UK.*

"Too often accounts of national responses to policy issues or governance problems focus on the same set of countries. This collection is genuinely international in drawing upon analysis from all corners of the world. For policy scholars and practitioners alike, this is an invaluable resource for understanding the reasons behind the diversity of governmental responses to a common problem."

Diane Stone, *School of Transnational Governance, EUI, Italy.*

POLICY STYLES AND TRUST IN THE AGE OF PANDEMICS

This book explores the reasons behind the variation in national responses to the COVID-19 pandemic. In doing so, it furthers the policy studies scholarship through an examination of the effects of policy styles on national responses to the pandemic.

Despite governments being faced with the same threat, significant variation in national responses, frequently of contradictory nature, has been observed. Implications about responses inform a broader class of crises beyond this specific context. The authors argue that trust in government interacts with policy styles resulting in different responses and that the acute turbulence, uncertainty, and urgency of crises complicate the ability of policymakers to make sense of the problem. Finally, the book posits that unless there is high trust between society and the state, a decentralized response will likely be disastrous and concludes that while national responses to crises aim to save lives, they also serve to project political power and protect the status quo.

This text will be of key interest to scholars and students of public policy, public administration, political science, sociology, public health, and crisis management/disaster management studies.

Nikolaos Zahariadis is Mertie Buckman Chair and Professor of International Studies at Rhodes College, USA.

Evangelia Petridou is Associate Professor of Political Science at Mid Sweden University, Sweden.

Theofanis Exadaktylos is Reader in European Politics at the Department of Politics, University of Surrey, UK.

Jörgen Sparf is Associate Professor in Sociology and a founding member of the Risk and Crisis Research Centre at Mid Sweden University, Sweden.

Routledge Studies in Governance and Public Policy

Middle Class and Welfare State
Making Sense of an Ambivalent Relationship
Marlon Barbehön, Marilena Geugjes, and Michael Haus

Localism and the Design of Political Systems
Rick Harmes

Varieties of Risk Analysis in Public Administrations
Problem-Solving and Polity Policies in Europe
Regine Paul

The Politics of Local Innovation
Conditions for the Development of Innovations
Edited by Hubert Heinelt, Björn Egner and Nikolaos-Komninos Hlepas

Municipal Territorial Reforms of the 21st Century in Europe
Paweł Swianiewicz, Adam Gendźwiłł, Kurt Houlberg and Jan Erling Klausen

Coping with Migrants and Refugees
Multilevel Governance across the EU
Edited by Tiziana Caponio and Irene Ponzo

Policy Styles and Trust in the Age of Pandemics
Global Threat, National Responses
Edited by Nikolaos Zahariadis, Evangelia Petridou, Theofanis Exadaktylos and Jörgen Sparf

For more information about this series, please visit: https://www.routledge.com

POLICY STYLES AND TRUST IN THE AGE OF PANDEMICS

Global Threat, National Responses

Edited by
Nikolaos Zahariadis, Evangelia Petridou,
Theofanis Exadaktylos and Jörgen Sparf

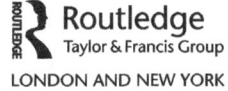

Routledge
Taylor & Francis Group

LONDON AND NEW YORK

Cover Image: © Martin Sanchez, Unsplash

First published 2022
by Routledge
4 Park Square, Milton Park, Abingdon, Oxon OX14 4RN

and by Routledge
605 Third Avenue, New York, NY 10158

Routledge is an imprint of the Taylor & Francis Group, an informa business

British Library Cataloguing-in-Publication Data
A catalogue record for this book is available from the British Library

Library of Congress Cataloging-in-Publication Data
A catalog record has been requested for this book

ISBN: 978-0-367-68396-2 (hbk)
ISBN: 978-0-367-68392-4 (pbk)
ISBN: 978-1-003-13739-9 (ebk)

DOI: 10.4324/9781003137399

Typeset in Bembo
by codeMantra

To the departed from COVID

CONTENTS

List of figures   *xiii*
List of tables   *xv*
Notes on contributors   *xvii*

I
Introduction   **1**

1 The Politics of National Responses to the COVID-19 Pandemic   3
   Nikolaos Zahariadis, Evangelia Petridou, Theofanis Exadaktylos
   and Jörgen Sparf

2 Policy Styles and Policymaking During Times of Crisis   17
   Nikolaos Zahariadis, Evangelia Petridou, Theofanis Exadaktylos
   and Jörgen Sparf

2
Centralized Responses   **39**

3 Policy Styles and the Chinese COVID-19 Response   41
   Stephen Ceccoli

4 Turkey's Response to the COVID-19 Pandemic   59
   Lacin Idil Oztig

5 Centralization and Lockdown: The Greek Response 79
Nikolaos Zahariadis and Vassilis Karokis-Mavrikos

6 Kenya's Response to COVID-19: Lockdown and Stringent
Enforcement 101
Shadrack W. Nasong'o

3
Centripetal Responses 117

7 Norwegian Corporatism: A Centripetal National Response
to the Pandemic 119
Jörgen Sparf

8 New Zealand COVID Response: Leadership,
Communication, and Trust 134
W. John Hopkins and Annick Masselot

4
Centrifugal Responses 155

9 Of "Herd Immunity" and Inoculation Investment: The
British Response to COVID-19 157
Theofanis Exadaktylos

10 The Breakdown of Cooperative Federalism: Brazil's
Response to the COVID-19 Pandemic 174
Valesca Lima and José de Arimatéia da Cruz

11 The U.S. Response to the COVID-19 Pandemic:
Incoherent Leadership, Fractured Federalism, and
Squandered Capacity 191
Kristin Taylor, Rob A. DeLeo, Deserai A. Crow and
Thomas A. Birkland

5
Decentralized Responses 209

12 Following the Public Health Agency's Guidelines:
The Swedish Approach to the COVID-19 Pandemic 211
Evangelia Petridou

6
Comparing Responses 229

13 Different Governments, Different Responses to the
   COVID-19 Pandemic? Concluding Remarks and the Way
   Forward 231
   Jale Tosun

Index *251*

FIGURES

1.1	A Typology of Policy Styles	11
2.1	A Typology of Policy Styles	28
4.1	New Daily Confirmed COVID-19 Cases in Turkey	70
4.2	Daily Deaths from COVID-19 in Turkey	70
5.1	New Daily Confirmed COVID-19 Cases in Greece	85
5.2	Regional Map of COVID-19 Cases per 100,000 of Population in Greece (October 19, 2020–October 29, 2020)	90
5.3	Greece's Response as a Function of Administrative Style and Fluctuating Political Trust	93
7.1	Notification and reporting lines in the health sector in the event of crises	124
9.1	Daily Cases Versus Stringency of Measures	161
9.2	Daily Recorded Deaths Versus Stringency of Measures	161
10.1	Approval Ratings for President Bolsonaro (June–November 2020)	182
13.1	Trust in Politicians, 2016/2017	234
13.2	Government Effectiveness, 2019	235
13.3	Reproduction Rate, 2020	236

TABLES

6.1   Hierarchy of Kenya's Health Institutions   104
10.1 Survey characteristics and overall adherence to mask-use for
      COVID-19 prevention in selected countries   183
11.1 Face-covering requirements by state as of February 17, 2021   203
12.1 Overview of Contagion Mitigation Measures   219

NOTES ON CONTRIBUTORS

Thomas A. Birkland is Professor of Public Policy in the School of Public and International Affairs at North Carolina State University, USA.

Stephen Ceccoli is Professor of International Studies, Rhodes College, USA.

Deserai A. Crow is Associate Professor of Public Affairs in the School of Public Affairs at the University of Colorado-Denver, USA.

José de Arimatéia da Cruz is Professor of International Relations and Comparative Politics at Georgia Southern University, Armstrong Campus, Savannah, Georgia, USA.

Rob A. DeLeo is an Associate Professor of Public Policy in the Department of Global Studies at Bentley University, USA.

Theofanis Exadaktylos is Reader in European Politics at the Department of Politics, University of Surrey, UK.

W. John Hopkins is a Professor of Law and Director of the Institute of Law, Emergencies and Disasters (LEAD), Faculty of Law, University of Canterbury, Aotearoa New Zealand.

Vassilis Karokis-Mavrikos is a PhD Candidate in European Public Policy at the Faculty of Arts and Social Sciences (FASS) of the University of Surrey, UK.

Valesca Lima is an Assistant Professor in Dublin City University at the Department of Law and Governance, Ireland.

Annick Masselot is Professor of Law, Faculty of Law, University of Canterbury, Aotearoa New Zealand.

Shadrack W. Nasong'o is Professor of International Studies at Rhodes College in Memphis, Tennessee, USA.

Lacin Idil Oztig is Associate Professor of International Relations at the Department of Political Science and International Relations, Yildiz Technical University, Istanbul, Turkey.

Evangelia Petridou is Associate Professor of Political Science at Mid Sweden University.

Jörgen Sparf is Associate Professor in Sociology and founding member of the Risk and Crisis Research Centre at Mid Sweden University.

Kristin Taylor is an Associate Professor in the Department of Political Science at Wayne State University, USA.

Jale Tosun is Professor of Political Science at the Institute of Political Science at Heidelberg University, Germany.

Nikolaos Zahariadis is Mertie Buckman Chair and Professor of International Studies at Rhodes College, USA.

I

Introduction

1

THE POLITICS OF NATIONAL RESPONSES TO THE COVID-19 PANDEMIC

Nikolaos Zahariadis, Evangelia Petridou,
Theofanis Exadaktylos and Jörgen Sparf

> *Please tell only who you must. I don't want to be responsible for a panic. And get to a boat*
> *quickly.*
>
> (Thomas Andrews, architect of the Titanic, played by
> Victor Garber, in the film *Titanic*)

When the *Titanic* hit an iceberg on that cold April morning of 1912, it caused great panic among passengers and crew. James Cameron brilliantly captured the subsequent confusion in his 1997 film of the same name by showing how people reacted to their impending doom. Some pushed and shoved their way to the lifeboats, others shot and were shot to death trying to escape, and still others wore their best clothes waiting patiently for the inevitable. Some wondered aimlessly, the band kept on playing as if nothing had happened, and others tried to help the less fortunate. Clearly, the same crisis elicited very different responses.

National governments behave in similar fashion. When the first cases of what we know now to be SARS-CoV-2 which causes COVID-19 emerged in China in early 2020, the Chinese government ignored available information to preserve the *status quo* in fear of appearing weak and indecisive (Ceccoli this volume; Mei 2020; Zahariadis, Ceccoli, and Petridou 2021). As a result, the coronavirus spread nationally and later internationally. Some governments immediately and proactively took measures to stop its spread, others waited for the dust to clear, while others downplayed the severity of the threat and kept on as if nothing had happened. Clearly, different governments responded to the same crisis in very different ways (Capano et al. 2020). Why?

In this book, we explore the variety of responses by national governments to the COVID-19 pandemic in 2020. More specifically, *we examine the effects of national policy styles and political trust, arguing they interact and systematically lead*

DOI: 10.4324/9781003137399-2

to predictable responses, which range from centralized to decentralized policies. National policy styles (Howlett and Tosun 2019; Richardson 1982) cast long shadows onto public policy, constraining and shaping not only normal policymaking, as the literature claims, but also policies under crisis conditions. Crises are plastic in the sense that they are moments of flux and extreme uncertainty. Their exposure of vulnerabilities often prompts political leaders to think outside the box to reassure citizens they are in control. At one level, if we can show that leader responses rely systematically upon stable patterns and "standard operating procedures" of policymaking, we have a critical case of the "least likely" variety, what some have called a "hard" test for theory (e.g., Flyvbjerg 2006). Extending, that is, the applicability of the concept beyond its usual limits adds more analytical tractability to its use and theoretical implications.

At another level, we contribute to the broader literature on policymaking by linking past administrative capacity to present conceptualizations of problems and solutions. Different countries develop variable administrative policy capacities over the years, which frame their ability to respond. What they do depends largely on what they can do, and the latter is to an extent a function of inheritance (Rose 1990). Policymakers inherit commitments, institutional arrangements, modes of deliberation, and a host of "standard operating procedures" and norms that constitute a country's policy style. But policy style does not directly affect response. Because the panoply of measures depends to a large extent on compliance, political trust crucially interacts with style to explain responses to the COVID-19 pandemic. Contributors to this volume assess this argument in ten national contexts spanning all continents. While the crisis caused by the COVID-19 pandemic is highly salient because it affects all aspects of social life and possibly unique because it is rare, implications about responses inform a broader class of crises beyond this specific context. Pandemics are here to stay, and as *The Economist* (2020) observed, responses to COVID-19 are pointing to a new state of affairs, one that we argue leads to a reconfiguration of the ways of managing pandemics both at national and international levels and of the policy responses available to national governments and international organizations.

The COVID-19 Pandemic as Crisis

Why do governments respond so differently to more-or-less the same threat? Before we lay out the answer in more detail, we first need to define the threat. What is a crisis, and how do we know it when we see it? Much ink has been spilled on this topic, but the literature generally defines crises as perceived threats causing consequential, sharp disruptions in organizational or political life, which appear to require far-reaching responses (Boin et al. 2017, 5). Crises are *disruptions* in that they represent a break in a system's operational rhythm. They cause or have the potential to cause significant change (Keown-McMullan 1997). As such, they are relatively rare and temporally bounded. When a crisis lasts a long period of time, its effects and any new equilibria tend to be normalized. They are *sharp* because they are urgent and turbulent. There is uncertainty and a paucity of useful information (Boin 2019). During crises, people not only look up to their national governments but also follow opinion leaders to make sense of the situation, reinforce their own beliefs, and form an understanding of what to do to help resolve the crisis (Capelos and Exadaktylos 2017). They are *consequential* because they represent stress tests for political systems and their leaders (Boin et al. 2017, 3). They often expose or create significant social or political rifts and generate material and (possibly) human losses that demand attention (Olson 2000). Finally, crises involve *perceived threats*, usually in the form of triggering events, to basic social values that, if left unchecked, heighten the probability of even bigger damages (Brecher and Wilkenfeld 1997, 3). Inability to cope with damages necessitates a *response* (Keown-McMullan 1997). Responses require not only effective measures to deal with the threat but also narratives that explain the causes, reassure people's safety, and uphold social values. The more salient the threat in terms of damage or cost of response, the deeper the sense of crisis will likely be.

Pandemics create crises and add more elements to the mix. They spread over a number of national boundaries and jurisdictions. They also represent complex transboundary problems which require considerable information production, coordination, and communication (Boin 2019). They often end up becoming fundamental crises, that is, crises that are hard to predict and hard to influence (Gundel 2005). As such, pandemics necessitate mobilization of highly skilled technical expertise that may identify the culprit and design effective treatments in addition to utilizing administrative capacity and political will. But responses constitute "walks on clouds" because preparedness, safety regulation, and countermeasures have to deal with high levels of uncertainty. As a result, the mix of responses often only treats symptoms, at least initially, involving problematic and undesired tradeoffs between public health, social conditions, and adverse economic consequences.

Pandemics also add dramaturgic and fundamentally political elements to the response ('t Hart 1993). As Rosenberg (1989, 2) asserts, pandemics[1] take "on the quality of pageant – mobilizing communities to act out proprietary rituals that incorporate and reaffirm fundamental social values and modes of understanding." As such, they combine politics with scientific expertise in what Rosenberg calls managing randomness, that is, the need to rationally understand the phenomenon in a way that promises control and minimizes vulnerability. But, more importantly, declaring a contagious disease a pandemic prompts decisive and visible public action. National response deploys, in turn, politically inspired collective rituals and familiar frames of community solidarity that provide both meaning and a sense of efficacy.

Pandemics create crises, and crises elicit policy responses of a fundamentally political character. Policy requires politics. Policies are ultimately made by politicians who occupy positions of formal authority. But their choices are not made in a vacuum. Somehow, the same policymakers need to produce support from bureaucracies who implement them, citizens who vote, and market actors who invest. If nothing else, responses to crises must generate compliance or even enthusiasm to minimize the cost of disruption and maximize the chances of recovery. Public campaigns of social distancing, lockdown, or inoculation are not only based on scientific evidence, but they are also framed in scientific terms to ensure compliance and political legitimacy.

COVID-19 has created such a crisis, replete with social rituals, political power plays, and costly community responses. It cuts across policy sectors and social classes, providing a rare glimpse into extraordinary policymaking. The crisis is important not simply in terms of salience—211.43 million confirmed cases worldwide (August 22, 2021) —or cost—4.43 million deaths (Johns Hopkins Coronavirus Resource Center 2021) and between $8.1 and $15.4 trillion in lost revenue globally (Dobson et al. 2020)—but also in terms of social values which are steeped in national traditions. Crises lay bare institutional (in)adequacies, leadership qualities, deep-seated social inequalities, and political (in)securities, and test the spirit of community as well as individual resilience. Therefore, national responses to pandemics reflect a dynamic and urgent interaction between individuals and the state; faith in the inherited capacity to deal with such threats and community trust toward the effectiveness of collective action. The urgent nature of the crisis does not leave much room for administrative reform, at least initially. Because different countries possess varying mixes of capacity, resources, and trust, national responses to the crisis caused by the COVID-19 pandemic should vary accordingly.

Big Village, High Fences

Even though it has created a global crisis by the very definition of pandemic, COVID-19 has prompted mostly national responses. Although global or regional institutions have not been successful at creating a worldwide systematic response, they have been instrumental in the dissemination of information, distributing medical materials to less affluent countries and caring for vulnerable social groups (such as immigrants, refugees, and domestic violence victims). Yet, at the same time, the pandemic has managed to reveal the inadequate levels of international cooperation and international organization funding, including the re-emergence of global cleavages and dormant alliances and enmities.

Additionally, the inability of transnational bodies to produce a successful coordinated response has exacerbated rifts among foes and allies, such as the war of words between China and the US (Gan 2020) and the eventual US withdrawal of funding from the World Health Organization (WHO)—as well as recriminations of unbecoming behavior between allies (Bouckaert et al. 2020). Additionally, in the middle of the first wave of the pandemic, Germany vocally complained to the US government of modern "piracy" for diverting masks and other personal protection equipment (PPE) to the US. In a similar vein, by imposing a ban on specific medical exports, the governments of France and Germany were accused by their Austrian, Swiss, and Italian counterparts of hoarding and economic nationalism (Tong 2020). In many ways, domestic politics has spilled over to the international level; COVID-19 has effectively nationalized policy responses.

For this reason, we seek answers at the national level of analysis. National borders have been used to defend against "foreign" carriers of the virus to prevent infection of local populations. Despite some pushback, heavy economic losses, and political recriminations, citizens in each country have more-or-less accepted national measures as legitimate and (in many cases) effective. To paraphrase an oft-used metaphor, we view the world as a "village" which is socially, technologically, and economically interdependent. But we notice high fences erected to protect some gated communities and, in all cases, individual houses. By exploring responses to the pandemic crisis at the national level, we elucidate differences and similarities and gain more insight into the effects of policy style and trust on policymaking under crisis conditions.

The Argument in Brief

We argue that the effects of the crisis caused by the pandemic are filtered through interactions between national policy styles and political trust, producing systematic variation in national responses. In countries with heavy administrative policy styles and low political trust in government, we observe top-down centralized response policies. In contrast, countries with more managerial policy styles and high political trust tend to adopt decentralized responses. We conclude that while national responses to crises aim to save lives, they also serve to project political power and protect the status quo. Serving as framing and political power contests (Boin et al. 2017), responses constitute political spectacles (Edelman 1988) that reflect and preserve the current distribution of power through symbolic politics ('t Hart 1993) and blame games (Hood 2011).

Choice of Time and Countries

To keep the study manageable and focused, we only analyze the responses to the first and second waves of COVID-19 cases from January 2020 to early January 2021. Focusing on short-term response plans, we set aside the preparedness and recovery phases of the crisis management cycle (Pursiainen 2018). This allows us to avoid examining policies aiming to slowly return social life back to some kind of normalcy, which pose different types of questions. Rather, our narrow focus provides for a sharper explanation of policy responses across ten countries.

The scope of this study is global, and for this reason, we chose countries that vary considerably in policy outcomes and in policy styles and trust, thereby increasing the generalizability of findings to a wider cohort of cases (Seawright and Gerring 2008). We conceptualize responses along a centralization continuum. China and Sweden represent the opposite ends: China adopted a highly centralized response with heavy concentration of steering capacity in the hands of a few national government agencies and very stringent lockdown measures while Sweden has pursued a far more decentralized approach with significant coordination across national agencies and no lockdown measures. Our sample includes democracies (and non-democracies) from all continents but Antarctica. Policy outcomes fall somewhere in-between the two extremes. Apart from China and Sweden, we compare responses in Greece, Norway, the United Kingdom, the United States, New Zealand, Turkey, Brazil, and Kenya.

We chose the countries using criteria of breadth and contrast. Our sample of national responses represents the full range of theoretically plausible variation, thus avoiding selection bias caused by truncation of the dependent variable (King, Keohane, and Verba 1994). Contrast ensures variation in styles and trust. Mapping them for each country avoids the pitfalls of idiosyncratic or only "great power" studies. To discount alternative explanations, we include democratic (and not) countries, industrialized states and developing countries, federal (and unitary) systems, and great (and not-so-great) powers. Each of these explanations—democracy, wealth, federalism, and power—affects the outcome. For example, centralized response is difficult to achieve in federal systems where subnational governments may constitutionally issue their own guidelines that address local, not national, effects. If we can replicate our findings (Yin 2018) with a series of structured, focused comparisons (George and Bennett 2005), we not only discount alternative explanations but also add analytical weight to our findings. We accept that there was a degree of lesson-drawing with some national responses having been inspired by developments in other countries. While the cases we chose may not be entirely independent, our large, for qualitative research, sample helps keep this pitfall to a minimum.

Demarcating the "National Response"

Crises responses may take many forms, raising the likelihood of idiosyncratic answers ('t Hart, Rosenthal, and Kouzmin 1993). To gain analytical leverage, we conceptualize the organizational structuring and policy orientation, the goals of decision-makers and citizen expectations, and the actual measures taken as aggregate constructs placed on a centralization–decentralization continuum. Centralization of the decision-making process during a crisis implies the concentration of power in the hands of a small number of executives at the national level (as opposed to subnational agencies or levels governance) and the tendency to seek strong leadership. For analytical purposes, we use the functional framework developed by the US Federal Emergency Management Agency (NIMS 2017). Responses contain three key components: command and coordination, communication and information management, and resource management. First, we expect national responses to differ in terms of the structure and amount of coordination. The main question we ask here is whether decision-making was concentrated in the hands of a few executives or diffused across many jurisdictions. Second, we expect variation in terms of communication strategies. The main questions we ask here concern the timeliness of the messages (whether they were anticipatory or reactive) and the consistency of communication. Finally, we examine the stringency of measures—managed resources expressed as an aggregate index of severity of lockdown and other measures taken. Taken concomitantly, more concentrated coordination, more synchronized messages, and more stringent measures constitute a more centralized response. Conversely, less concentrated coordination, less synchronized messages, and less stringent measures constitute a more decentralized response. In cases where the policy mix steers in both directions—that is, two components point in one while the other points in the opposite direction—we talk about centripetal or centrifugal responses, respectively. Explaining variation in national responses thus involves analyzing policy mixes containing not only dissimilarities in decision-making structures and processes but also fluctuations in message and in the intensity of applicable measures found in different countries.

Policy Styles, Political Trust, and National Responses

Why do countries respond to the same crisis in very different ways? We summarize our argument in the form of two propositions. It specifies what government can do and what citizens expect and pressure it to do.

1   *National responses to the COVID-19 crisis vary systematically based on national policy styles.*

At its core, policy style selectively examines the institutional arrangements within which policy deliberations take place and the actors and ideas present in such deliberations. Policy styles begin with how institutional structure and norms interact with actor behavior in a given political system to shape what Crawford and Ostrom (1995) called "a grammar of institutions." Styles, in turn, facilitate and constrain policymaking to produce historically rooted patterns of decisions (Pierson 2004). The point is that path dependence in public policy does not flow only from previous decisions but also persistent modes of deliberation. Richardson (1982) conceptualized policy style as interactions between

- the government's approach to problem-solving (anticipatory vs. reactive); and
- state-society relations in terms of aiming to reach consensus or not.

From these two dimensions, four styles emerged and different countries fell within each quadrant. More recently, Howlett and Tosun (2019) have adapted and applied the concept beyond Europe to incorporate major developing and developed countries.

We retain the two dimensions of policy style but update and adapt them as follows: *pattern of administrative arrangements* and *state-society relations*. We begin with the claim that policymaking is strongly affected by existing administrative arrangements, especially during pandemics, because the structure of bureaucratic agencies remains largely unchanged. Their interactions determine the government's approach to problem-solving because institutions create opportunities and help shape the strategic opportunities and alternative options available (Weaver and Rockman 1993). The dimension of administrative arrangements is operationalized as administrative policy capacity (Peters 2015). Capacity ensures that policy actions are technically sound to attain the intended goals, they are aligned with the necessary resources to make them implementable, and they may obtain and sustain the needed political support to legitimate them. It describes the human and organizational resources governments have at their disposal when dealing with pandemics (Capano et al. 2020, 298).

Peters (2015) adds nuance by elaborating on three dimensions of administrative policy capacity: autonomy, staffing, and aspirations. Autonomy refers to the agency legal and organizational ability to craft their own decisions or shirk political pressure. It is a function not only of legal rules but also of political resources and permanence of status. Staffing refers to adequate number and quality of technical expertise and knowledge of clientele in the policy domain within which agencies work. Aspirations relate to patterns of cooperation and respect between the bureaucracy and their political masters. As Peters (2015, 265) states, "although political leaders in general desire to control policy they may also respect the expertise of the bureaucracy and want to utilize that expertise rather than to oppose it." Higher autonomy, more expert staffing, and more cooperative aspirations indicate higher policy capacity.

State-society relations refer to accommodative (or not) patterns of interest mediation (Howlett and Tosun 2019). An important consideration of style is the degree of inclusiveness of social actors in policymaking and its level of formalization. Where social actors are traditionally included in policymaking, the political system seeks a reasonable consensus before policy is made to minimize political conflict during implementation. Other systems exhibit a more top-down imposition style with minimal social consultation. The reasons behind the development of such relations may be administrative and historical, reflecting a way of ameliorating conflict. We operationalize state-society relations by degree of inclusiveness. Systems where social actors are routinely consulted and listened to throughout the policy process are characterized as more inclusive. We acknowledge the fact that crisis conditions may shorten the consultation process, but this is precisely our argument. Policy styles cast long shadows so that inclusiveness is likely to lead to different national responses to crises—policy actions that are more widely accepted and less perceived as imposed.

The two dimensions of national policy style, administrative policy capacity, and inclusiveness yield a matrix with four cells (Figure 1.1). We label cases of:

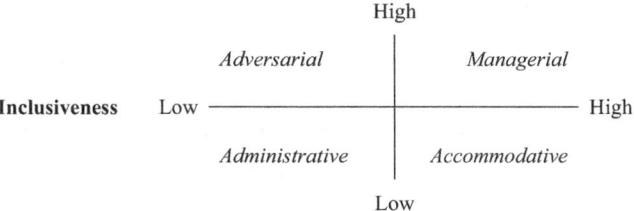

FIGURE 1.1   A Typology of Policy Styles.

- Lower administrative policy capacity and lower inclusiveness as "administrative."
- Higher administrative policy capacity and lower inclusiveness as "adversarial."
- Lower administrative policy capacity and higher inclusiveness as "accommodative."
- Higher administrative policy capacity and higher inclusiveness as "managerial."

2   *The effects of policy styles under crisis conditions depend on level of political trust.*

Citizen expectations (captured by the concept of political trust) are also important in understanding and explaining national responses. The protracted, highly personal, and embodied dimensions of the pandemic necessitate a public that makes a conscious choice to comply to measures issued by the public sector. Lack of voluntary compliance makes for stringent measures and foments the use of "sticks" rather than "carrots," including hefty fines for breaking lockdown rules (Petridou, Zahariadis, and Ceccoli 2020). Thus, it makes a difference in whether citizens comply with harsh measures perceived as imposed (Cairney and Wellstead 2021). While the range of measures differs across countries, their stringency makes them very hard to enforce, especially in democratic societies. Some countries have a more legitimate and efficient public administration system than others, likely determined by the amount of trust citizens have in the bureaucracy in their country. If the level of trustworthiness and legitimacy of the bureaucracy is low, implementing public policy becomes an arduous process. Moreover, low levels of political trust decrease administrative capacity and increase problem intractability (Exadaktylos and Zahariadis 2014; Rothstein 2012).

Public administrators are not elected officials; traditionally, their role has been to implement public policy based on their impartial and depoliticized professional expertise. However, given the increased and inescapable political nature of policy implementation including citizen demands for safety during crises, the role of non-elected officials and the power they wield has expanded (Cooper 2006). This is the reason why legitimacy and political trust (trust in the system of administration) are important, especially at a time when palpable mistrust of professionals and experts is evidenced in a number of countries worldwide.

To claim that trust is an important catalyst for action is not novel. Our contribution lies in specifying the way political trust interacts with policy styles to shape national responses. Trust affects and is affected by policy style, and both have a significant impact on responses. Higher trust in government and health practitioners, as expressed in public opinion polls, widens citizen acceptance of government measures. In systems with higher policy capacity and higher inclusiveness in decision-making, trust magnifies agency capabilities leading to decentralized responses.

Citizens trust the ability of policymakers to design effective plans and the competence of the bureaucracy to execute them. This is especially true under conditions of crises, when urgency and uncertainty necessitate "walks on blind faith." Without much time to collect enough information and consult with social partners, individual accountability and faith in the policy system's capacity to pursue responsible action are important ingredients of national response.

Conversely, in systems with lower policy capacity and lower inclusiveness citizens lack faith in the system and expect central authority to take over. Lack of trust weakens the effects of policy capacity because it pushes and pulls in two opposite directions (Exadaktylos and Zahariadis 2014). It lowers willingness to act while it increases political conflict within the administration. The lack of clear guidance from central authority gives discretion to implementing agents to frame issues the way they see fit. The problem is the same element that empowers agents also paralyzes them because it pinpoints responsibility. In the presence of ambiguous roles, political responsibility for adverse effects is shifted to agents. If the rules call for stringent and politically costly measures, such as a lockdown, agents have no incentive to act. Hence, central authority takes over control of crisis response.

When the values of policy style and trust are mixed, the effects of the interaction are amplified by institutional capacity. That is, in cases where higher policy capacity coincides with low trust, the tendency is not to trust policymakers to make the right calls but rather to place faith in policy capacity (i.e., health system and bureaucratic coordination) to handle the crisis. From a policymaker's perspective, a politically expedient and profitable course of action is to pursue a more centrifugal response which has the added advantage of blame avoidance (Hood 2011). When there is higher trust but lower policy capacity, policymakers and citizens know that the health system cannot handle the crisis if left without strong political direction. Past behavior is an important signal of commitment to future repercussions in cases of failure. This is especially true in cases where the stakes are high in terms of possible human losses. The higher the trust, the more important policy capacity becomes in effective implementation and the higher the cost will be in case of failure. Hence, policymakers are more likely to pursue a centripetal response because it is politically more profitable. It gives central authority more control over outcomes, maximizing political benefits and minimizing blame.

There are four more types that are theoretically possible but practically improbable. Regardless of policy capacity, it is very unlikely to have a high inclusive policy style but low trust. Inclusiveness presupposes responsibility and faith in the system. Using similar logic, it is highly unlikely to have cases of low inclusion but high trust. Policy actors and citizens are less likely to trust the system if they have little input in it. For this reason, we find it unlikely to consider the hypotheses linking high trust to administrative and adversarial policy styles and low trust to accommodative and managerial styles. The only possible exception is China. Its high policy capacity (but not accessible uniformly throughout the country), low inclusiveness, and generally, high trust point to the direction of adversarialism and high trust. However, it is highly doubtful that China's policy style can be characterized as adversarial given strong centralized control and the absence of pluralism. In addition, one cannot be certain of how genuine trust may be in such an environment. Rather than fit reality to our theoretical scheme, we let the empirical evidence speak for itself. We also recognize that crises are dynamic events. As they evolve, perhaps policy style (capacity or inclusiveness) and especially trust change, leading to fluctuations in national responses. Rather than characterize national responses statically, we tease the implications empirically.

We summarize the effects of policy style and trust in the form of the following hypotheses. During crises, conditions of:

- Administrative policy style and lower trust prompt the construction of more centralized response plans (H1).
- Adversarial policy style and lower trust prompt the construction of more centrifugal response plans (H2).
- Accommodative policy style and higher trust prompt the construction of more centripetal response plans (H3).
- Managerial policy style and higher trust prompt the construction of more decentralized response plans (H4).

Structure of the Book

In this book, we examine the interaction of national policy styles and political trust to explain differences across national contexts. Dominant styles of "normal" policymaking cast long shadows on crisis management, while institutional and behavioral elements that underpin the approach spill over and frame responses during crises. However, when policymakers decide on the appropriate course of action, the acute turbulence, uncertainty, and urgency of crises complicate their ability to make sense of the problem and alter calculations and estimates of consequences. The tendency to centralize response plans is shaped by how style legacy interacts with underlying low trust. Centralization raises citizen expectations for strong, coordinated, and effective government response. Decentralized plans place the onus on individuals to take appropriate measures and bear responsibility for slowing down the spread of the virus.

Chapter 1 has introduced the policy puzzle and addressed broad theoretical concerns. After explaining our research design, we presented the argument in brief. The short duration of the time period, roughly one year, prevents a full examination of recovery or preparedness policies. But enough variation exists among our sample of countries, enabling us to capture the first and second waves of the pandemic in rich empirical detail. Even though the crisis caused by the COVID-19 pandemic is novel, national responses contain familiar patterns of making policy, heavily laden in political conflict and dramaturgic rituals.

Chapter 2 begins by reviewing the literature on policy styles. After adding trust to model the interactions, we specify hypotheses on national response effects. Despite strong involvement by health professionals to combat the pandemic and a heavy toll on local populations, policy decisions are fundamentally political. They aim to address public health goals while upholding social values and bolstering the political fortunes of those in power.

Chapters 3–12 constitute the empirical portion of our study. Each country gets its own treatment in a separate chapter. National responses are tentatively divided in four parts, representing four possible outcomes. While contributors are free to structure chapters as they deem appropriate, each chapter provides empirical analysis of three elements: policy style, political trust, and how their interaction affects (or not) the degree of centralization of national response.

Chapter 13 puts the findings in comparative perspective and draws out implications for the usefulness of policy styles and trust in public policy. The findings are also placed in broader perspective deriving implications for theories of policy making and crisis management.

Note

1 Although Rosenberg talks about the AIDS epidemic, his argument applies equally well to pandemics.

References

Boin, Arjen. 2019. "The Transboundary Crisis: Why We Are Unprepared and the Road Ahead." *Journal of Contingencies and Crisis Management* 27: 94–99.

Boin, Arjen, Paul 't Hart, Eric Stern, and Bengt Sundelius. 2017. *The Politics of Crisis Management: Public Leadership under Pressure.* 2nd ed. Cambridge: Cambridge University Press.

Bouckaert, Geert, Davide Galli, Sabine Kuhlmann, Renate Reiter, and Steven Van Hecke. 2020. "European Coronationalism? A Hot Spot Governing a Pandemic Crisis." *Public Administration Review* 80 (5): 765–73.

Brecher, Michael, and Jonathan Wilkenfeld. 1997. *A Study of Crisis.* Ann Arbor: The University of Michigan Press.

Cairney, Paul, and Adam Wellstead. 2021. "COVID-19: Effective Policymaking Depends on Trust in Experts, Politicians, and the Public." *Policy Design and Practice* 4 (1): 1–14.

Capano, Giliberto, Michael Howlett, Darryl S. L. Jarvis, M. Ramesh, and Nihit Goyal. 2020. "Mobilizing Policy (In)Capacity to Fight COVID-19: Understanding Variations in State Responses." *Policy and Society* 39 (3): 285–308.

Capelos, Tereza, and Theofanis Exadaktylos. 2017. "Feeling the Pulse of the Greek Debt Crisis: Affect on the Web of Blame." *National Identities* 19 (1): 73–90.

Crawford, Sue, E. S., and Elinor Ostrom. 1995. "A Grammar of Institutions." *American Political Science Review* 89 (3): 582–600.

Dobson, Andrew P. et al. 2020. "Ecology and Economics for Pandemic Prevention." *Science* 369 (6502): 379–81. At https://science.sciencemag.org/content/369/6502/379.

The Economist. 2020. "Covid-19 Is Here to Stay. The World Is Working out How to Live with It." July 4. At https://www.economist.com/international/2020/07/04/covid-19-is-here-to-stay-the-world-is-working-out-how-to-live-with-it.

Edelman, Murray. 1988. *Constructing the Political Spectacle*. Chicago: The University of Chicago Press.

Exadaktylos, Theofanis, and Nikolaos Zahariadis. 2014. "*Quid pro Quo*: Political Trust and Policy Implementation in Greece during the Age of Austerity." *Politics & Policy* 42 (1): 160–83.

Flyvbjerg, Bent. 2006. "Five Misunderstandings about Case-Study Research." *Qualitative Inquiry* 12 (2): 219–45.

Gan, Nectar. 2020. "Coronavirus has Created a Rift between the US and China that may Take a Generation to Heal." CNN.com. May 8. At https://www.cnn.com/2020/05/08/asia/us-china-relations-nationalism-intl-hnk/index.html.

George, Alexander L., and Andrew Bennett. 2005. *Case Studies and Theory Development in the Social Sciences*. Cambridge, MA: The MIT Press.

Gundel, Stephan. "Towards a New Typology of Crises." *Journal of Contingencies and Crisis Management* 13 (3): 106–15.

't Hart, Paul. 1993. "Symbols, Rituals and Power: The Lost Dimensions of Crisis Management." *Journal of Contingencies and Crisis Management* 1 (1): 36–50.

't Hart, Paul, Uriel Rosenthal, and Alexander Kouzmin. 1993. "Crisis Decision Making: The Centralization Thesis Revisited." *Administration & Society* 25 (1): 12–45.

Hood, Christopher. 2011. *The Blame Game: Spin, Bureaucracy, and Self-Preservation in Government*. Princeton: Princeton University Press.

Howlett, Michael, and Jale Tosun, eds. 2019. *Policy Styles and Policy-Making: Exploring the Linkages*. New York: Routledge.

Johns Hopkins Coronavirus Resource Center. 2021. Global Map. August 22. At https://coronavirus.jhu.edu/map.html.

Keown-McMullan, Caroline. 1997. "Crisis: When does a Molehill Become a Mountain?" *Disaster Prevention and Management: An International Journal* 6 (1): 4–10.

King, Gary, Robert O. Keohane, and Sidney Verba. 1994. *Designing Social Inquiry: Scientific Inference in Qualitative Research*. Princeton: Princeton University Press.

Mei, Ciqi. 2020. "Policy Style, Consistency and the Effectiveness of the Policy Mix in China's Fight Against COVID-19." *Policy and Society* 39 (3): 309–25.

Olson, Richard Stuart. 2000. "Toward a Politics of Disaster: Losses, Values, Agendas and Blame." *International Journal of Mass Emergencies and Disasters* 18 (2): 265–87.

Patrick, Stewart. 2020. "When the System Fails: COVID-19 and the Costs of Global Dysfunction." *Foreign Affairs* (July–August). At https://www.foreignaffairs.com/articles/world/2020-06-09/when-system-fails.

Peters, B. Guy. 2015. "Policy Capacity in Public Administration." *Policy and Society* 34 (3–4): 219–28.

Petridou, Evangelia, Nikolaos Zahariadis, and Stephen Ceccoli. 2020. "Averting Institutional Disasters? Drawing Lessons from China to Inform the Cypriot Response to the COVID-19 Pandemic." *European Policy Analysis* 6 (2): 318–27.

Pierson, Paul. 2004. *Politics in Time: History, Institutions, and Social Analysis.* Princeton: Princeton University Press.

Pursiainen, Christer. 2018. *The Crisis Management Cycle: Theory and Practice.* New York: Routledge.

Richardson, Jeremy, ed. 1982. *Policy Styles in Western Europe.* London: Allen & Unwin.

Rose, Richard. 1990. "Inheritance Before Choice in Public Policy." *Journal of Theoretical Politics* 2 (3): 263–91.

Rosenberg, Charles E. 1989. "What Is an Epidemic? AIDS in Historical Perspective." *Daedalus* 118 (2): 1–17.

Rothstein, Bo. 2012. "Political Legitimacy for Public Administration." In *The Sage Handbook of Public Administration*, eds. B. Guy Peters and Jon Pierre. Thousand Oaks, CA: Sage, 357–69.

Schmitt, Eric. 2004. "Iraq-Bound Troops Confront Rumsfeld Over Lack of Armor." *New York Times.* December 8. At https://www.nytimes.com/2004/12/08/international/middleeast/iraqbound-troops-confront-rumsfeld-over-lack-of.html.

Seawright, Jason, and John Gerring. 2008. "Case-Selection Techniques in Case Study Research: A Menu of Qualitative and Quantitative Options." *Political Research Quarterly* 61(2): 294–308.

Tong, Scott. 2020. "Countries Race to Limit, Ban Exports of Masks, Ventilators, Other Gear." March 30. At https://www.marketplace.org/2020/03/30/countries-race-to-limit-ban-exports-of-masks-ventilators-other-gear/.

Yin, Robert K. 2018. *Case Study Research and Applications: Design and Methods.* 6th ed. Thousand Oaks, CA: Sage.

Zahariadis, Nikolaos, Stephen Ceccoli, and Evangelia Petridou. 2021. "Assessing the Effects of Calculated Inaction on National Responses to the COVID-19 Crisis." *Risks, Hazards, & Crisis in Public Policy* 12 (3): 328–45. https://doi.org/10.1002/rhc3.12230.

2

POLICY STYLES AND POLICYMAKING DURING TIMES OF CRISIS

Nikolaos Zahariadis, Evangelia Petridou, Theofanis Exadaktylos and Jörgen Sparf

> *The emergence of COVID-19 was characterized by **a mix of some early and rapid action, but also by delay, hesitation,** and **denial,** with the net result that an outbreak became an epidemic and an epidemic spread to pandemic proportions.*
>
> (The Independent Panel 2021, 21; emphasis in the original)

In the 1975 classic film *Jaws*, Police Chief Martin Brody (Roy Scheider) famously quips upon catching a glimpse of the shark: "We are going to need a bigger boat." Startled by the size of the beast, he realizes at that moment that the town's response to their predicament was wholly inadequate. Following warning signs earlier in the film, Mayor Larry Vaughn (Murray Hamilton) overruled Chief Brody's recommendation to close the beaches, fearing that the loss of tourist revenue would financially cripple the town. The town's inability to make sense of the threat, coupled with the mayor's decision to reject the evidence-based, expert advice of Chief Brody, led to a highly ineffective response that cost lives. The situation with COVID-19 shares many similarities with the town's predicament as the above quote aptly illustrates. Why did some countries respond efficiently and effectively to the crisis while others did not?

Understanding the societal and political dimensions of the COVID-19 pandemic necessitates intellectual engagement from disciplines beyond the health sciences and medicine. With policy sciences as a theoretical departure point, Weible et al. (2020) argue for an integrated consideration of several policy perspectives as a tool for understanding the COVID-19 pandemic, including domestic and global policymaking, crisis response and management, policy networks, policy implementation, knowledge and expertise, emotions, narratives, learning, and policy success and failure.

DOI: 10.4324/9781003137399-3

In this volume, we tackle the question of the effects of policy style on shaping crisis response to the COVID-19 pandemic. We first survey the literature on national responses to the COVID-19 pandemic. We then trace, present, and operationalize our generalized conceptualization of national policy style, which serves as one of the two variables we use to answer our research puzzle. After expounding on the second variable, trust in government, we explain the interaction between trust and policy style with a view toward understanding national policy responses to the COVID-19 pandemic.

National Responses to the COVID-19 Pandemic

As fundamentally devastating as this pandemic has been, the universal character of this complex and multifaceted policy problem constitutes a natural experiment, a fruitful empirical field for research with the aim to understand and explain the variation of national responses to the pandemic (Capano et al. 2020). Bouckaert et al. (2020) show a nationally oriented dimension and several similarities (centered on containment logic, activation of risk management procedures, and increasing hospital capacity) in the pandemic responses of Belgium, France, Germany, and Italy, despite the overall diversity of the responses within European Union (EU) member states, which, at least partly, is a corollary of their political and administrative systems.

Divergence of varying degree was also observed in within-country, albeit federal, contexts. In the United States, the response to the pandemic was left entirely to the states. Kettl (2020) finds that the pandemic response at the state level was not correlated to the seriousness of the problem; rather, differences were partisan-based and consistent with a set of policy decisions made over a long period of time, including expanding Medicaid as part of the Affordable Care Act (ACA) and prior investment to the health care system in that state. Indicatively, Republican governors and state legislatures were averse to stringent measures and generally delayed the implementation of physical distancing measures (Adolph et al. 2021; Huberfeld, Gordon, and Jones 2020; Rocco, Béland, and Waddan 2020). Additionally and depending on social cleavages, increased intergovernmental friction and lack of federal support result in perpetuating inequalities and disproportionately harm small, recourse-poor local governments (Dzigbede, Gehl, and Willoughby 2020). Conversely, Canadian federalism exhibited a more cooperative policy process, resulting in a more centralized approach vis-à-vis non-crisis conditions, though still allowing for divergence among the provinces (Migone 2020).

An analysis by Capano et al. (2020) finds that the diversity of responses concerns not only the kinds of policy instruments or the combination of instruments different countries used but also differences in the timing, sequence, and speed of adoption of measures as well as the stringency of these measures. Notably, considerable divergence characterizes the national pandemic response of politically and culturally similar and geographically proximate countries such as the Scandinavian countries. Whereas the Swedish response privileged voluntary guidelines rather than mandating a lockdown, the closing of schools, retail stores, and gyms masking when in public, the national approaches of Denmark, Finland, and Norway were considerably more stringent in that they included mandated closures to varying degrees and some form of lockdown for some period of time (Christensen and Lægreid 2020; Giritli Nygren and Olofsson 2020; Petridou 2020). These responses were also more centralized than the Swedish response. A segment of the literature on national responses to COVID-19 sought to explain these, treating the policy response as the dependent variable, while other research sought to explore other issues, focusing on the ways the pandemic has exacerbated existing societal cleavages, including the role of actors and institutions in the policy response, as well as implications for leadership and crisis management. We provide an overview in the section that follows.

COVID-19 National Response as the Dependent Variable

Several factors have been shown to inform national responses. Policy learning (within- and cross-country) is credited with the formulation (and implementation) of a successful South Korean response. Lee, Hwang, and Moon (2020) argue that a quadruple-loop learning model that incorporates past experiences, the political and social context, and the specificities of the policy problem furthered organizational learning. This not only informed the initial Korean response, but also continues to inform the country's long-term strategy. Conversely, Petridou, Zahariadis, and Ceccoli (2020) show how the Cypriot response was shaped partly through indirect lesson drawn from China, the first country to deal with the virus and the ensuing pandemic. In the absence of learning and prior experience with large societal crises in combination with low administrative capacity, countries (Italy in particular) tended to favor incremental measures at the outset of the pandemic (Capano 2020).

Structural factors offer explanations for the understanding of national responses. Petridou (2020) argues that the dualism in the Swedish administrative system, with a highly autonomous bureaucracy and technocratic policymaking tradition, explained the liberal Swedish response, while Sager and Mavrot (2020) find that the Swiss response is largely consistent with that country's power sharing, consensus narrative, even if there is evidence that there was a shift toward a predominance of executive power. In China, Mei (2020) combines the concepts of policy style and policy mix to shed light on the governmental response, whereas Bakir (2020), in contrast, argues against deterministic explanations and sheds light on the Turkish response by claiming that the pandemic created exceptional circumstances that deviated from the path dependency of authoritarian, centralized policies.

COVID-19 and Social Inequality

Crises tend to unravel existing disparities, and they can also "reproduce and greatly exacerbate these disparities […]" (Gotham and Greenberg 2014, 223). The pandemic is no exception. These disparities and the (in)adequacy of responses to tackle them has been the focus of some recently published scholarship, with special attention paid on gender and racial cleavages. A preliminary examination of COVID-19-related crisis communication reveals "military masculinity" and gender insensitivity, leading to ineffectiveness (Subert 2020, 1). Moreover, the COVID-19 experience has shed light on persistent and longstanding health inequities in the American context that require a long-term response targeting these inequities at the local level, including constructing a continuous dialogue on the role of public administration and equity in health policy; monitoring health disparities; paying attention to scientific knowledge; investing in addressing health needs at the local level; facilitating access to healthcare; bolstering the infrastructure of community health workers; and generally daring to integrate social equity in policy planning by taking into account the needs of all population groups (Gadson 2020; Gaynor and Wilson 2020; Martin-Howard and Farmbry 2020; see also Deslatte, Hatch, and Stokan 2020; Lynch 2020).

Actors and Institutions and Implications for Leadership and Crisis Management

Fundamental structural changes to counteract disparities notwithstanding, administrative capacity and the role of public administrators are crucial in the long-term managing of crisis. Given the imperative for coordination (Boin, 't Hart, Stern, and Sundelius 2017), several salient competences for public managers emerge: engaging stakeholders; responding to, and activating politicians, building, maintaining, and leveraging collaborative networks, as well as learning and knowledge transfer from previous crises (Grizzle, Goodin, and Robinson 2020; Shomaker and Bauer 2020; van der Wal 2020). In terms of political leadership, a comparative study of the national responses of Turkey and Greece revealed similarities in the strategies employed by the leaders of the two countries, pointing to a renewed attention to credit claiming vis-à-vis blame avoidance, while transparency was used as both a legitimizing and rhetorical device (Zahariadis, Petridou, and Oztig 2020).

In summary, the current scholarship in policy and public administration on governmental responses to COVID-19 seeks to explain these policy responses at the national and subnational levels, focuses on inequalities that the pandemic has exposed, and attempts to identify strategies conducive for effective crisis management. The examination of national responses has consisted mostly of single case studies and less so of studies with comparative design. Explanations are often based on institutional factors; however, they tend to be monocausal, paying less attention to variables that may interact with institutional factors.

Democracy, Public Policy, and Policy Community

It is perhaps ironic but not at all surprising that the literature on public policy-making under conditions or crisis would look for inspiration to work that was done in the 1970s. During that tumultuous decade, policy scholarship sought to better understand how policy was made when government appeared over-loaded with wicked problems. As Samuel Huntington (1975, 23) claimed at the time, who governs is important, but one needs to ask an even more important question: "does anyone govern?" Writing about the UK, Tony King (1975, 284) claims exasperated:

> It was once thought that Britain was an unusually easy country to govern, its politicians wise, its parties responsible, its administration efficient, its people docile. Now we wonder whether Britain is not perhaps an unu-sually difficult country to govern, its problems peculiarly intractable, its people increasingly bloody-minded.

It was a lack of faith, the absence of trust in governing institutions, high expecta-tions, rising social complexity, and interdependency; in short, a crisis, a crisis of democracy (Crozier, Huntington, and Watanuki 1975).

Partly as a result of this crisis and lack of trust in governing institutions, scholarship turned to examining the process of governance as the antidote. Dissatisfied with the study of formal institutions, the competitive electoral process, and majoritarian politics as the main explanatory variables of public policy outcomes, scholars, such as Heclo and Wildavsky (1981), Heclo (1974), and Richardson and Jordan (1979), began to look for answers away from majoritarian politics and parliamentary democracy in less visible arenas where specialists and interest groups interacted away from the lime light to negotiate agreements and make policy that formal institutions like parliaments only appeared to ratify or at least replicate. The reason was simple: most policy decisions are effectively beyond the reach or interest of politicians. The size of government, complex-ity of issues, citizen expectations for speedy resolution, and the general policy environment necessitate decomposing policy down into issues that may be more effectively managed by a smaller number of interested and knowledgeable participants. Therefore, for Richardson and Jordan (1979), most public policy is conducted primarily through specialist policy communities which process issues at a sub-systemic level of government not particularly visible or interesting to the public, Parliament, or senior policymakers.

In parallel to this argument, Heclo (1978) developed his concept of issue networks, spelling out a similar idea: an actor-centered, relational perspective on policy that describes the highly intricate webs of influence among "invisible" actors who shape American public policy. Like Richardson and Jordan, Heclo uncovered greater continuity than change in a series of resource-interdependent relations among bureaucrats, interest groups, think tanks, members of the media, business lobbyists, and union representatives. Inclusion into this network does not follow organizational boundaries but the development of personal trust, re-gard by others as important and knowledgeable, and the emergence of a culture of loose agreement on the unwritten rules of debating public problems and for-mulating policy solutions.

Developing the Concept of Policy Style

These ideas evolved into the concept of policy style. Placed within the broader policy studies literature, policy styles refer to a particular mode of deliberating on public problems and solutions among policy actors within nationally designed and inherited institutional arrangements. Patterns of deliberation crystallize over time to create a distinctive way of addressing public problems, given the administrative tools and innovative capacity that a country has at its disposal. As Howlett and Tosun (2019, 5) maintain:

> The general idea is that policy making tends to develop in such a way that the same actors, institutions, instruments, and governing ideas dominate policy making for extended periods of time, infusing policy with both a consistent content and a set of typical policy processes or procedures and actors.

Such a notion is not only empirically plausible but also tends to be relatively efficient and effective in specific cultural settings. A policy style is enduring and efficient because it reduces the transaction costs of debate, decreases uncertainty as to who should be consulted or at least answered, increases collaboration among actors, and reduces the likelihood of policy conflict thereby augmenting performance with similar inputs. A style is effective because major issues are addressed in politically acceptable ways. The widening scope of government along with its complex programs and the expectation for results inevitably have given rise to issue experts and policy advocates, who make policy more technocratic and politically "objective."

The trigger to develop such a concept stems from the observation that different countries handle essentially similar problems very differently. If policy communities represented "an alternative approach to comparative government" (Richardson and Jordan 1979, 163), the implication was that there could be a wider and systematic examination of (European at the time) policymaking along those lines. Aggregating to the national level, Richardson (1982) argued that similar norms, institutions, and standard operating procedures tended to characterize national policymaking despite some variation within each country or policy sector. Not all policy decisions would be explained this way, but there would be a tendency toward convergence of style within countries (assuming some variance across sectors and time), and policy styles would diverge systematically across national borders. Extrapolating from (West) European cases, Richardson went on to argue that analysts can predict how individual countries will deal with environmental or health policy problems, for example, by reference to the stable patterns of interaction encapsulated in the notion of national policy style.

Interestingly, although the concept was developed as applying first to the UK and then elsewhere in Europe amidst a general conception of crisis and ungovernability, it related primarily to "normal" policymaking. This entails policies being made on an everyday basis addressing common problems under ordinary circumstances. In other words, there is no conceptualization of policymaking under extreme conditions of urgency, turbulence, uncertainty, or ambiguity, elements that characterize crises (Boin 2019). Quite the contrary, the aim has been to specify the "standard operating procedures" of political systems (Richardson et al. 1982, 2). And this is part of our contribution to policy theory: we argue that the concept of style may explain both normal and extraordinary policymaking. With some adjustments and adaptations, the people, tools, and institutions who make and within which policy is made remain largely the same under crisis conditions. Policy styles cast long shadows in many directions.

How has the Concept of Policy Style been Used in the Literature?

Despite criticism, research utilizing the concept of policy style has remained robust. Apart from general national applications (e.g., Howlett and Tosun 2019; Richardson 1982), policy styles have been extended to regulatory regimes (e.g., Adam et al. 2017; Halffman 2005; Vogel 1986) and administrative traditions (e.g., Knill 2001), but it must be said that most studies seek to specify policy style rather than assess its effects.

At its core, policy style selectively examines the institutional arrangements within which deliberations take place and the actors, ideas, and mode present in such deliberations. It steers scholarship away from the study of formal institutions toward informal arrangements. Most policymakers recognize the value of building on past policies and seek to bargain and compromise. In very few cases, and certainly in highly salient issues such as privatization, will they expend political capital and resources to impose their preference for a specific pet solution. Because they also operate within the context of shared norms and conceptualization about the nature of policy problems and their solutions, so the argument went regarding the UK (Richardson and Jordan 1979), it was rare for policymakers to reject established knowledge that supports existing policy. Consequently, in most instances, the policy style literature expects incremental change and few changes in punctuation.

Examining democratic European countries, Richardson et al. (1982, 13) conceptualized policy style as the interaction between two dimensions: (a) the government's approach to problem-solving (anticipatory vs. reactive) and (b) state-society relations, that is, whether actors aim to reach consensus or not. From these two dimensions, four styles emerged, and different countries fell within each quadrant. For example, Germany was found to have an anticipatory but consensual style, whereas the UK was more reactive but also consensual. Underpinning the interactions are core normative values that guide actual behavior. These often represent deep-rooted social principles that permeate many policy arenas and point to an ideal, national policy behavior. For example, Sweden is a country where policy consultation among many public actors is highly valued, often buttressed by an assumed individual responsibility to the community as a whole (Pierre 2016). Not every individual actor behaves like this, and policy does not always follow this ideal. But there is a tendency to converge around this ideal across policy sectors.

The dimension of anticipatory versus reactive style refers to a government's approach to problem-solving. Governments across political systems build institutions and encourage particular ways of policy participation and deliberation. There is constant planning, scanning, participation, and consultation to design policies and anticipate problems. The idea is that anticipation increases up front administrative costs, including significant specialization costs, but lowers response costs once problems arise. The idea has found considerable currency in disaster management policy where governments build resilience to anticipate risk and be better prepared to deal with disasters (DeLeo 2016). Another example is health care. The health care system of some countries, such as France, is built on prevention, not treatment. Considerable emphasis and resources are spent on anticipating and lessening the cost of health issues so that treatments are far less frequent and less costly.

The second dimension deals with state-society relations. Is there an interest by government officials to actively invite participation in policymaking and how wide is this participation? Less participation leads to greater tendency toward the state imposing policy decisions onto society while more participation by policy actors indicates an effort to seek consensus. In some countries, participation and consultation are mandated by law. Of course, the existence of consultation does not necessarily entail meaningful participation, as Richardson et al. (1982, 2) were keenly aware. The plethora of committees and forums may serve to hide the real locus of decision or simply be used *pro forma*. Policymakers may quickly dismiss the recommendations as unreasonable, too costly, or simply politically unacceptable. In this case, participation looks more like a political spectacle, a ritual of the exercise of power, how policy should be made rather than how it actually is (Edelman 1988; Kertzer 1988; Lukes 1975). The dimension has two polar opposites. In some countries, policymaking aims toward consensus, while in others, it is imposed. Authors in the Richardson (1982) volume placed (West) European political systems on points in-between these ideals.

Subsequent work has elucidated but also criticized the concept. Knill (2001) focuses more narrowly on administrative style and argues that national administrative traditions hold the key to understanding policymaking. Investigating the interplay of national administrative traditions and European policy implementation, the author finds distinct differences across national contexts, which he calls administrative styles, and shows how these differences affect and are affected by European requirements. Extending the concept to international organizations, Knill et al. (2019) still talk about "style" but define it as constituting an entrepreneurial style in policy initiation, a strategic approach to policy formulation and a mediating implementation style. Van Waarden (1995) stresses the degree of formalization of interaction as the building block of national policy style. Any cross-national variation is due to structural foundations, such as the legal and administrative systems, that are resistant to radical change. In essence, he maintains that despite strong international pressure exerted by economic globalization, advances in technology, and, in his case, the EU, policy styles across sectors will tend toward convergence within national borders, leading to a magnification of distinct national styles.

Research on policy styles is not without critics as the concept of style has been seen as a variant of cultural explanations or too general to be analytically useful (e.g., Richardson 2018, 3) and even more useful at the sectoral than the national level (e.g., Freeman 1985). Moreover, empirical studies have revealed idiosyncrasies in specific countries like China (Qian 2019), variation within countries like the UK (Cairney 2009), or even fluctuation across time within the same country (Richardson 2018). This last point is important because it raises a fundamental question: if policy styles refer to relatively stable and persistent values, norms, and modes of policy deliberation, can styles change over time? The answer is only glacial, but some punctuations must be noted. Certainly, Margaret Thatcher's tenure in power in the 1980s was not only tumultuous but also heavily skewed toward breaking off from traditional modes of policymaking. She intentionally sought to isolate and, in some cases, ignore certain groups from policy communities, mainly labor unions, in order to steer deliberations toward views of public problems and solutions that were closer to her point of view. In short, she broke off from the consensus-seeking tradition that characterized much of policymaking in the UK. Still, does the UK's policy style look the same now, more or less, as it did 40 years ago when the concept was first introduced? The answer depends on how one conceptualizes the government's approach to problem-solving.

What does anticipatory policymaking look like in practice, and does it imply that countries do not also follow a reactive style as well? In other words, can countries follow both at the same time or at least a mix of both depending on the issue? It is a question that the literature has difficulty answering. Atkinson and Coleman (1992) find consistency over time, and the either/or hypothesis is highly implausible. The answer may have to do partly with the range and scope of problems at hand, the ability of government to craft adequate solutions, and external constraints. As long as the range is somewhat limited and adequate resources can be mobilized to address public issues, policymaking may continue along familiar paths of deliberation with minimal perturbations. However, when resources dry up in cases where constraints are lifted or imposed, or when the number of problems multiplies exponentially, a reactive policy style is a likely outcome for two reasons. First, anticipation requires what organization theorists call slack or idle resources to be encumbered in case a problem occurs. However, in resource famines, slack is too precious and politically untenable. Second, as the number of problems grows, the ability to address them diminishes unless capacity also grows. The ability to address problems in an anticipatory environment presupposes planning and flexible tools that cover many different conditions. Because there are limits to public policy tools but limitless public problems, the capacity to address problems is likely to diminish rather than grow. As the latter is a function of resources, it follows that more problems lead to more reactive policymaking.

A Generalized Conceptualization of Policy Style

Cognizant of the above limitations and the concept's circumscribed capacity to travel beyond Western Europe, Howlett and Tosun (2019) have successfully adapted and specified policy styles in major developing and developed countries. We pick up where they leave off to examine how policy styles in different countries cast long shadows and affect policymaking during crises. We still retain the model of two dimensions of policy style but update and adapt it following Howlett and Tosun's (2019) lead. They replace the anticipatory/reactive dimension with the *key actors* involved in policymaking and the consensus/imposition dimension with *state-society relationships*. We keep their second dimension but consider the first, key actors, as unsatisfactory in an analytical and descriptive sense. Identifying key actors does not necessarily describe or even hint at their mode of deliberation. Instead, we use the following two dimensions: *administrative arrangements* and *state-society relations*.

We begin with the claim that policymaking is strongly affected by administrative arrangements, which involve key policy actors but also go beyond identification toward the more dynamic view of how they relate to one another. They determine the government's approach to problem-solving because institutions help shape perceptions of problems and, more importantly, the various tools used to address those problems (Weaver and Rockman 1993). We stay within the contours of the original conceptualization of the anticipatory/reactive dimension because bureaucrats and experts are the key actors who, often in consultation with other policy actors, develop instruments to anticipate or react to particular public problems in specific ways. In this way, we continue stressing the point that prompted the development of the concept of policy style. Policy is often made not so much in formal public institutions, such as parliament, but in informal institutional arenas, called policy communities (or networks) by "invisible" policy actors who deliberate, learn, broker, persuade, and sometimes impose their ideas and public problem frames onto other interested actors (Kingdon 1995).

We operationalize administrative arrangements as administrative policy capacity (Peters 2015). Policy capacity is defined as "the set of skills and resources—or competences and capabilities—necessary to perform policy functions" (Wu et al. 2015). Capacity performs three important functions in public policy. First, capacity ensures that policy actions are technically sound to attain the intended objectives. The term technical refers to administrative technology, that is, pulling together available legal, organizational, and human competences that are available at a given time in a particular national setting. For example, hospitals need to be equipped with appropriate technology, space, equipment, and staff to perform their function effectively. Second, capacity refers to resource adequacy. One may wish for many laboratories to experiment on new medicines and ways for delivering them to patients, but are there resources to make this happen on a sustained basis? Third, behind the use of capacity, there has to be political support to legitimate it. To stay with the health policy examples, institutionalizing the family doctor in any health system facing vocal opposition by health professionals and insurance companies makes it a politically risky and probably ineffective proposition.

Capacity reveals, facilitates, and constrains opportunities and actions in the policy process. Because we deal with the COVID-19 crisis, we will use examples mainly from the health sector although the points apply to other policy sectors as well. For example, in countries where agency autonomy is constitutionally prescribed, such as Sweden, policy responses to problems tend to be more aligned with what bureaucracies are capable of doing and not what politicians want them to do. Peters (2015) adds nuance to this possibility by elaborating on three dimensions of administrative policy capacity: autonomy, staffing, and aspirations. Different countries maintain a different mix of them and even though summary values may be the same in the aggregate, important differences will surface at the sub-systemic level. Autonomy refers to an agency's legal and organizational ability to craft its own decisions or shirk political pressure. It is a function not only of formal legal rules but also of political resources and durability of status. Staffing refers to the number of technical expertise in the policy domain within which agencies work and knowledge of its clientele. Aspirations refer to patterns of cooperation and deference between the bureaucracy and political masters. Sometimes, relations between the two may be cooperative and other times not. Even when politicians desire to control policy and the bureaucracy, as Peters (2015, 265) explains, "they may also respect the expertise of the bureaucracy and want to utilize that expertise rather than to oppose it." Higher autonomy, more expert staffing, and more cooperative aspirations indicate higher policy capacity. The particular mix differs across countries.

State-society relations refer to accommodative (or not) patterns of interest mediation (Howlett and Tosun 2019). The reasons behind their development may be administrative and historical and do not necessarily reflect efficiency or effectiveness; rather, they reflect a national way of ameliorating or bypassing social conflict (Skocpol 1987). As Richardson (1982) makes clear, at the core of policy style rests the degree of social participation: there can be no consensus-seeking without participation. Conversely, imposition of decisions presupposes the substantive absence of participation. Therefore, an important consideration of style is the degree of inclusiveness of social actors in policymaking and its level of formalization. In some political systems, such as Sweden and Norway, social actors are traditionally included in the policymaking process aiming for a reasonable consensus before decisions are made to minimize political conflict during implementation and uphold individual responsibility and social cohesion as important political values (Einhorn and Logue 2003). Other political systems, such as Greece, owing to their Napoleonic administrative traditions and despite some variation across sectors and Europeanization pressures, tend to follow a more top-down, imposition style with minimal social consultation (Dimitrakopoulos and Passas 2004; Spanou 2008). The idea is not that inclusion never or always happens. The image of a totalitarian system that is completely insulated from society or a totally inclusive political system is of course a caricature. Even in authoritarian China where the communist party has control over many aspects of social and political life, central government decisions still need to take into account, incentivize, and bring along regional and community actors (Chen et al. 2020; Qian 2019). There are obviously degrees of inclusion.

We operationalize state–society relations by degree of inclusiveness. Systems where social actors routinely and substantively participate, be it by law or as a matter of tradition, are labeled as more inclusive. We are sensitive to the fact that crisis conditions may shorten, but usually don't eliminate the consultation/participation process. But this is precisely our argument. Policy styles cast long shadows even in times of crises. Inclusiveness (or not) affects compliance, minimizes political conflict, and is consequently likely to lead to more effective measures during a crisis.

The two dimensions of national policy style, administrative policy capacity and inclusiveness, yield a matrix with four cells (Figure 2.1). We label cases of:

- Lower administrative policy capacity and lower inclusiveness as "administrative."
- Higher administrative policy capacity and lower inclusiveness as "adversarial."
- Lower administrative policy capacity and higher inclusiveness as "accommodative."
- Higher administrative policy capacity and higher inclusiveness as "managerial."

Trust (Also) Matters

While policy style sets the scene for political decision-making, we should also take into account the nature of the relationships between those governing and being governed: the polity and the citizen. These relationships essentially concern expectations. The government expects the bureaucracy to impartially implement the decided measures, and it also expects the citizen to accept and comply with them; bureaucratic institutions expect the government to allocate resources and make decisions that facilitate the fulfillment of its obligations and the citizen to act responsibly so as to not hamper policy implementation. Finally, the citizen expects the government to apply strategies and measures that protect the

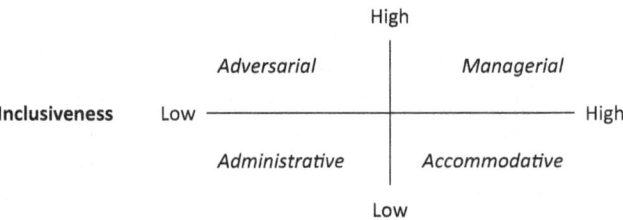

FIGURE 2.1 A Typology of Policy Styles.

population and the bureaucracy to fulfill its obligation by implementing these measures. In reality, of course, state-society and principal-agent relationships are complicated, especially when considered under different policy styles and in a crisis situation with high levels of uncertainty.

In order to understand how these relationships combined with policy style in the context of crisis management of the COVID-19 pandemic result in different national responses, we add *political trust* as an explanatory factor. While acknowledging the overlapping of *social trust* (generalized trust in others) and *political trust* (trust in government and the democratic system) (Zmerli and Newton 2017) as well as interaction effects between them (Jackman and Miller 1998; Levi and Stoker 2000; Rothstein and Stolle 2008) not least in times of crisis (Esaiasson et al. 2021), we choose here to focus on the latter, simply because our analytical construct concerns the governmental-bureaucratic system rather than peoples' abiding by social norms (Vallier 2019).

In the remainder of this section, we will first unpack trust and political trust by pointing to some of the most relevant aspects to consider in the case at hand and then discuss the interaction between policy style and political trust.

Trust

Regardless of whether we understand trust as a way of coping with uncertainty (Luhmann 1988; Simmel 1978) and the inherent complexity of late modernity (Giddens 1990), as a lubricant of the society (Arrow 1974; Axelrod 1984; Coleman 1990; Gambetta 1988; Leibenstein 1987), as a form of knowledge and social intelligence (Yamagashi 2003), or as a suspension of time and space (Möllering 2001; Sparf 2014), trust is fundamentally relational and situational (van der Meer and Zmerli 2017). In its most general form, trust conveys the expectations of social actors about their future actions, with no or limited power to influence each other's actions. This limitation of influential power ushers forth trust as a remedy for the potential risk or vulnerability in the social relationships (Levi and Stoker 2000). This remedial idea is based on trust as a crucial factor for the societal unity and integration (Misztal 2011a, 2011b; Parsons 1951) or, as Bok (1979, 26) conversely puts it: "when trust is destroyed, societies falter and collapse." Rarely is the unity and solidarity among people tried as much as during extended times of crisis involving great uncertainty and collective vulnerability. In such circumstances, expectations, decisions, power, and action become crucial.

In practice, trust is really about choosing one of many possible future scenarios (Luhmann 1979), the one that seems the most appropriate at that point in time (Sztompka 1999). It is a social mechanism to control and reduce uncertainties about the future (Bachmann 2001; Luhmann 2005). From this perspective, trust has a double function in helping us manage a "perennial epistemological gap" (Sztompka 1999, 19). The first function of trust is to *reduce uncertainty* through the judgment and expectations of the alternatives and their attendant risks. The second function is to *let go of the problem*; once the decision is made, we can move forward with confidence knowing that the best possible option was chosen.

The lack of knowledge, security, and control over the potential consequences of our own actions and those of others can be particularly problematic for individuals and institutions in crises and volatile situations. In addition to *expectation*, Guido Möllering (2001) explains the function of trust as a process also consisting of *interpretation* and *suspension*. Expectation, according to Möllering (2001), is preceded by the interpretation of the potential results from different options which, in turn, is based on, in addition to rationality, on emotions, values, and morals. Since the interpretation is ontologically based, trust has a suspending function, meaning that the risk and uncertainty following the decision are temporarily neutralized. "Suspension: the bracketing of the unknowable," as Möllering (2001, 417) puts it.

Further theorizing expectation, Sztompka (1999) distinguishes between three types of expectations involved in uncertain decisions. The first one is amoral *instrumental trust*, that is, trust without any connection to moral values but rather about previously achieved results and the actor's competence. The second is *axiomatic trust* which is about the actor's inclination to follow normative rules. The third type of expectation is *fiduciary trust* which concerns the actor's impartiality and completion of tasks regardless of vested interests. The point of this distinction is that the expectations on different actors vary according to the type of actor.

Political Trust

The conceptual scope of political trust is wide. It may refer to all aspects of political life from national identities, core regime principles, and values (e.g. democratic ideals) (Norris 2017) through "the core institutions of liberal democracy, – such as parliament, government and the justice system as well as the civil service, the police and the military [...][and] incumbent political office-holders, such as party leaders, legislators and public officials" (van der Meer and Zmerli 2017, 4) and particular public administration agencies (Vigoda–Gadot et al. 2010). Despite this wide scope, political trust essentially refers to the political institutions that link overarching democratic principles to everyday actors and policies. Ken Newton and Pippa Norris (2000, 53) argue that this understanding of political trust is "the central indicator of the underlying feeling of the general public about its polity."

From the perspective of the citizen, Rothstein and Stolle (2002, 20) find that "citizens make distinctions between types of confidence in institutions [...][and] do not view all institutions in a similar way," while they also "develop different levels of trust dependent on their institutional experiences" (Rothstein and Stolle 2002, 27) which nuances the understanding of van der Meer and Zmerli's (2017) situational approach mentioned above. Moreover, Bauer and Freitag (2017) stress that trust changes over time. This may potentially complicate the trust relationships even further in an extended crisis, reflecting differentials in the time horizon among the short-term policy outcomes, evaluations of leaders and institutions, and the public's expectations toward their governments and institutions. Indeed, Levi and Stoker (2000, 496) urge scholars to "expand their inquiries beyond the traditional focus on citizens' trust in 'government' in general, by studying the causes and consequences of citizens' trust in specific political actors, organizations, or institutions."

A brief review of the literature on public trust in the healthcare system reveals two broad trajectories. The first consists of the political and administrative functions of the healthcare system such as the level of acceptance of priority setting in health policy (Brall et al. 2019)—referring to the idea that "policy-makers who act according to values that are in line with public values are more trusted than others" (Gille and Brall 2020, 233)—and level of vaccine coverage (Ozawa and Stack 2013). It also pertains to technical issues such as setting up secure databases with patient records (van Staa, Godacre, Buchan, and Smeeth 2016), genome projects, and biobanks (Gille Smith and Mays 2021) as well as trust in non-discriminatory and fair health practices (Bonner, Ferrans, Moore Burke, and Gorelick 2005; Tarn et al. 2005). Gilson (2003) refers to this trajectory as 'macro-relationships.'

The second trajectory, which Gilson (2003) refers to as 'micro-relationships,' consists of the individual's encounters within healthcare and the "past experiences, present perceptions and future expectations" (Gille and Brall 2020, 233). This is a wide research field in itself and beyond the scope of this chapter (see, e.g., Birkhäuer et al. 2017; Goold 2002; Hall, Dunga, Zheng, and Mishra 2001). While some studies indicate a general decrease in trust in the healthcare system (Abelson, Miller, and Giacomini 2009), health professionals are still one of the most trusted professions. While acknowledging the importance of micro-relationships in healthcare and the interaction effects between different levels, in this volume, we focus on the systemic macro level where trust is crucial in ensuring societal impact through met expectations and increasing influence. It is worth noting that the public trust in the healthcare system is a complex concept formed "not only by the health care system itself, individuals' experiences of it and its media image but also by discourse in the public sphere about individuals' experiences and the system as a whole" (Gille, Smith, and Mays. 2017, 25). In a comparative study, van der Schee et al. (2007), reporting on Germany, the Netherlands, and England and Wales shows that both interpersonal trust (patient doctor) and public trust (in the healthcare system) are deeply influenced by media, and the authors suggest that the different levels of trust between the countries can be explained by cultural differences.

In Conclusion: The Interaction of Trust and Policy Styles—National Responses to COVID-19

Essentially, trust helps policymakers and citizens cope with uncertainty. Trust is fundamentally relational; its introduction to the policy styles literature ushers the aspect of the consumers of public policy. Citizen compliance has proven to be of salience in crisis situations in general and in the aftermath of the pandemic in particular. In fact, Marien and Hooghe (2011) show that citizens with low levels of political trust are significantly more likely to tolerate non-compliance with the law and illicit behavior. Political trust, viewed as a set of expectations (both by the polity and by the citizens), sidesteps uncertainty in policymaking through the analytical parsing of the concept in three categories mentioned elsewhere in this section: instrumental, axiomatic, and fiduciary. Instrumental trust is based on past performance: how has the public sector performed in the past? Largely, this is a question of professional competence and may be operationalized as administrative policy capacity. The issue here is whether the institutional structure of the public sector is staffed with professionals and able to formulate, implement, and evaluate public policies. Axiomatic trust is normative—one trusts the public sector because it is the right thing to do—or is it? The issue here is a matter of historical contingencies. Fiduciary trust is at the heart of inclusiveness—are diverse interests accommodated?

The contribution of this edited volume lies in specifying the way political trust interacts with policy styles to shape national responses. Trust affects and is affected by policy style, and both have a significant impact on responses. Higher trust in government and health practitioners increases the legitimacy of governmental responses and results a wider acceptance of government measures. In systems with higher policy capacity and higher inclusiveness in decision making, trust magnifies agency capabilities leading to decentralized responses. In such systems, citizens trust the ability of policymakers to design effective plans and the competence of the bureaucracy to execute them. This is especially salient under conditions of crises underpinned by urgency and uncertainty. Individual accountability and faith in the policy system's capacity to pursue responsible action are important ingredients of the national response.

Conversely, in systems with lower policy capacity and lower inclusiveness, citizens lack faith in the system and expect central authority to take over. Lack of trust weakens the effects of policy capacity because it pushes and pulls in two opposite directions (Exadaktylos and Zahariadis 2014). It lowers willingness to act while it increases political conflict within the administration. The lack of clear guidance from central authority gives discretion to implementing agents to frame issues the way they see fit. The problem is the same element that empowers agents also paralyzes them because it pinpoints responsibility. In the presence of ambiguous roles, political responsibility for adverse effects is shifted to agents. If the rules call for stringent and politically costly measures, such as a lockdown, agents have no incentive to act. Hence, central authority takes over control of crisis response.

References

Abelson, Julia, Fiona A. Miller, and Mita Giacomini. 2009. "What Does It Mean to Trust a Health System? A Qualitative Study of Canadian Health Care Values." *Health Policy* 91: 63–70.

Adam, Christian, Steffen Hurka, and Christoph Knill. 2017. "Four Styles of Regulation and their Implications for Comparative Policy Analysis." *Journal of Comparative Policy Analysis* 19 (4): 327–44.

Adolph, Christopher, Kenya Amano, Bree Bang-Jensen, Nancy Fullman, and John Wilkerson. 2021. "Pandemic Politics: Timing State-Level Social Distancing Responses to Covid-19." *Journal of Health Politics, Policy and Law* 46 (2): 211–33.

Arrow, Kenneth J. 1974. *The Limits of Organization.* New York: Norton.

Atkinson, Michael M., and William D. Coleman. 1992. "Policy Networks, Policy Communities and the Problems of Governance." *Governance* 5 (2): 154–80.

Axelrod, Robert. 1984. *The Evolution of Cooperation.* New York: Basic Books.

Bachmann, Reinhard. 2001. "Trust, Power and Control in Trans-Organizational Relations." *Organization Studies* 22 (2): 337–65.

Bakir, Caner. 2020. "The Turkish State's Responses to Existential Covid-19 Crisis." *Policy and Society* 39: 424–41.

Bamberger, Walter. 2010. *Interpersonal Trust – Attempt of a Definition.* München: Technische Universität. Retrieved 12 August 2014 from http://www.ldv.ei.tum.de/en/research/fidens/interpersonal-trust/

Bauer, Paul C., and Markus Freitag. 2017. "Measuring Trust." In *The Oxford Handbook of Social and Political Trust*, ed. Eric M. Uslaner, Part I. Oxford: Oxford University Press. doi.10.1093/oxfordhb/9780190274801.013.1.

Bauhr, Monika. 2007. "Explaining Public Trust in Institutions. The Role of Consensual Expert Ideas." In *From Kyoto to the Town Hall: Making International and National Climate Policy Work at the Local Level*, eds. Lennart J. Lundqvist and Anders Biel, 27–42. London: Earthscan.

Birkhäuer Johanna, Jens Gaab, Joe Kossowsky, Sebastian Hasler, Peter Krummenacher, and Christoph Werner. (2017) "Trust in the health care professional and health outcome: A meta-analysis." *PLoS One* 12(2): e0170988.

Boin, Arjen, Paul 't Hart, Eric Stern, and Bengt Sundelius. 2017. *The Politics of Crisis Management: Public Leadership under Pressure.* 2nd ed. Cambridge: Cambridge University Press.

Boin, Arjen. 2019. "The Transboundary Crisis: Why we are Unprepared." *Journal of Contingencies and Crisis Management* 27 (1): 94–99.

Bok, Sissela. 1999. *Lying: Moral Choice in Public and Private Life.* New York: Vintage Books.

Bonner, Gloria J., Carol Estwing Ferrans, Edna F. Moore-Burke, and Philip Gorelick. 2005. "Determinants of Trust and Mistrust in Physicians Identified by African American Family Caregivers." *African American Research Perspectives* 11 (1): 89–102.

Bouckaert, Geert, Davide Galli, Sabine Kuhlmann, Renate Reiter, and Steven Van Hecke. 2020. "European Coronationalism? A Hot Spot Governing a Pandemic Crisis." *Public Administration Review* 80: 765–73.

Cairney, Paul. 2009. "The 'British Policy Style' and Mental Health: Beyond the Headlines." *Journal of Social Policy* 38 (4): 1–18.

Capano, Giliberto, Michael Howlett, Darryl S. L. Jarvis, M. Ramesh, and Nihit Goyal. 2020. "Mobilizing Policy (in)Capacity to Fight Covid-19: Understanding Variations in State Responses." *Policy and Society* 39: 285–308.

Capano, Giliberto. 2020. "Policy Design and State Capacity in the Covid-19 Emergency in Italy: If You Are Not Prepared for the (Un)Expected, You Can Be Only What You Already Are." *Policy and Society* 39: 326–44.

Cheng, Yuan, Jianxing Yu, Yongdong Shen, and Biao Huang. 2020. "Coproducing Responses to COVID-19 with Community-Based Organizations: Lessons from Zhejiang Province, China." *Public Administration Review* 80 (5): 866–73. doi:10.1111/puar.13244.

Christensen, Tom, and Per Lægreid. 2020. "Balancing Governance Capacity and Legitimacy: How the Norwegian Government Handled the Covid-19 Crisis as a High Performer." *Public Administration Review* 80: 774–79.

Coleman, James S. 1990. *Foundations of Social Theory*. Cambridge, MA: Harvard University Press.

Crozier, Michael J., Samuel P. Huntington, and Joji Watanuki. 1975. *The Crisis of Democracy: Report on the Governability of Democracies to the Trilateral Commission*. New York: New York University Press.

DeLeo, Rob A. 2016. *Anticipatory Policymaking: When Government Acts to Prevent Problems and Why Is It So Difficult*. New York: Routledge.

Deslatte, Aaron, Megan E. Hatch, and Eric Stokan. 2020. "How Can Local Governments Address Pandemic Inequities?" *Public Administration Review* 80: 827–31.

Devos, Thierry, Dario Spini, and Shalom H. Schwartz. 2002. "Conflicts among Human Values and Trust in Institutions." *British Journal of Social Psychology* 41 (4): 481–94.

Dimitrakopoulos, Dionyssis, and Argyris G. Passas. 2004. "Conclusion: Europeanisation and the Greek Policy Style: National or Sectoral?" In Greece in the European Union, eds. Dionyssis Dimitrakopoulos and Argyris G. Passas, 139–47. London: Routledge.

Edelman, Murray. 1988. *Constructing the Political Spectacle*. Chicago: University of Chicago Press.

Edlund, Jonas. 2006. "Trust in the Capability of the Welfare State and General Welfare State Support: Sweden 1997–2002." *Acta Sociologica* 49 (4): 95–417.

Einhorn, Eric S., and John Logue. 2003. *Modern Welfare States: Scandinavian Politics and Policy in the Global Age*. 2nd ed. Westport, CT: Praeger.

Esaiasson, Peter, Jacob Sohlberg, Marina Ghersetti, and Bengt Johansson. 2021. "How the Coronavirus Crisis Affects Citizen Trust in Institutions and in Unknown Others: Evidence from 'the Swedish Experiment'." *European Journal of Political Research* 60 (3): 748–60. https://doi.org/10.1111/1475-6765.12419.

Exadaktylos, Theofanis, and Nikolaos Zahariadis. 2014. "*Quid pro Quo*: Political Trust and Policy Implementation in Greece during the Age of Austerity." *Politics & Policy* 42 (1): 160–83. doi:10.1111/polp.12058.

Federal Emergency Management Agency. 2017. *National Incident Management System*, 3rd ed. Washington, DC: US Department of Homeland Security. Retrieved from https://www.fema.gov/media-library-data/1508151197225-ced8c60378c3936-adb92c1a3ee6f6564/FINAL_NIMS_2017.pdf

Freeman, Gary P. 1985. "National Styles and Policy Sectors." *Journal of Public Policy* 5 (4): 467–96.

Gadson, Danielle N. 2020. "Advancing Equity in Public Administration: Prioritizing Equality of Outcomes in the Covid-19 Crisis." *Risk, Hazards & Crisis in Public Policy* 11 (4): 449–57.

Gambetta, Diego. 1988. "Can we Trust Trust?" In *Trust: Making and Breaking Cooperative Relations*, ed. Diego Gambetta, 213–37. Oxford: Basil Blackwell.

Gaynor, Tia Sherèe, and Meghan E. Wilson. 2020. "Social Vulnerability and Equity: The Disproportionate Impact of Covid-19." *Public Administration Review* 80: 832–38.

Gilson, Lucy. 2003. "Trust and the Development of Health Care as a Social Institution." *Social Science & Medicine* 56: 1453–68.

Giddens, Anthony. 1990. *The Consequences of Modernity*. Cambridge: Polity in Association with Blackwell.

Gille, Felix, and Caroline Brall. 2020. "Public Trust: Caught between Hype and Need." *International Journal of Public Health* 65: 233–34.

Gille, Felix, Sarah Smith, and Nicholas Mays. 2017. "Towards a Broader Conceptualisation of 'Public Trust' in the Health Care System." *Social Theory & Health* 15 (1): 25–43. http://dx.doi.org.proxybib.miun.se/10.1057/s41285-016-0017-y

Gille, Felix, Sarah Smith, and Nicholas Mays. 2021. "What Is Public Trust in the Healthcare System? A New Conceptual Framework Developed from Qualitative Data in England." *Social Theory & Health* 19: 1–20.

Giritli Nygren, Katarina, and Anna Olofsson. 2020. "Managing the Covid-19 Pandemic through Individual Responsibility: The Consequences of a World Risk Society and Enhanced Ethopolitics." *Journal of Risk Research* 23 (7–8): 1–5.

Goold, Susan Dorr. 2002. "Trust, Distrust and Trustworthiness: Lessons from the Field." *Journal of General Internal Medicine* 17 (1): 79–81.

Gotham, Kevin Fox, and Miriam Greenberg. 2014. *Crisis Cities: Disaster and Redevelopment in New York and New Orleans.* New York: Oxford University Press.

Grizzle, David, Amy Goodin, and Scott E. Robinson. 2020. "Connecting with New Partners in Covid-19 Response." *Public Administration Review* 80: 629–33.

Halffman, Willem. 2005. "Science-Policy Boundaries: National Styles?" *Science and Public Policy* 32 (6): 457–67.

Hall, Mark A., Elizabeth Dugan, Beiyao Zheng, and Aneil K. Mishra. 2001. "Trust in Physicians and Medical Institutions: What Is It, Can It Be Measured, and Does It Matter?" *Milbank Quarterly* 79: 613–39.

Hardin, Russell. 1998. "Trust in Government." In *Trust and Governance*, eds. Valerie A. Braithwaite and Margaret Levi, 9–27. New York: Russell Sage Foundation.

Heclo, Hugh. 1974. *Modern Social Politics in Britain and Sweden.* New Haven: Yale University Press.

Heclo, Hugh. 1978. "Issue Networks and the Executive Establishment." In *The New American Political System*, ed. Anthony King, 87–124. Washington, DC: American Enterprise Institute for Public Policy Research.

Heclo, Hugh, and Aaron Wildavsky. 1981. *The Private Government of Public Money: Community and Policy inside British Politics.* 2nd ed. London: Macmillan.

Howlett, Michael, and Jale Tosun, eds. 2019. *Policy Styles and Policy-Making: Exploring the Linkages.* New York: Routledge.

Huberfeld, Nicole, Sarah H. Gordon, and David K. Jones. 2020. "Federalism Complicates the Response to the Covid-19 Health and Economic Crisis: What Can Be Done?" *Journal of Health Politics, Policy and Law* 45 (6): 951–65.

Huntington, Samuel P. 1975. "The Democratic Distemper." *The Public Interest* 41 (Fall): 9–38.

Jackman, Robert W., and Ross A. Miller. 1998. "Social Capital and Politics." *Annual Review of Political Science* 1 (1): 47–73.

Kertzer, David I. 1988. *Ritual, Politics & Power.* New Haven, CT: Yale University Press.

Kettl, Donald F. 2020. "States Divided: The Implications of American Federalism for Covid-19." *Public Administration Review* 80: 595–602.

King, Anthony. 1975. "Overload: Problems of Governing in the 1970s." *Political Studies* XXIII: 284–96.

Kingdon, John W. 1995. *Agendas, Alternatives, and Public Policies.* 2nd ed. New York: Harper Collins.

Knill, Christoph. 2001. *The Europeanisation of National Administrations: Patterns of Institutional Change and Persistence.* Cambridge: Cambridge University Press.

Knill, Christoph, Louisa Bayerlein, Jan Enkler, and Stephan Grohs. 2019. "Bureaucratic Influence and Administrative Styles in International Organizations." *The Review of International Organizations* 14: 83–106.

Kumagai, Saki, and Federica Iorio. 2020. *Building Trust in Government through Citizen Engagement*. Working Paper. Washington, DC: World Bank. http://hdl.handle.net/10986/33346

Lee, Sabinne, Changho Hwang, and M. Jae Moon. 2020. "Policy Learning and Crisis Policy-Making: Quadruple-Loop Learning and Covid-19 Responses in South Korea." *Policy and Society* 39: 363–81.

Levi, Margaret. 1998. "A State of Trust." In *Trust and Governance*, eds. Valerie A. Braithwaite and Margaret Levi, 77–101. New York: Russell Sage Foundation.

Levi, Margaret, and Laura Stoker. 2000. "Political Trust and Trustworthiness." *Annual Review of Political Science* 3 (1): 475–507.

Luhmann, Niklas. 1979. *Trust and Power: Two Works*. Chichester: J. Wiley.

Luhmann, Niklas. 1998. *Observations on Modernity*. Stanford: Stanford University Press.

Lukes, Steven. 1975. "Political Ritual and Social Integration." *Sociology* 9 (2): 289–308.

Lynch, Julia. 2020. "Health Equity, Social Policy, and Promoting Recovery from Covid-19." *Journal of Health Politics, Policy and Law* 45 (6): 983–995.

Marien, Sophie, and Marc Hooghe. 2011. "Does Political Trust Matter? An Empirical Investigation into the Relation between Political Trust and Support for Law Compliance." *European Journal of Political Research* 50: 267–91.

Martin-Howard, Simone, and Kyle Farmbry. 2020. "Framing a Needed Discourse on Health Disparities and Social Inequities: Drawing Lessons from a Pandemic." *Public Administration Review* 80: 839–44.

Mei, Ciqi. 2020. "Policy Style, Consistency and the Effectiveness of the Policy Mix in China's Fight against Covid-19." *Policy and Society* 39: 309–25.

Migone, Andrea Riccardo. 2020. "Trust, but Customize: Federalism's Impact on the Canadian Covid-19 Response." *Policy and Society* 39: 382–402.

Miller, Arthur H., and Ola Listhaug. 1999. "Political Performance and Institutional Trust." In *Critical Citizens: Global Support for Democratic Governance*, ed. Pippa Norris, 204–16, Oxford: Oxford University Press.

Misztal, Barbara A. 2011a. *The Challenges of Vulnerability: In Search of Strategies for a Less Vulnerable Social Life*. Basingstoke: Palgrave Macmillan.

Misztal, Barbara A. 2011b. "Trust: Acceptance of, Precaution Against and Cause of Vulnerability." *Comparative Sociology* 10 (3): 358–79.

Möllering, Guido. 2001. "The Nature of Trust: From Georg Simmel to a Theory of Expectation, Interpretation and Suspension." *Sociology* 35 (2): 403–20.

Newton, Kenneth, and Pippa Norris. 2000. "Confidence in Public Institutions: Faith, Culture, or Performance?" In *Disaffected Democracies. What's Troubling the Trilateral Countries?* eds. Susan J. Pharr and Robert D. Putnam, 52–73. Princeton, NJ: Princeton University Press.

Norris, Pippa. 2017. "The Conceptual Framework of Political Support." In *Handbook on Political Trust*, eds. Sonja Zmerli and Tom W. G. van der Meer, 19–32. Cheltenham, UK: Edward Elgar.

Ozawa, Sachiko, and Meghan L. Stack. 2013. "Public trust and vaccine acceptance-international perspectives." *Human vaccines & immunotherapeutics* 9(8): 1774–1778.

Parsons, Talcott. 1951. *The Social System*. NY: The Free Press of Glencoe.

Peters, B. Guy. 2015. "Policy Capacity in Public Administration." *Policy and Society* 34 (3–4): 219–28.

Petridou, Evangelia, Nikolaos Zahariadis, and Stephen Ceccoli. 2020. "Averting Institutional Disasters? Drawing Lessons from China to Inform the Cypriot Response to the Covid-19 Pandemic." *European Policy Analysis* 6: 318–27.

Pierre, Jon. 2016. "Introduction: The Decline of Swedish Exceptionalism." In *The Oxford Handbook of Swedish Politics*, ed. Jon Pierre, 1–16. Oxford: Oxford University Press.

Pierre, Jon. 2020. "Nudges against Pandemics: Sweden's Covid-19 Containment Strategy in Perspective." *Policy and Society* 39: 478–93.

Qian, Jiwei. 2019. "Policy Styles in China: How to Control and Motivate Bureaucracy." In *Policy Styles and Policy-Making: Exploring the Linkages*, eds. Michael Howlett and Jale Tosun, 201–21. New York: Routledge.

Richardson, Jeremy, and Grant Jordan. 1979. *Governing Under Pressure: The Policy Process in a Post-Parliamentary Democracy*. Oxford: Robertson.

Richardson, Jeremy, ed. 1982. *Policy Styles in Western Europe*. London: Allen & Unwin.

Richardson, Jeremy, Gunnel Gustafsson, and Grant Jordan. 1982. "The Concept of Policy Style." In *Policy Styles in Western Europe*, ed. Jeremy Richardson, 1–16. London: Allen & Unwin.

Rocco, Philip, Daniel Béland, and Alex Waddan. 2020. "Stuck in Neutral? Federalism, Policy Instruments, and Counter-Cyclical Responses to Covid-19 in the United States." *Policy and Society* 39: 458–77.

Rothstein, Bo, and Dietlind Stolle. 2002, August. "How Political Institutions Create and Destroy Social Capital: An Institutional Theory of Generalized Trust." In *98th meeting of the American Political Science Association in Boston, MA*. Retrieved from http://www.academia.edu/download/33629039/2003winner.pdf

Rothstein, Bo, and Dietlind Stolle. 2008. "The State and Social Capital: An Institutional Theory of Generalized Trust." *Comparative Politics* 40 (4): 441–59. https://doi.org/10.5129/001041508X12911362383354

Sasaki, Masamichi. 2011. "Trust: Comparative Perspectives." *Comparative Sociology* 10 (2): 161–65.

van der Schee, Evelien, Peter P. Groenewegen, and Roland D. Friele. 2006. "Public Trust in Health Care: A Performance Indicator?" *Journal of Health Organization and Management* 20: 468–76.

Schomaker, Rahel M., and Michael W. Bauer. 2020. "What Drives Successful Administrative Performance During Crises? Lessons from Refugee Migration and the Covid-19 Pandemic." *Public Administration Review* 80: 845–50.

Simmel, Georg. 1978. *The Philosophy of Money*. London: Routledge.

Skocpol, Theda. 1987. "A Society without a 'State'? Political Organization, Social Conflict, and Welfare Provision in the United States." *Journal of Public Policy* 7 (4): 349–71.

Spanou, Calliope. 2008. "State Reform in Greece: Responding to Old and New Challenges." *International Journal of Public Sector Management* 21 (2): 150–73.

Sparf, Jörgen. 2014. *Tillit i samhällsskyddets organisation: Om det sociala gränssnittet i risk – och krishantering mellan kommunen och funktionshindrade (Trust in Civil Protection and Preparedness. On the Social Interface in Risk and Crisis Management Between Disabled People and the Municipal Organization)*. Mid Sweden University Doctoral Thesis 202.

van Staa, Tjeerd-Pieter, Ben Goldacre, Iain Buchan, and Liam Smeeth. 2016. "Big Health Data: The Need to Earn Public Trust." *British Medical Journal* 354: i3636.

Sztompka, Piotr. 1999. *Trust: A Sociological Theory*. Cambridge: Cambridge University Press.

Tarn, Derjung M., Lisa S. Meredith, Marjorie Kagawa-Singer, Shinji Matsumura, Seiji Bito, Robert K. Oye, Honghu Liu, Katherine L. Kahn, Shunichi Fukuhara, and Neil S. Wenger. 2005. "Trust in One's Physician: The Role of Ethnic Match, Autonomy, Acculturation, and Religiosity among Japanese and Japanese Americans." *Annals of Family Medicine* 3: 339–47.

The Independent Panel for Pandemic Preparedness and Response. 2021. *Covid-19: Make It the Last Pandemic*. Retrieved from https://theindependentpanel.org/wp-content/uploads/2021/05/COVID-19-Make-it-the-Last-Pandemic_final.pdf

Vallier, Kevin. 2019. *Social and Political Trust: Concepts, Causes, and Consequences*. Retrieved from Niskanen Center, https://www.niskanencenter.org/wp-content/uploads/old_uploads/2019/05/Vallier-Social-and-Political-Trust-Niskanen.pdf

van der Meer, Tom W. G., and Sonja Zmerli. 2017. "The Deeply Rooted Concern with Political Trust." In *Handbook on Political Trust*, eds. Sonja Zmerli and Tom W. G. van der Meer, 1–15. Cheltenham, UK: Edward Elgar.

van der Wal, Zeger. 2020. "Being a Public Manager in Times of Crisis: The Art of Managing Stakeholders, Political Masters, and Collaborative Networks." *Public Administration Review* 80: 759–64.

van Waarden, Frans. 1995. "Persistence of National Policy Styles." In *Convergence or Diversity? Internationalization and Economic Policy Response*, eds. B. Unger and F. Van Waarden, 333–72. Aldershot, UK: Avebury.

Vigoda-Gadot, Eran, Aviv Shoham, and Dana R. Vashdi. 2010. "Bridging Bureaucracy and Democracy in Europe: A Comparative Study of Perceived Managerial Excellence, Satisfaction with Public Services, and Trust in Governance." *European Union Politics* 11 (2): 289–308. https://doi.org/10.1177%2F1465116510363657

Vogel, David. 1986. *National Styles of Regulation: Environmental Policy in Great Britain and the United States*. Ithaca, NY: Cornell University Press.

Weaver, R. Kent, and Bert Rockman, eds. 1993. *Do Institutions Matter? Government Capabilities in the United States and Abroad*. Washington, DC: Brookings Institution.

Weible, Christopher M., Daniel Nohrstedt, Paul Cairney, David P. Carter, Deserai A. Crow, Anna P. Durnová, Tanya Heikkila, Karin Ingold, Allan McConnell, and Diane Stone. 2020. "Covid-19 and the Policy Sciences: Initial Reactions and Perspectives." *Policy Sciences* 53: 225–41.

Wu, Xun, M. Ramesh, and Michael Howlett. 2015. "Policy Capacity: A Conceptual Framework for Understanding Policy Competences and Capabilities." *Policy and Society* 34 (3–4): 165–71.

Yamagashi, Tosho. 2003. "Cross-societal Experimentation on Trust." In *Trust and Reciprocity: Interdisciplinary Lessons for Experimental Research*, eds. Elinor Ostrom and James Walker, 352–70. Russell Sage Foundation.

Yang, Kaifeng. 2006. "Trust and Citizen Involvement Decisions: Trust in Citizens, Trust in Institutions, and Propensity to Trust." *Administration & Society* 38 (5): 573–95.

Zmerli, Sonja, and Ken Newton. 2017. "Objects of Political and Social Trust: Scalers and Hierarchies." In *Handbook on Political Trust*, eds. Sonja Zmerli and Tom W. G. van der Meer, 104–24. Cheltenham, UK: Edward Elgar.

2

Centralized Responses

3

POLICY STYLES AND THE CHINESE COVID-19 RESPONSE

Stephen Ceccoli

Examining China's COVID-19 response through a policy styles prism presents several opportunities and challenges. China's inclusion in this volume's comparative research design, for instance, addresses a notable "deficiency" in a policy styles typology focusing almost exclusively on Western democracies (Freeman, 1985: 476). This traditionally narrow scope reflects a "democratic prism" (Reny, 2011) prioritizing the study of democracies while often imposing democratic lenses on non-democracies. A policy styles approach also offers valuable crisis policymaking insights, particularly given the cross-national COVID-19 outcome disparities. During the pandemic's first and second waves (i.e., January through November 2020), China reported 93,329 cases, 4,750 deaths, and 3 cumulative deaths per million population (World Health Organization, 2020), the latter rivaling New Zealand and Vietnam among the world's lowest.[1] By April 8, 2020, with the pandemic still ravaging the globe, Chinese authorities reported just a trickle of new infections and no COVID-19 deaths as daily life converged toward normalcy capping a tumultuous 100-day period.

Analytically, challenges arise as China's mix of policy styles characteristics do not divide neatly and clearly relative to other country cases. Using this volume's theoretical framework, China represents an adversarial policy style given its combination of high policy capacity and relatively low actor inclusiveness. High policy capacity, reflected in the ability to "make intelligent collective choices" and direct "scarce resources to public ends" (Painter and Pierre, 2005: 2), emanates from substantial Chinese human and material resources as well as centralized political leadership. Conversely, the ruling party's outsized role in dominating the country's political space traditionally limits the depth and scope of policymaking participation. Although more widespread than commonly presumed, particularly since the 1980s "deliberative turn" in Chinese political

DOI: 10.4324/9781003137399-5

development (He and Warren, 2011), the absence of Western-style legislative and electoral institutions implies low actor inclusiveness.

Evidence suggests a two-tiered Chinese COVID-19 response. Initially, a short-lived centrifugal response featured loosely concentrated decision-making and implementation, inconsistent messaging, and clumsy resource mobilization. Yet, following a critical January 20 turning point, a highly centralized response based on the party-state's concentrated steering capacity, stringent lockdown measures, strategically coordinated messaging, and substantial resource marshaling soon suppressed the virus. Underscoring the turning point, one of this volume's primary contributions lies in specifying how political trust interacts with policy styles to shape national COVID-19 responses.[2] Fukuyama (2020) asserts that the "crucial determinant" in pandemic performance lies in "the state's capacity and, above all, trust in government." Thus, independent of regime type, Fukuyama (2020) contends that "citizens have to believe that the executive knows what it is doing." Therefore, we should anticipate that policy style critically interacts with political trust and citizen confidence in the executive, particularly in a crisis response situation. In this case, adversarial policy styles combine with lower trust tend to prompt centrifugal responses, whereas higher trustworthiness facilitates greater centralization as the polity becomes less prone to question implementation tactics or motives.

This chapter begins by reviewing Chinese policy styles, emphasizing longstanding traditions of centralized leadership, fragmented authority, and policy experimentation. This approach, interacting with a hierarchical sense of political trust, shaped the country's COVID-19 response, examined here by focusing on three key components: (a) command and coordination, (b) communication and information management, and (c) resource management. *New York Times* columnist Nicholas Kristoff (2021) perhaps summed up the Chinese response best, writing, "China badly bungled its initial handling of the coronavirus outbreak, but then moved heaven and earth to halt the virus and save hundreds of thousands of lives … China is a complex and contradictory place, not a caricature."

China and Policy Style: Power, Centralized Leadership, and Fragmented Authoritarianism

As "the interaction" between governmental problem-solving approaches and relationships among policy process actors, policy styles encapsulate both the institutional arrangements shaping policy deliberations and the actors and ideas engaged in such deliberations (Richardson et al., 1982: 13). In specific terms, Howlett and Tosun (2018) classify China as a "closed-centralist" policy styles type featuring bureaucrats and experts in active policymaking roles (relative to politicians and the public) and relatively limited societal actor involvement in decision processes. While seemingly plausible, given China's single-party hegemonic authoritarianism, this categorization remains contestable. For instance, while Chinese bureaucrats undoubtedly play key implementation roles, top party officials and policymakers monopolize consequential decision-making, while embodying leadership priorities of maintaining stature, authority, and power and political survival (Lieberthal and Oksenberg, 1988). Moreover, far from closed, the system features a vast network of complex and often overlapping relationships across several dimensions, including party and state, vertical and horizontal, and formal and informal.

Qian (2018) contends that China's policy styles exhibit two predominant characteristics: a hierarchical approach and a reactive tendency. The former reflects China's rich imperial history, Confucian political culture, and ancient cosmological view of *tian xia* (literally, 'all under heaven'). For centuries, Chinese emperors derived legitimacy from a 'Heavenly Mandate' based on righteous rule (rather than a religious connotation) coupled with the Confucian understanding that if one followed the rules, the 'Great Harmony' could be achieved. In the People's Republic era, the Maoist "mass line" perhaps best characterizes both centralized interests and local initiative as cadres apprise leaders of citizen policy demands. The system's reactive rather than proactive tendency stems from several institutional and agency-based considerations. Institutionally, the party-state's hierarchical bureaucratic structure fosters a 'stove-piping' tendency with various ministries conditioned and incentivized to share information vertically, though not horizontally across other ministries, bureaucracies, or geographic units.

An adversarial style reflects the combination of high policy capacity and low actor inclusiveness. Though distinct from understandings of adversarial in Western contexts, separate decision-making structures maintained by the government of the People's Republic of China (PRC) and the Communist Party of China (CPC) constitute perhaps the most fundamental differentiating characteristic of Chinese policy style. While some PRC and CPC governing bodies overlap in terms of function, authority and personnel, the Party remains "the organized expression of the will of society," so its authority remains supreme, not the state's (Schurmann, 1968: 110).[3] Modeled in principal-agent terms and reflecting inherent adversarial relations, the Party functions as principal with the state acting as the agent (Shirk, 1992).[4] Consequently, the Chinese political system's greatest concentration of power lies with the seven-member Politburo Standing Committee (PSC), the country's ultimate decision-making body, led by CPC General Secretary Xi Jinping.

A related capacity feature reflects the informal nature of power at the party's highest levels. Specifically, *ad hoc* administrative vehicles known as Leading Small Groups (LSGs), whose agendas and memberships are usually secretive, maintain implementation responsibilities for major PSC policy decisions (Miller, 2017). Typically led by a PSC member and featuring an interlocking nature of appointments, party-directed LSG's facilitate inter-agency coordination that tempers the "structural rigidity" associated with the Chinese bureaucracy. Gore contends that LSG's provide "the missing 'joint' that allows the otherwise 'fragmented and disjointed' bureaucracy to function" (2019: 179).

Though bargaining between Chinese officials takes place at all levels (i.e., national, provincial, municipal, county, and township), central state actors engage in critical decision-making, leaving implementation responsibilities to provincial and local authorities. While policy generally reflects the leaders' problem understandings and political interests, implementation often reflect "differentiated understandings" of the problems among those involved (Lieberthal and Oksenberg, 1988: 15). Consequently, as Mertha observes, policy outcomes often remain both "increasingly malleable" and "at a considerable variance" with the top leaders' initial policymaking goals (2008: 5, 2009: 996). This phenomenon has propelled "fragmented authoritarianism" (FA) as the Chinese politics literature's predominant policymaking framework (Landry, 2012; Lieberthal and Lampton, 1992; Lieberthal and Oksenberg, 1988; Mertha, 2008, 2009).

Bridging the gap between policymaking and implementation, particularly for local authorities in implementing central government policies, remains a perennial policy challenge (Zhao and Peters, 2009). FA is based on a "dual rule" bureaucratic agency logic derived from the Soviets' "vertical and dual subordination" approach (Schurmann, 1968: 188). Effectively, agencies engage in dual relationships, referred to as *tiao* and *kuai*, with *tiao-tiao* relations depicting vertical (functional) relationships between superior and subordinate entities and *kuai-kuai* relations connecting horizontal (geographic) relationships between administrative, legislative, and other agencies within the same jurisdictions (Mertha, 2005; Schroeder, 1992). According to Schroeder (1992: 286–87), "The relative power of *tiao-kuai* authorities changes with time and with different functional systems." Lacking effective monitoring and oversight from an independent legislature exposes bureaucratic agencies to multiple principal-agent problems since dual rule "means multiple rather than single channels of command and information" (Schurmann, 1968: 189).

Heilmann and Perry's (2011) depiction of "guerilla policy style," the most compelling account of Chinese policy style to date, well captures these top-down, reactive, and adversarial qualities. As with CPC revolutionary strategies confronting Chinese nationalists and foreign imperial powers a century ago, guerilla policy style, they argue, has "proved capable of generating an array of creative — proactive as well as evasive — tactics for managing sudden change and uncertainty" (2011: 7). Unlike "the stability oriented 'anticipate-and-regulate' norm of modern constitutional government," Heilmann and Perry characterize "a change-oriented 'push-and-seize' style" (2011: 13). Effectively, this approach sacrifices ostensibly desirable tradeoffs like predictability, consistency, and procedural stability in exchange for a mode of operation based on "an acceptance of pervasive uncertainty, a readiness to experiment and learn…, an agility in grasping unforeseen opportunities, a singlemindedness in pursuing strategic goals, a willingness to ignore ugly side effects, and a ruthlessness in eradicating unfriendly opposition" (2011: 21–22). These features, coupled with the interaction of political trust, figure prominently in understanding China's COVID-19 response.

Political Trust: Hierarchical Trust and Policy Memories

At the capacity-inclusion-trust nexus, the Chinese system remains exceptional relative to this volume's other cases. Despite comparatively low inclusiveness, high administrative capacity is augmented by hierarchical trust in the administrative system. Unlike countries where individuals trust local and provincial governments more than central ones, China remains a rare exception. Li (2016) uses the term "hierarchical trust" to describe the Chinese case where individuals trust the national government more than local governments. Wu and Wilkes (2018) demonstrate that unlike other Asian countries, two in three Chinese respondents exhibit greater levels of trust in national institutions relative to local ones. Moreover, they find China as the only Asian country where a majority of respondents trust national institutions. Importantly, those who exhibit hierarchical trust are also less likely to be satisfied by political democracy (Li, 2016).

Beyond centralized leadership and bureaucratic mobilization, Mei (2020) asserts that policy memories associated with the handling of previous health crises also remain an integral Chinese policy style component. Consequently, trust affects and is affected by policy style, and both can have significant impact on crisis response. Higher trust in government and health practitioners widens citizen acceptance of government measures. Yang and Tang (2010) demonstrate that levels of institutional trust remain high in China, particularly across the three dimensions of administrative, legal, and societal trust and argue that trust is more than simply a product of traditional Chinese values and cultural traditions (see also Tong, 2011). Others contend that "performance legitimacy"—particularly in light of several decades of rapid economic growth—is the driving factor behind such trust (Zhao, 2009).

Beyond political trust, horizontally directed social trust among citizens also remains crucial in suppressing a pandemic. As Schrad (2020) argues, there must be "a broad sense of societal trust that others will act responsibly, too: that they'll self-isolate and look out for one another as much as they look out for themselves."

China's COVID-19 Response: From "Badly Bungled" to "Moved Heaven and Earth"

A policy styles interpretation of China's COVID-19 response anticipates high levels of policy capacity intersecting with substantial hierarchical trust. Coupled with the high costs of failure, central authorities will pursue centripetal responses seeking to ensure greater control over outcomes, maximum political benefits (and minimal blame), and ultimately preventing a situational crisis from metastasizing into an institutional one ('t Hart, 2014; Petridou et al., 2020). Yet, despite the top-down style, reactive disposition, and high capacity, factors such as fragmented implementation, myriad principal-agent entanglements, and initial trust concerns (and conflicting incentives) in regional and local authorities exposed significant capacity gaps as the crisis ensued.

Successfully containing the spread of infectious diseases requires a combination of prevention, detection, and response. The discussion below focuses primarily on three key response components: (a) command and coordination, (b) communication and information management, and (c) resource management. Evidence suggests that the party-state's crisis response over the first three weeks featured loosely concentrated decision-making and uncoordinated implementation, inconsistent messaging and information suppression, and an initially slow resource mobilization.

Following the detection of an 'unknown pneumonia,' local health authorities in the central city of Wuhan issued an epidemiological alert on December 31, 2019. Yet, nearly a month following the alert and by then with at least 3,000 known infections, January 20 marks a key turning point both publicly and behind the scenes. First, and most prominently, President Xi Jinping publicly acknowledged the epidemic for the first time and offered "important instructions" on how to "make every effort to prevent and control" the outbreak (Xinhuanet, 2020) and the next day the CPC's main newspaper, *The People's Daily*, provided its first virus coverage, running six separate stories. Also on January 20, renowned pulmonologist Zhong Nanshan, a national hero from battling SARS who holds no formal government role, appeared on state television to confirm for the first time person-to-person virus transmission, something Wuhan doctors had been discussing for weeks and a move Mei suggests was "approved by the highest authority to signal the center's intervention" (2020: 315). The same day, the National Health Commission began issuing daily updates on case numbers, and authorities announced an almost immediate quarantine of Wuhan, which shortly later extended to more than 50 million people in surrounding Hubei province and nearly 760 million nationwide.

Critical state and party-directed actions unfolded behind the scenes on January 20 as well. Notably, the State Council, the state's highest administrative organ, convened a teleconference for planning disease control efforts and its executive committee created the State Council Joint Prevention and Control Mechanism (known as the 'joint mechanism'), which would coordinate more than 30 sectors (deLisle and Kui, 2020; Mei, 2020). Chaired by Vice Premier Sun Chunlan, the only female Politburo member and whose portfolio included public health, the joint mechanism coordinated both the regime's national response (e.g., conducting daily press conferences, establishing guidelines and standards) and its on-the-ground response in Wuhan and Hubei province (e.g., dispatching medical teams and allocating supplies) (State Council, 2020). Shortly later, the PSC formed a nine-member Leading Small Group for Epidemic Response (known as "Coronavirus Leading Small Group," or CLSG) headed by Premier Li Keqiang and comprised exclusively of Politburo and CPC Central Committee members (Dotson, 2020). Signaling the regime's appreciation of the situational gravity, Swaine (2020a) points out that relative to the LSG created years earlier in response to SARS, the CLSG "has fewer members, is of a far higher party rank, lacks any health specialists or experts in epidemics, and is directly under the

PSC." Collectively, the state's joint mechanism and the party's CLSG would coordinate COVID-19 response initiatives.

Following the January 20 turning point with the public acknowledgment and behind the scenes machinations, the party-state's highly centralized response, strategically coordinated messaging and muscular propaganda efforts, and substantial mobilization efforts effectively suppressed the virus by April 8, capping a 100-day crisis. Mei (2020) argues that the "early chaos" associated with the government's initial response was the product of the exogenous shock of the virus spread that magnified policy inconsistencies by multiple Chinese policy actors operating at disparate policy levels (e.g., the National Health Commission, the National Center for Disease Control, and the Wuhan city government). The "turning point," he argues, was the "heavy hand" intervention of the central government, which served to "break the existing policy logics of both local governments and the NHC" (2020: 315).

Command and Coordination

At the crisis onset, top leaders remained largely behind the scenes as President Xi first publicly acknowledged the virus (January 20) three weeks following the initial epidemiological alert. Pei (2020a) recounts Xi's whereabouts and public statements throughout the month of January and little suggests an urgent response. Perhaps, modeling "strategic evasion" (Boin et al., 2017: 53), Xi remained publicly quiet during the critical threat defining stages, including a January 17 state visit to Myanmar and visiting troops in Yunnan province when he made the January 20 announcement. Moreover, Xi dispatched Premier Li Keqiang to Wuhan in early February while not visiting Wuhan himself until March 10 in a "carefully choreographed victory lap" (Fifield, 2020) as he praised residents and medical personnel for their "heroic" efforts once the situation was clearly stabilizing. Had the crisis worsened, Xi presumably would have someone to blame.[5] Later, in a February 3 Politburo speech "that smacked of damage control," Xi acknowledged both his awareness of the virus as early as January 7 and that the epidemic served as "a big test of China's governance system and capabilities" (Pei, 2020b). Pre-empting potential criticism, he conceded, "We must sum up experience and learn lessons … in response to the shortcomings and deficiencies exposed in this epidemic response."[6]

Coupled with Xi's public acknowledgment, the January 20 turning point set into motion several critical administrative developments, some state-directed and others party-led. Under the 2003 Health Emergency Regulations, the State Council maintains responsibility for leading the nationwide public health crisis response.[7] Atop China's public health architecture, the National Health Commission (NHC) serves as the primary body for drafting national health policies, laws, and regulations as well as coordinating and guiding regional health planning. The Hubei Province Health Commission, whose offices are located in Wuhan, provides similar functions at the provincial level, while in the public health hierarchy's third tier, the Wuhan Municipal Health Commission serves as the city's primary health agency. With a population of just over 11 million, Wuhan is divided into 13 districts, and each district has its own health bureau.

Key laws dealing with public health emergencies and related national crises include the 1989 Law on the Prevention and Treatment of Infectious Diseases (aka, the Infectious Disease Law) and the 2007 Emergency Response Law as well as the 2003 Health Emergency Regulations. Conventionally, such laws and regulations remain critical because they are "how the state 'talks to itself' – a significant channel mechanism that a regime's leaders use to communicate with lower-level officials and structure their incentives" (deLisle and Kui, 2020: 70). Collectively, such laws distinguish China from most of the other countries in this volume since the Chinese regime "operates in a permanent, but almost never declared, state of emergency" (2010: 342).

As the highest profile state vehicle, the Sun-led joint mechanism was substantively and symbolically critical. Substantively, the NHC became the leading coordinating department, and once the joint mechanism was established, the NHC was "no longer a disadvantaged professional leader in a system dominated by horizontal local governments" (Mei, 2020: 316). The NHC classified the "unknown pneumonia" caused by the novel coronavirus as a Class B infectious disease, but the State Council on January 21 authorized approval to treat the unknown virus as a category A disease under the Infectious Disease Law, leading to stricter prevention, isolation, and control measures as well as more rapid reporting requirements.[8] The Infectious Disease Law, which grew in the aftermath of the 2003 SARS crisis, calls for "suspected patients be isolated for treatment at designated places until a definite diagnosis is made" while the government provides the daily necessities for those isolated (Du, 2020). In addition to the impending lockdown, authorities later amended the PRC Health and Quarantine Law, opening the way for mandatory quarantines.

Parallel to the joint mechanism, the CLSG functioned as the party's primary response vehicle with Premier Li in charge, a delegation decision which Dotson (2020) suggests was an "unusual move for such a high-profile policy issue." The CLSG soon established a "central guidance group" to manage the crisis and potentially punish local officials. Swaine (2020a) contends that the central guidance group, also headed by Sun Chunlan, was created to "establish firm central control over the handling of the virus in Hubei" and also "to mollify the growing public criticism of the handling of the virus."

On January 27, just four days after the lockdown, Wuhan Mayor Zhou Xianwang acknowledged on CCTV state television what was becoming apparent to many about the tightening up of the country's command and coordination response: "We are not allowed to publish information about the epidemic outbreak without [higher-level] authorization" (Li et al., 2020, 18). Two weeks later, his superior, Wuhan party leader Ma Guoqiang, as well as Hubei party secretary Jiang Chaoliang were removed, the latter replaced by former Shanghai Mayor Ying Yong, a close associate of President Xi. Several other local and provincial officials were replaced in the early days of the virus outbreak. For instance, the Hubei Provincial Health Commission's two leading officials, Party Secretary Zhang Jin and Director Liu Yingzi, were removed from their positions on February 11. These sackings, along with Mayor Zhou's CCTV concession and public offer to resign, illustrate how trust interacts with capacity and sends a principal-agent signal that central leaders remain in control. On one hand, the central government can deploy "lightning rods" to receive much of the blame for health crises, while "insulating the top-tier leadership" (Baekkeskov and Rubin, 2017, 425). On the other hand, provincial and local officials are forced into what deLisle and Kui (2020: 84) describe as a "fess up or cover up" choice.

Communication and Information Management

Epidemic outbreaks require at least three distinct elements of crisis communication and information management: information reporting (e.g., new case detection), releasing and announcing information, and individual information sharing (e.g., an individual's right to report) (Liu, 2005). The 2002–2003 SARS epidemic, which originated in China's Guangdong province during a time of leadership transition elevating Hu Jintao as president and Wen Jiabao as premier, provided authorities with important crisis response lessons and a valuable public health communication reference point. Namely, officials were slow to react and initially withheld critical information fearing economic losses and reputational damage. For instance, SARS was first detected in November 2002, but public notification occurred notified nearly two months later, with the WHO epidemiological alert issued four months later and major city quarantines not imposed until the following April.[9]

Information Reporting. Prior to January 20, health authorities did not fully disclose the extent of emerging case numbers, a charge implicating both local and national authorities, and it is in this regard that Swaine (2020a) contends, "the system clearly failed." Reasons for such omissions are many, ranging from the seeking to avoid disruptions to the upcoming January 25 New Year holiday, the busiest travel period of the year, to the "fess up or cover up" principal-agent logic of local officials. From January 5 to 17, for instance, a span overlapping with the annual "two sessions" municipal and provincial People's Congress and People's Political Consultative Conference meetings, the Wuhan Municipal Health Commission (WMHC) reported no new cases. Moreover, Wuhan's leading commercial newspaper "did not feature the outbreak on its front page for two weeks, between January 6 and January 19" (Hancock and Wong, 2020).

Further, as later reported, "internal documents" revealed that NHC head Ma Xiaowei acknowledged in a January 14 "confidential teleconference" with provincial health officials that "The epidemic situation is still severe and complex, the most severe challenge since SARS in 2003, and is likely to develop into a major public health event" (Associated Press, 2020a). Yet, "Ma demanded officials unite around Xi and made clear that political considerations and social stability were key priorities" (Associated Press, 2020a), and he was quoted as saying, "Emphasize politics, emphasize discipline, emphasize science" (Associated Press, 2020b).

Releasing and Announcing Information. At least two critical communication missteps were made in the early crisis response with respect to suppressing the flow of critical epidemiological information related to human transmission and genome sequencing. First, the intentional delays in publicly confirming human-to-human transmission—amid repeated government denials in early January—would carry profound consequences beyond triggering extreme health and economic repercussions. In early January, Dr. Wang Guangfa, a respiratory expert sent to Wuhan as part of a medical team from Beijing, claimed that the virus was "preventable and controllable," insisting that virus could not be spread by human-to-human contact. Less than two weeks later, Dr. Wang acknowledged that he had contracted the virus, and his case came to "symbolize how slowly China recognized the urgency of the outbreak" (Stevenson, 2020).

On the January 20 turning point when finally confirming person-to-person transmission on state television, Dr. Zhong also acknowledged resulting infections among medical workers, a reliable transmission marker. According to Da (2020), Zhong's presence was largely for symbolic purposes since medical authorities had already known about the virus' human transmission properties. Da (2020) alludes to the critical intersection of capacity and trust by contending that Dr. Zhong

> was brought into the picture because there was no way to really and truly turn the tide without the appearance somehow of a third party with sufficient credibility to break through the paper windows of reporting on the epidemic to that point.

Further, as Meng conceded about Dr. Zhong's television appearance:

> Nothing could be done to hold back [the truth about the outbreak]. Our best bet was to have Old Dr. Zhong, this great god, come out and reveal something of the real facts of the situation, and try to calm people's nerves.
> *(as quoted in Da, 2020)*

Second, scientists at the Wuhan Institute of Virology had genetically mapped the novel coronavirus by January 2 shortly following the initial epidemiological alert, but the NHC on the following day "issued a confidential notice ordering labs with the virus to either destroy their samples or send them to designated institutes for safekeeping" (Associated Press, 2020c). The order prevented lab authorities from sharing warnings about such findings or publishing them without government authorization. Days later, the coronavirus genome was independently mapped by two other state labs and at least two other medical laboratories, but not shared with global health authorities until January 12 (Page et al., 2020).

Yet, any potential public health rewards stemming from "probably the earliest, fastest roll-out of a genome in association with an outbreak we have ever seen" (McCarthy, 2020) were lost as a result of the decision to delay in sharing the scientific findings with global health authorities such as the World Health Organization until January 12 (Page et al., 2020) despite the genome results being reported days earlier in the *Wall Street Journal*. The government's release of the genetic map occurred only after its independent release on a virologist website, a move, according to reports, that "angered Chinese CDC officials" and led health authorities to temporarily shutter the offending lab (Associated Press, 2020c). Moreover, although government authorities confirmed the presence of the novel coronavirus to global health officials, these scientific findings would not be shared with the Chinese people for yet another week.

In referring to the rapid achievement of sequencing the coronavirus genome, the China CDC's Meng Xin conceded, "originally [the government] had one ace card" (Da, 2020), enabling epidemiologists to quickly isolate the disease and develop test reagents. Yet, according to Meng:

> The ace card was ... played very poorly, because at the first opportunity politics came into play and directed strict confidentiality requirements – this can't be talked about ... we must maintain stability ... so the test reports were locked into the safety deposit box.
>
> *(as quoted in Da, 2020)*

Reflecting the considerable unifying authority of the Communist Party as leading from the center, Zeng Guang, a chief China CDC scientist lamented that unlike the US Centers for Disease Control, the China CDC "has no power ... It is not allowed to talk about an epidemic without authorization" (Li et al., 2020). Thus, this particular communication lapse reinforces the notion that when it comes to health crises, secrecy remains "China's general default blame–avoidance approach" (Baekkeskov and Rubin, 2017, 440).

Individual Information Sharing. Article 22 of the Infectious Disease Law asserts that government officials, medical personnel, and those involved in epidemic prevention and surveillance "shall not withhold the truth about or make a false report on the epidemic situation or inspire others to do so." This provision gives authorities greater ability to solidify trust, control narratives, and prevent 'rumor spreading'. Prior to Dr. Zhong's human transmission confirmation, scores of citizens—from front-line Wuhan health professionals to so-called Chinese netizens throughout the country—were discredited and punished for spreading rumors. The day following President Xi's January 20 virus acknowledgment, the Party's main political and legal affairs organ warned, "Anyone who deliberately delays and hides the reporting of [virus] cases ... will be nailed on the pillar of shame for eternity" (Zheng and Lau, 2020). These Article 22 provisions offer authorities great pandemic fighting tools while substantially curtailing individual rights. Such provisions invoke a nationwide sense of legal consciousness, defined as "the ways in which individuals interpret and mobilize legal meanings and signs" (Sibley, 2001: 8624). At the intersection of policy and trust, Jacobs (2007: 516) refers to legal consciousness as "a form of cultural practice where beliefs and attitudes about legal rights affect practices and what people do, which in turn shape beliefs and attitudes."

Arguably, the case of Wuhan ophthalmologist Li Wenliang, whose initial targeting and detention as a 'rumor spreading' whistleblower best personifies the problems associated with individual information sharing. Dr. Li's subsequent virus-related death triggered an outpouring of national grief, suspicion, and anger. Shortly following his death, a private Chinese firm's research report prepared for CPC officials that tracked the tone and volume of Chinese public's social media responses to Dr. Li's illness and death was leaked (Demick, 2020). The report indicated that the prevailing Sina Weibo (considered "China's Twitter") chatter leading up to Dr. Li's death involved primarily expressions of sadness, but the user mood quickly was replaced by anger upon news of his death and reached a "flood-level event" on the day of his February 7 death (Rudolph, 2020). It was at this point where the regime was closest in terms of letting a situational crisis devolve into an institutional crisis and a pivotal point to merge trust with capacity in pursuing a centralized response.

Resource Management

The January 20 turning point triggered a substantial bureaucratic mobilization involving a wide range of vertical and horizontal responses. Beyond comprehensive non-pharmaceutical interventions such as case identification and isolation, social distancing, and contact-tracing, numerous mitigation measures such as mask-wearing and temperature checks remain familiar to Chinese citizens as a result of SARS and other previous health crises.[10] Other mitigation measures such as community policing[11] and the use of a neighborhood grid system, intercity travel prohibitions, and reimbursement for rail and airfare lost as a result of the early quarantine are embedded into provisions of the Health Emergency Regulations and Infectious Disease Law. Still others such as the use of smart phone tracking apps (e.g., cell phone monitoring) and QR code scans in public places for monitoring individual movements reflect the combination of innovative technology and policy experimentation, enabled by a top-down policy style.

Vertically, the state marshaled substantial material resources, including the unprecedented lockdown of Wuhan and surrounding Hubei province, which included the suspension of flights and trains as well as road blockades. Tremendous administrative capacity was also demonstrated through the erection of several 'instant hospital' facilities and the conversion of more than a dozen large-scale public venues such as gymnasiums and exhibition centers for patient isolation and mild case treatment. On January 23, construction began on the 1,000-bed Huoshenshan hospital (meaning Fire God Mountain), completed in a remarkable nine days, while the 1,500-bed Leishenshan (Thunder God Mountain) Hospital opened a few days later. As one observer put it, the CPC's "ability to build big things is one of its few expressions of control amid a spiraling epidemic … and when disaster strikes, it is speed that matters most" (Chia, 2020). Construction on the Huoshenshan facility was live-streamed by Xinhua, the state news agency, which also flooded the internet with video updates.

Horizontally, the central state relied on personnel and resources from provinces across China. More than 42,000 medical workers were mobilized as 'medical assistance teams' sent to the virus epicenter. Centralized relief efforts early in the crisis led to bottlenecks and resource misallocation. Drawing from its prior 2008 Wenchuan earthquake relief efforts, the NHC decentralized coronavirus assistance on February 7 through a process known as "counterpart assistance" (Zhang and Xu, 2020), which paired Chinese provinces and municipalities with various Hubei cities in most need. Such a targeted pairing generates added efficiencies by enabling recipients to communicate resource needs directly with donors. As Zhang and Xu (2020) point out, this program was modified slightly on February 10 by retaining the recipient cities, but modifying the donor list, suggesting some degree of on the ground updating.

Additional resources, particularly seeking trust building, were soon deployed in various other capacities. First, state propaganda efforts quickly accelerated. Following Xi's February 3 Politburo speech, the state dispatched more than 300 journalists to Wuhan to cover the crisis with "positive energy" in Xi's attempt to strengthen 'publicity work' and "let the masses know more about what the party and government are doing" (Zhong, 2020). The narrative soon turned to the offensive as well, with Xi describing a "people's war" against the epidemic. As one analyst notes, "Wars invite people to cast aside their squabbles and dissent and to come together … [they] make heroes – and heroes are the stuff propaganda thrives upon" (Moritsugu, 2020).

Second, the case of Dr. Li Wenliang is again instructive. On the day he died, Dr. Li's name "was the most heavily censored term on Weibo" (Shih, 2020a). Sensing rising political discord, Beijing authorities promptly sent a team from the country's leading anti-corruption agency, the National Supervisory Commission, to Wuhan to investigate Dr. Li's death "in response to issues raised by the masses" (Jiang, 2020). Six weeks following his death, Beijing investigators determined that the Wuhan police acted inappropriately. Two police officers were reprimanded, the government offered a "solemn apology" to his family, and Dr. Li was bestowed with the title of state martyr as one who gave his life for the country. Such efforts were clearly consistent with the party-state's emphasis on trust building and "stability maintenance." As Barmé (2020) points out, the stability maintenance process is cyclical: "A new crisis generates new dissent, followed by repression — and then more dissent."

Conclusion

The Chinese response during the first and second waves considered in this volume reflects a tale of two responses. The first three weeks of crisis response demonstrated a combination of disjointed decision-making, inconsistent messaging, information suppression, and coordination bottlenecks and ineffi-ciencies. Yet, following a January 20 turning point, the party-state's highly cen-tralized response led to more coordinated vertical and horizontal interactions, strategically coordinated messaging efforts, and the amassing of substantial na-tional resources to suppress the virus.

China's response, especially following January 20, illustrates the critical inter-section of high policy capacity, low inclusiveness, and hierarchical trust. Rather than serving as a "China's Chernobyl" as some analysts had speculated early on (Tharoor, 2020), President Xi's incumbent regime not only emerged from the crisis with strengthened governing authority but also, since the outbreak China increased its share of global trade, regained its status as world's top foreign in-vestment destination and was the only major economy not to have contracted (Hancock and Curran, 2021). Moreover, despite its initial stumbles and trust-related concerns, "China's ultimate success in managing the spread of the virus may actually build popular trust in the government, rather than undermining it" (Chen, 2020).

More broadly, from Mao's "permanent revolution" to Deng's "crossing the river by feeling the stones" reformist approach to Xi's current prioritization on "modernizing governance," China's policy styles remain focused on "finding innovative policy *instruments*, rather than defining *objectives*, which remains the prerogative of the Party leadership" (Heilmann, 2008a: 3, italics in original). Collectively, combined effects of party-state relations, central-local interaction, formal–informal arrangements, a top-down style, and reactive disposition con-tribute to a policy style reflecting the highly adaptive nature of Chinese policy-making, which Heilmann calls "experimentation under hierarchy" (2008b: 2) and "maximum tinkering under the shadow of hierarchy" (2009: 458).

Empirically, China's centralized response, coupled with a better theoretical understanding of the capacity-inclusiveness-trust nexus, become particularly sa-lient in light of cautionary words of Dr. Michael Ryan, the WHO's Executive Director of WHO's Health Emergencies Program:

> This pandemic has been very severe … but this is not necessarily the big one. This is a wake-up call. If there is one thing we need to take from this pandemic, with all of the tragedy and loss, is we need to get our act together. We need to honour those we've lost by getting better at what we do every day.
>
> *(as quoted in Davey, 2020)*

Notes

1 During the same span, 61.86 million cases, 1.45 million deaths, and 186 deaths per million population were reported worldwide, including 12.94 million cases, 262,736 deaths, and 794 deaths per million in the United States.
2 Wu and Wilkes define political trust as "the belief that government leaders and insti-tutions serve the people's interest" (2018: 437). Alternatively, Li defines political trust

as "citizens' belief that the political system, government and politicians will work to produce outcomes consistent with their expectations" (2016: 101).
3 Technically, PRC constitution Article 57 establishes the National People's Congress as "the highest organ of state power."
4 Lieberthal and Lampton (1992: 61) contend, "The Party's authority over the government is based primarily on its authority to appoint and promote government officials (*nomenklatura*). The Party also sets the general policy line (*luxian*), which the government implements, and oversees the work of the government."
5 The Party's official virus account in the People's Daily praises Xi for his bravery, mentioning him 83 times, but mentions Li just once (Meyers and Buckley, 2020).
6 For speech text, see: http://www.qstheory.cn/dukan/qs/2020-02/15/c_1125572832.htm?mod=article_inline.
7 Provincial emergency headquarters maintain responsibility for crisis response within their own jurisdictions. See LOC: Legal Report (2020) for a description of China's Public Health Crisis Management System.
8 The 1989 Infectious Disease Law categorizes infectious diseases into three categories, including category A (plague and cholera) and category B infectious diseases (including SARS, HIV/AIDS, and two dozen other diseases).
9 See deLisle (2010), Liu (2005), and Jacobs (2007) on the government's SARS response.
10 For a timeline and description of the Chinese response, see State Council (2020).
11 For instance, Article 55 of the 2007 Emergency Response Law empowers "residents' committees, villagers' committees and other organizations in the place where an emergency occurs" to "help maintain social order."

References

Associated Press. 2020a. "China Didn't Warn Public of Likely Pandemic for 6 Key Days." April 15. https://apnews.com/article/68a9e1b91de4ffc166acd6012d82c2f9

Associated Press. 2020b. "Takeaways from Internal Documents on China's Virus Response." April 16. https://apnews.com/article/a75e4e452f5a2d0ecaa241ca2045599e

Associated Press. 2020c. "China Delayed Releasing Coronavirus Info, Frustrating WHO." June 1. https://apnews.com/article/3c061794970661042b18d5aeaaed9fae

Baekkeskov, Erik and Olivier Rubin. 2017. "Information Dilemmas and Blame-Avoidance Strategies: From Secrecy to Lightning Rods in Chinese Health Crises." *Governance: An International Journal of Policy, Administration, and Institutions*. 30(3): 425–43.

Barmé, Geremie. 2020. "China's Coronavirus Crisis Is Just Beginning." *New York Times*. March 3. https://www.nytimes.com/2020/03/03/opinion/coronavirus-china-xi-jinping.html

Boin, Arjen, Paul 'Hart, Eric Stern, and Bengt Sundelius. 2017. *The Politics of Crisis Management: Public Leadership under Pressure*. 2nd ed. Cambridge: Cambridge University Press.

Chen, Dan. 2020. "China's Coronavirus Response Could Build Public Support for Its Government." *Washington Post*. March 27. https://www.washingtonpost.com/politics/2020/03/27/chinas-coronavirus-response-could-build-public-support-its-government/

Chia, Jasmine. 2020. "The Message Behind China's Insta-Hospital." February 6. *The Diplomat*. https://thediplomat.com/2020/02/the-message-behind-chinas-insta-hospital. Accessed 14 May 2020.

Da, Shiji. 2020. "The Truth about 'Dramatic Action'." *China Media Project*. January 27. https://chinamediaproject.org/2020/01/27/dramatic-actions/

Davey, Melissa. 2020. "WHO Warns COVID-19 Pandemic Is 'Not Necessarily the Big One'." *The Guardian*. December 29. https://www.theguardian.com/world/2020/dec/29/who-warns-COVID-19-pandemic-is-not-necessarily-the-big-one deLisle, J. 2010. "States of Exception in an Exceptional State: Emergency Powers Law in China." In A. Thiruvengadam and V. Ramraj (eds.) *Emergency Powers in Asia: Exploring the Limits of Legality.* Cambridge: Cambridge University Press, 342–90.

deLisle, Jacques and Shen Kui. 2020. "Lessons from China's Response to COVID-19: Shortcomings, Successes, and Prospects for Reform in China's Regulatory State." *Faculty Scholarship at Penn Law.* 2239: 66–149. https://scholarship.law.upenn.edu/faculty_scholarship/2239

Dotson, John. 2020. "The CCP's New Leading Small Group for Countering the Coronavirus Epidemic—and the Mysterious Absence of Xi Jinping. Jamestown Foundation." February 5. https://jamestown.org/program/the-ccps-new-leading-small-group-for-countering-the-coronavirus-epidemic-and-the-mysterious-absence-of-xi-jinping/

Du, Guodong. 2020. "China's Infectious Diseases Regulatory Framework: From SARS to Novel Coronavirus." *China Justice Observer.* January 30. https://www.chinajustice-observer.com/a/chinas-infectious-diseases-regulatory-framework

Fifield, Anna. 2020. "As Coronavirus goes Global, China's Xi Asserts Victory on First Trip to Wuhan Since Outbreak." *Washington Post.* March 10. https://www.washingtonpost.com/world/asia_pacific/chinas-xi-attempts-a-coronavirus-victory-lap-with-visit-to-wuhan/2020/03/10/ca585ddc-6281-11ea-8a8e-5c5336b32760_story.html

Fukuyama, Francis. 2020. "The Thing that Determines a Country's Resistance to the Coronavirus." *The Atlantic.* March 30. https://www.theatlantic.com/ideas/archive/2020/03/thing-determines-how-well-countries-respond-coronavirus/609025/

Hancock, Tom and Enda Curran. 2021. "A Year after COVID-19 Began, China's Economy Is Beating World." *Japan Times.* January 15. https://www.japantimes.co.jp/news/2021/01/15/business/economy-business/china-economy-beating-world/

He, Baogang and Mark Warren. 2011. "Authoritarian Deliberation: The Deliberative Turn in Chinese Political Development." *Perspectives on Politics.* 9(2): 269–89.

Heilmann, Sebastian. 2008a. "From Local Experiments to National Policy: The Origins of China's Distinctive Policy Process." *The China Journal.* 59: 1–30.

Heilmann, Sebastian and Elizabeth J. Perry. 2011. "Embracing Uncertainty: Guerrilla Policy Style and Adaptive Governance in China." In Heilmann, Sebastian and Elizabeth J. Perry, (eds.) *Mao's Invisible Hand: The Political Foundations of Adaptive Governance in China.* Cambridge, MA: Harvard University Press. 1–29.

Howlett, Michael and Jale Tosun, eds. 2018. *Policy Styles and Policy-Making, Exploring the Linkages.* New York: Routledge.

Huang, Yanzhong. 2020. "China's Public Health Response to the COVID-19 Outbreak." *China Leadership Monitor.* June 1. https://www.prcleader.org/huang

Jacobs, Lesley. 2007. "Rights and Quarantine During the SARS Global Health Crisis: Differentiated Legal Consciousness in Hong Kong, Shanghai, and Toronto." *Law & Society Review.* 41(3): 511–51.

Kristof, Nicholas. 2021. "Biden's Nightmare May Be China." *New York Times.* January 30. https://www.nytimes.com/2021/01/30/opinion/sunday/foreign-policy-china.html?searchResultPosition=1

Landry, Pierre 2012. *Decentralized Authoritarianism in China: The Communist Party's Control of Local Elites in the Post- Mao Era.* Cambridge: Cambridge University Press.

Li, Lianjiang. 2016. "Reassessing Trust in the Central Government: Evidence from five national surveys." *The China Quarterly.* 225(3): 100–21.

Lieberthal, K. G. 1992. "Introduction: The 'Fragmented Authoritarianism' Model and Its Limitations." In Kenneth G. Lieberthal and David M. Lampton (eds.) *Bureaucracy, Politics, and Decision Making in Post-Mao China.* Berkeley: University of California Press, 1–30.

Lieberthal, Kenneth and Michel Oksenberg 1988. *Policy Making in China: Leaders, Structures, and Processes*. Princeton, NJ: Princeton University Press.

LOC Legal Report. 2020. "China: Legal Responses to Health Emergencies." *Library of Congress*. December 30. https://www.loc.gov/law/help/health-emergencies/china.php#_ftn30

Mei, Ciqi. 2020. "Policy Style, Consistency, and the Effectiveness of the Policy Mix in China's Fight Against COVID-19." *Policy and Society*. 39(3): 309–25.

Mertha, Andrew. 2005. "China's 'Soft' Centralization: Shifting the Tiao/Kuai Authority Relations." *The China Quarterly*. 184(11): 791–810.

Mertha, Andrew. 2008. *China's Water Warriors: Citizen Action and Policy Change*. Ithaca: Cornell University Press.

Mertha, Andrew. 2009. "Fragmented Authoritarianism 2.0': Political Pluralization in the Chinese Policy Process." *The China Quarterly*. 200: 995–1012.

Meyers, Steven Lee and Chris Buckley. 2020. "In China's Crisis, Xi Sees a Crucible to Strengthen His Rule." *New York Times*. May 20. https://www.nytimes.com/2020/05/20/world/asia/coronavirus-china-xi-jinping.html

Moritsugu, Ken. 2020. "China's Effort to Regain Trust: A 'People's War' Against a Virus." *Christian Science Monitor*. March 9. https://www.csmonitor.com/World/Asia-Pacific/2020/0309/China-s-effort-to-regain-trust-A-people-s-war-against-a-virus.

Page, Jeremy, Wenxin Fan, and Natasha Page. 2020. "China's Early Missteps Fed Epidemic." *Wall Street Journal*. March 7, A1.

Painter, Martin and Jon Pierre. 2005. "Unpacking Policy Capacity: Issues and Themes." In Martin Painter and Jon Pierre. (Eds.) *Challenges to State Policy Capacity*. Palgrave Macmillan, London. 1–18.

Pei, Minxin. 2020a. "How Has the Coronavirus Crisis Affected Xi's Power: A Preliminary Assessment." *China Leadership Monitor*. June 1. https://www.prcleader.org/pei-1

Pei, Minxin. 2020b. "Coronavirus has the Power to Topple China's One-party Regime." *MarketWatch*. 4 March. https://www.marketwatch.com/story/coronavirus-has-the-power-to-topple-chinas-one-party-regime-2020-03-04

Petridou, Evangelia, Nikolaos Zahariadis, and Stephen Ceccoli. 2020. "Averting Institutional Disasters? Drawing Lessons from China to Inform the Cypriot Response to the COVID-19 Pandemic." *European Policy Analysis* 6: 318–27.

Qian, Jiwei. 2018. "Policy Styles in China: How to Control and Motivate Bureaucracy." In Michael Howlett and Jale Tosun (eds.) *Policy Styles and Policy Making*. New York: Routledge, 201–21.

Reny, Marie-Evie. 2011. "Review Essay: What Happened to the Study of China in Comparative Politics?" *Journal of East Asian Studies*. 11: 105–35.

Richardson, Jeremy, Gunnel Gustafsson, and Grant Jordan 1982. "The Concept of Policy Style." In Jeremey Richardson (ed.) *Policy Styles in Western Europe*. George Allen & Unwin. 1–16.

Schrad, Mark Lawrence. 2020. "The Secret to Coronavirus Success is Trust." *Foreign Policy*. April 15. https://foreignpolicy.com/2020/04/15/secret-success-coronavirus-trust-public-policy/

Schroeder, Paul. 1992. "Territorial Actors as Competitors for Power: The Case of Hubei and Wuhan." In Lieberthal, Kenneth G. and David M. Lampton. (eds.) *Bureaucracy, Politics, and Decision Making in Post-Mao China*. Berkeley: University of California Press, 283–307.

Schurmann, Franz. 1968. *Ideology and Organization in Communist China*. 2nd ed. Berkeley and Los Angeles: University of California Press.

Shirk, Susan 1992. "The Chinese Political System and the Strategy of Economic Reform." In Lieberthal, Kenneth G. and David Lampton (eds.) *Bureaucracy, Politics, and Decision Making in Post-Mao China*. Berkeley: University of California Press, 59–91.

Silbey, Susan. 2001. "Legal Culture and Consciousness." In Smelser, N. and Baltes, P. (eds.) *International Encyclopedia of the Social and Behavioral Sciences*. Amsterdam: Elsevier Science, 8623–29.

State Council Information Office (China.) 2020. "Fighting COVID-19: China in Action." June 7. White Paper. http://sc.china-embassy.org/eng/zxhd/t1787248.htm

Swaine, Michael. 2020. "Chinese Crisis Decision Making –– Managing the COVID-19 Pandemic Part One: The Domestic Component." *China Leadership Monitor*. June 1. https://www.prcleader.org/swaine

Tharoor, Ishaan. 2020. "China's Chernobyl? The Coronavirus Outbreak Leads to a Loaded Metaphor." *Washington Post*. February 11. https://www.washingtonpost.com/world/2020/02/12/chinas-chernobyl-coronavirus-outbreak-leads-loaded-metaphor/

Tong, Yangqi. 2011. "Morality, Benevolence, and Responsibility: Regime Legitimacy in China from Past to the Present." *Journal of Chinese Political Science*. 16: 141–59.

World Health Organization. 2020. Weekly Epidemiological Report – 1 December 2020. https://www.who.int/publications/m/item/weekly-epidemiological-update---1-december-2020

Wu, Cary and Rima Wilkes. 2018. "Local–national Political Trust Patterns: Why China Is an Exception." *International Political Science Review*. 39(4): 436–54.

Xinhuanet. 2020. "Xi Jinping made Important Instructions on the Pneumonia Epidemic caused by the New Coronavirus, Emphasizing that the Safety and Health of the People should be put First, Resolutely Curbing the Spread of the Epidemic, Li Keqiang Issued Instructions." January 20. http://www.xinhuanet.com/politics/leaders/2020-01/20/c_1125486561.htm

Yang, Qing and Wenfang Tang. 2010. "Exploring the Sources of Institutional Trust in China: Culture, Mobilization, or Performance?" *Asian Politics and Policy*. 2(3): 415–36.

Zhang, Xiaobo and Lihe Xu. 2020. "China's 'Counterpart Assistance' Approach to Coronavirus: Lessons from the Wenchuan Earthquake Response." *CGD Note*. Center for Global Development. February. https://www.cgdev.org/sites/default/files/chinas-counterpart-assistance-approach-coronavirus-lessons-wenchuan-earthquake-response.pdf

Zhao, Dingxin. 2009. "The Mandate of Heaven and Performance Legitimation in Historical and Contemporary China." *American Behavioral Scientist*. 53: 416–33.

Zhao, Yongfei and B. Guy Peters. 2009. "The State of the State: Comparing Governance in China and the United States." *Public Administration Review*. December. 69: S122–S128.

Zheng, William and Mimi Lau. 2020. "China's Credibility on the Line as It Tries to Dispels Fears It Will Cover Up Spread of Wuhan Virus." *South China Morning Post*. 21 January. https://www.scmp.com/news/china/politics/article/3046984/china-warns-cadres-cover-spread-virus-and-be-nailed-pillar

Zhong, Raymond. 2020. "China Clamps Down on Coronavirus Coverage as Cases Surge." *New York Times*. 5 February. https://www.nytimes.com/2020/02/05/world/asia/china-coronavirus-censorship.html

4

TURKEY'S RESPONSE TO THE COVID-19 PANDEMIC

Lacin Idil Oztig

Introduction

This paper examines the structural and behavioral dynamics in Turkey's policy-making to test the argument that policy style and political trust interact to determine Turkey's response to the COVID-19 pandemic. More specifically, it looks at whether Turkey's administrative policy style that shapes normal policymaking through norms, "standard operating procedures," and institutional arrangements is reflected in the management of the pandemic which is classified as extraordinary policymaking (Chapter 1 in this book). This paper is informed by the premise that politico-administrative decision-making processes are affected by the structure of administrative organization (Clemens and Cook 1999; Howlett and Tosun 2019).

Turkey traditionally follows a top-down, imposition style with respect to political decision-making. Turkey's top-down approach has been bolstered under the Justice and the Development Party (JDP) rule through increased political control over bureaucracy and deliberate exclusion of a wide range of societal actors from decision-making processes. Turkey maintained its policymaking style in the management of the pandemic by adopting a centralized response plan that is implemented through circulars issued by the Ministry of Interior. The Presidency, the Ministry of Interior, the Ministry of Health, and the Scientific Advisory Board (SAB) played major roles in policymaking processes during the pandemic. President Erdogan's instructions (given in view of the recommendations of the SAB) in cabinet meetings were issued as the circulars of the Ministry of Interior and then implemented at provincial and local levels.

As this chapter shows, Turkey's imposition style coupled with low inclusiveness of social actors (administrative policy style) explain why the pandemic has been managed by a few policymakers and health experts and major medical

DOI: 10.4324/9781003137399-6

associations have been excluded from policymaking processes. Lower trust in government throws light on the rationale behind the creation of the SAB and the enforcement of public health rules through monetary fines. On the other hand, Turkey's anticipatory approach to the pandemic coupled with a centralized response plan led to the effective handling of the pandemic.

The remainder of the chapter is as follows. This first section examines patterns of administrative arrangement in Turkey. As the main focus of analysis is Turkey's response to the pandemic, this section also gives a frontal place to Turkish health system including recent health sector reforms. The second section examines the dynamics of state-society relations and sheds light on the degree of political inclusiveness. The third section describes the degree of Turkish citizens' political trust to the government by relying on a number of surveys. The fourth section examines the trajectory of Turkey's response to the pandemic from January 2020 to the beginning of the vaccine roll-out on January 14, 2021. The final section discusses the ways in which Turkey's policy style coupled with political trust has affected the policy outcome with respect to the pandemic.

Turkey's Administrative Policy Capacity

Turkey inherited the legacy of the Ottoman state that had a social structure based on the conspicuous distinction between the rulers (the sultan and his servants) and the ruled. Civil servants were subservient to the sultan who had the absolute authority (Heper 1985), and local politics was only limited to the implementation of the rules determined by the center (Koker 1995). Modern Turkey maintained the Ottoman tradition of a centralist state (Ahmad 1993) as well as the distrust for the periphery (Koker 1995). It was established on the basis of a state-centered, elite-directed modernization project that ordered state-society relations in a hierarchical way, leaving little room for pluralism and political inclusiveness (Keyder 1997; Cinar 2006). Even though the ruling elites in the early Turkish Republic worked toward achieving top-down modernization of the society and cultural homogeneity, the Turkish society has been characterized by different lines of division in terms of ethnicity (Turks-Kurds), religion (Sunnis-Alevis), ideology/politics (secularists-conservatives), and culture (urbanized modernist Turks-rural traditionalist Turks) (Ozbudun 2014).

Turkey's central administration consists of central administrative institutions (ministries and governmental agencies) and provincial administration. Provincial administration operates as an extension of central administration (Ustuner and Yavuz 2017). Turkey has 81 provinces, each of which is administrated by a governor. Governors act as a bridge between the central authority and local administration. Provinces are divided into districts, each of which governed by district governors (Tan 2014). Local administration (municipal, village, and special provincial administration) is under the administrative tutelage of the central government (Ustuner and Yavuz 2017). Turkey's administrative tradition fits into the Napoleonic tradition (Bolukbasi and Ertugal 2019) under which the state is "conceived as a means of integrating society, and subsuming social differ-ence in the general entity that is the overarching source of governance" (Peters 2008, 121). In this state-centric conception of governance, the state is ascribed the role of defending the society, while the society is ascribed less autonomous role (Peters and Pierre 2002; Peters 2008, 2015).

Differing strikingly from the consensus model that disperses and limits power in numerous ways, in the majoritarian model, political power is concentrated in the hands of a majority (Lijphart 2012). In this respect, the majoritarian form of government is "exclusive, competitive, and adversarial" (Lijphart 2012, 2). As underlined by Lijphart (2012), in societies characterized by ideological, cultural, and ethnic cleavages, the majoritarian rule might sow the seeds of authoritarian-ism through prolonged exclusion of non-majoritarian groups from policymaking processes.

Turkey fits into the majoritarian model conceptualized by Lijphart. Turkey's majoritarianism is visible in the formation of government apparatus and in the way the executive dominates the legislative process (Lord 2012; Bolukbasi and Ertugal 2019). Its unitary and centralized structure results in the concentration of executive power (Lord 2012). The 10% electoral threshold introduced after the 1980 coup has led to the underrepresentation of small parties and overrep-resentation of big parties (Tosun 2015). Majoritarianism has been bolstered since the JDP came to power. In light of Lijphart's criteria, the period under the JDP rule in Turkey can be evaluated as "the most majoritarian in Turkey's history of multiparty politics" (Lord 2012, 235).

The 2010 constitutional amendments, that changed the composition of the Constitutional Court and the High Council of Judges and Public Prosecutors and limited military privileges and immunities, can be considered important stepping stones in the JDP's consolidation of power, as they decreased the power of the military and judicial actors (Ozbudun 2014). The 2017 constitutional amendments, on the other hand, are milestones in Turkey's majoritarianism (Bolukbasi and Ertugal 2019) as a result of which the Turkish political system was transformed from a parliamentary into a presidential system, strengthening further one-man rule.

Presidentialism has increased the president's power, also paving the way for an increased centralization of the state and bureaucracy (Ustuner and Yavuz 2017). The power of the executive has been expanded at the expense of the non-core executive and the legislature (Bolukbasi and Ertugal 2019). Under the new sys-tem, the president appoints ministers, high-level civil servants, four members of the Board of Judges, and Prosecutors and selects 12 members of the Con-stitutional Court. Moreover, he has the right to bypass legislation, send laws back to the parliament, and dissolve the parliament (Yilmaz 2020). While in the previous system, governors reported to the Ministry of Interior, in the new system, they are directly tied to the Presidency. As the president's control over judicial appointments has expanded, the courts' ability to provide checks and balances on the executive has shrunk accordingly (Kirisci and Sloat 2019). All in all, the president's powers have been increased at the detriment of the protection of civil rights, separation of powers, democratic public life (Yilmaz 2020). This is a diversion from the post–1980 coup political and institutional tradition that is based on the neutrality of the president who was expected to play a symbolic and ceremonial role in politics (Zafer 2020). Bakir (2020) uses the terms "the presidentialisation of the executive branch" and "presidential bureaucracy" to describe the new system.

Traditionally, bureaucrats are not active participants in policymaking in Turkey. Frequent coup d'états, that destroyed the country's democratic potential since 1960, rendered bureaucratic institutions weak (Ozen 2013). Bureaucratic recruitment and promotion are dominated by patronage networks. Under the JDP rule, the politicization of bureaucracy and increased favoritism further undermined the agency of the bureaucracy and deteriorated quality and efficiency of bureaucratic functioning (Ustuner and Yavuz 2017). Using Peter's (2015) terminology, the Turkish bureaucracy can be characterized by a lack of *autonomy*, lack of expert *staffing* (due to prevailing favoritism), and lack of *cooperative aspirations* (due to hierarchical relationship between policymakers and bureaucrats).

Turkey's administrative policy capacity and style are concretized in numerous indexes. For example, according to the Government Effectiveness Index (World Bank 2018), Turkey ranks 86th out of 193 countries, with the sharpest declines in scores taking place between 2012 and 2016. According to the Rule of Law Index (World Justice Project 2020a), Turkey ranks 107th out of 128 countries (World Justice Project 2020). According to the Corruption Perception Index (2019), Turkey ranks 91st out of 191 countries.

Turkish health care system lags behind developed countries when a number of indicators are considered. As of 2018, Turkey has 9,2 infant and maternal deaths per 1,000 live births (the second highest number among OECD countries after Mexico), an important indicator that reflects health service accessibility (Kisa, Younis, and Kisa 2007). As of 2018, in Turkey, there are 1,88 physicians per 1,000 people, the lowest figure among OECD countries. As of 2019, Turkey ranks the lowest among OECD countries with respect to health expenditures (OECD 2019a). On the other side of the spectrum, compared to some developed countries, the health care is more affordable in Turkey (Aslan, Cinar, and Ozen 2014).

Furthermore, significant improvements took place in Turkish health care system after the JDP came to power, with considerable increases in public investment in health infrastructure; the number of medical personnel, hospital beds as well as intensive care unit beds (Tatar et al. 2011; Burki 2017). Economic growth in the first electoral term of the JDP created permissive conditions for an increase in health spending (Okem and Cakar 2015). In 2000, there were 21 hospital beds per 10,000 people. This number increased to 28.5 in 2018 (World Health Organization 2020a). The JDP also encouraged private sector to invest more on health as a result of which the number of private hospitals increased (Okem and Cakar 2015). The digitalization of health services, that began in the 1990s, gained momentum throughout 2000s. The digitalization of health services includes the Central Physician Appointment System (online doctor appointment system); the Pharmaceutical Tracking System (that tracks supply and demand for medicines); e-Pulse (an application that enables citizens to manage their health information as well as gain access to health data collected from health institutions); and the digitization of the hospitals (Şahiner and Ozer 2020).

Before 2005, the Turkish health system was fragmented with the provision of health care by various public organizations to which different rules and regulations applied. In 2005, all these facilities were transferred to the Ministry of Health by virtue of which the Ministry became the dominant provider in the system.[1] Through General Insurance Scheme, different health insurance schemes were unified, covering the majority of the population (Tatar et al. 2011). While in 2010, 96.2% of the population was covered public or private health insurance, it increased to 98.5% in 2018 (OECD 2019). In 2010, family practice was introduced as the primary system of health care which resulted in improved access to health care (Yaman and Gunes 2016). Along with health reforms, many natural and human-induced disasters played an important role in the strengthening of the health system (World Health Organization 2020b).

Taken all together, policymaking system in Turkey is highly centralized and hierarchical. Bureaucratic actors do not play an active role in policymaking. Especially after the 2017 constitutional amendments, political power is concentrated in the hands of the president. In general, the Turkish political behavior is characterized by reactive (short-sighted) approach to problem-solving, antithetical to anticipatory problem-solving that is based on the identification of, and taking action against, future problems (Richardson 1982, 2018).[2] The standardization of construction rules only after the devastating 1999 earthquake epitomizes Turkey's reactive approach to problem-solving.

State-Society Relations in Turkey

In Turkey, policies are decided without minimum social consultation and implemented even when some interest groups voice their opposition. Consistent with the Napoleonic tradition to which Turkey belongs, interest groups are seen as a threat to the state's autonomy; as such, they are not integrated into the formal policymaking process (Peters 2008). There are interactions between state and societal actors during the policy implementation phase, but state-society relationship is hierarchical and not consensual (Bolukbasi and Ertugal 2019). As underlined by Ozbudun (2011), hierarchical state-society relationship is engrained in the Turkish constitutional system that is built upon the protection of the state against individuals rather than the other way around. Professional organizations such as bar associations, engineers and architects associations, medical associations, etc. are, in principle, autonomous, but they are under the strict control of the central authority (Ozbudun 2011). Especially under the rule of the JDP, their role exponentially shrank.

The first period of the JDP (2002–2007) was characterized by commitment to the EU process, liberal reforms, and the amelioration of the economy. The party received support from people across the political spectrum, including liberals, conservatives, and nationalists. During this period, the JDP actualized a number of public sector reforms geared toward enhancing accountability and citizen participation in public administration. For example, the 2004 law on the right to information enables individuals and legal persons to seek information from public authorities (Ustuner and Yavuz 2017). The law of municipalities, adopted in 2005, established city councils that bring local residents and civil society organizations together with representatives of the municipalities and province (Yalçın-Riollet 2019). This mechanism was designed to encourage greater citizen participation in local decision-making processes. Overall, these reforms increased optimism regarding the country's prospect for democratization, accountability, and improved state-society relations.

Nevertheless, especially after the second term of the JDP, the democratization process was reversed (Bolukbasi and Ertugal 2019). The role of city councils proved to be insignificant due to the dominant role played by the municipal council members and financial problems (Ustuner and Yavuz 2017). The civil society witnessed politization, as new networks were established with the aim of harnessing political support for the JDP. The Civil Solidarity Platform (created with the support of approximately 500 pro-government civil society organizations in 2010) is a case in point (Esen and Gumuscu 2016). With the 2014 Internet law, the governmental surveillance over the internet intensified. The party tightened its grip over the media by encouraging pro-government business people to buy major media outlets (Kirisci and Sloat 2019).

Through a number of mechanisms of capital accumulation (such as public spending and privatization of state-owned enterprises), the JDP ensured the support of the pro-government business class. The pro-government businessmen financed the Civil Solidarity Platform that actively lobbied in favor of the JDP. On the other hand, the party used taxation, debt collection, and trusteeship to weaken its opponents among entrepreneurs (Esen and Gumuscu 2018). While the party alienated further its opponents by playing a zero-sum game, the alliance it established with liberal democrats and religious conservatives gradually ended (Şahin 2018).

The Supreme Election Council rejected the complaints from the opposition parties that concerned President Erdogan's campaign rallying (despite his constitutionally neutral status) before the 2015 parliamentary elections (Esen and Gumuscu 2016). Opposition parties frequently complain about the limitations imposed on their electoral campaigns. Overall, the JDP has been criticized for its uneven access to media and resources (Esen and Gumuscu 2016). Gezi park protests, the coup attempt in 2016, and the subsequent purging of Gulenists exacerbated political and social polarization. After the failed coup, the state of emergency was declared, and more than 100,000 public officials were either suspended or sacked (Esen and Gumuscu 2018). The state of emergency was extended seven times until 2018 and supported by a range of emergency decrees that covered almost all aspects of public life (Yilmaz 2020). The state of emergency resulted in the malfunctioning of legislative and judiciary processes (Yilmaz 2020). Further restrictions were imposed on the media through the closure of hundreds of media outlets and the arrest of journalists (Esen and Gumuscu 2018).

Overall, under the JDP rule, state-society relations increasingly gained conflictual character. While, initially, the JDP had appealed to large segments of society by enacting liberal reforms and adopting distributive economic policies (Oniş 2015), it started lose supporters from across political spectrum with its increasing authoritarian tendencies. The party's initial populist rhetoric that operated on a dichotomy between victimized masses versus the ruling elites gradually evolved into a polarizing one, deepening the lines of division within the society (Ozbudun 2014).

Since the JDP came to power, secularists, ultra-nationalists, and the Kurds have been suspicious of the party's policies (Oniş 2012). Erdogan further alienated his opponents by describing them "as traitors and collaborators of external forces seeking to undermine Turkey's prosperity and stability" (quoted in Kirisci and Sloat, 6). The party's exclusionary policies reflect Erdogan's understanding of democracy that is based on the idea that "if you have the mandate of an electorate that grants you a comfortable majority in Parliament, you then have the right to govern without any respect for checks and balances" (quoted in Oniş 2015, 27).

Starting from the JDP's second term, citizen participation no longer dominated the agenda of the parliament (Yalçın-Riollet 2019). For instance, the absence of referendums on issues concerning the social and economic situations of ordinary Turkish citizens is reflective of policymakers' reluctance to involve citizens in decision-making processes. Constitutional referendums, on the other hand, were held in 2007, 2010, and 2017, respectively. Furthermore, that almost 49% of the voters rejected the changes to the constitution in the 2017 referendum is a testament to deep political divisions within the society.

The JDP's growing authoritarian tendencies are reflected in Turkey's democracy and freedom rankings. While between 2002 and 2017, Turkey was evaluated as partially free by Freedom House Index (2020), its status descended to non-free in 2018. According to the World Press Freedom of 2020, Turkey ranks 154th out of 180 countries (Reporters without Borders 2020). With respect to transparency and citizen participation in public policy deliberations, Turkey ranks 97th out of 128 countries (World Justice Project 2020).

Trust in Government and the Health System

While political trust to the government in Turkey is above the average of many developed countries, it has decreased considerably over the years. According to the survey conducted by the Eurobarometer in 2005, 76% of the respondents expressed their trust to the government in 2005 (above the EU average which is

34%) (Eurobarometer 2005). In 2009, only 51% of the respondents thought that the government was trustworthy (Eurobarometer 2009). A year later, 52% of the respondents expressed their distrust toward the government (Eurobarometer 2010). According to the survey conducted by Statista in 2018, 51% of people reported their distrust toward the government (Statista 2021). The survey conducted by European Social Survey in 2016 shows that 36.8% of the respondents believe that they have a say in what the government does (OECD 2019b).

According to the Pew Research Survey, conducted in 2015, the majority of people (54%) are dissatisfied with the way things are going in Turkey, while 44% are satisfied. Between 2012 and 2015, while favorable opinions of Erdogan decreased from 59% to 39%, negative views increased from 33% to 39%. As of 2015, while 48% of the respondents hold negative views of the government, only 45% think that the government has a good influence on the way things are going in Turkey (Poushter 2015).

Approximately 40% of survey participants to the Pew Research Survey stated that health care are top problems in Turkey, while the majority of respondents cited inflation, crime, and inequality as top problems (Poushter 2015). According to the survey conducted by Eurostat (2018), approximately 7% of Turkish respondents reported unmet needs for medical examination or treatment (below the EU average which is 3.2%). However, a significant increase is observed in citizen satisfaction with the healthcare system from 2007 to 2016 (OECD 2017), alluding to parallels between recent public health reforms and citizens' experience with the health care provision. According to the Trustworthiness Index (2019), scientists and doctors are seen as the most trustworthy in Turkey, a stark contrast to government ministers and politicians who are seen the least trustworthy.

Turkey's Response to the COVID-19 Pandemic

Differing from many countries, Turkey adopted an anticipatory approach toward the COVID-19 pandemic. The Ministry of Health had been mapping out plans and making preparations for large-scale outbreaks and pandemics since 2004. These efforts came to fruition with "the national preparation plan for pandemic influenza" (prepared by professors of medicine and medical experts) that came into force with a presidential circular in 2019. The plan specified preemptive measures to be taken at land and maritime borders; risk communication; public health rules; relevant institutions' responsibilities; plans and strategies; infection control; the treatment and vaccination procedures; the organization of social and economic life in case of a pandemic (The Ministry of Health 2019).

Against the backdrop of a sophisticated pandemic preparedness plan, Turkey responded to the COVID-19 pandemic through an adaptive and agile decision-making. Turkey's response to the pandemic includes a combination of preemptive and restrictive measures. Immediately after WHO Health Emergencies Programme published a rapid risk assessment report regarding atypical pneumonia cases in the world on January 6, Turkey accelerated its readiness actions.

Emergency Operations Centre in Ankara began monitoring the developments in the world, working on a 24/7 basis (World Health Organization 2020b). Soon after, institutional mechanisms were set up as part of emergency measures. The SAB, headed by the Health Minister Fahrettin Koca, was established on January 10. The SAB consists of university professors and medical experts specialized in pulmonology, virology, infectious diseases, clinical diseases, and a legal advisor.

A few days after its establishment, the SAB published a COVID-19 disease guide so as to inform citizens about the virus and public health rules. The disease guide determined the main parameters of Turkey's response to the pandemic. The guideline was updated in light of new information and developments with respect to the virus (World Health Organization 2020b). In February 2020, Turkey urged its citizens not to travel to China unless necessary. Passengers who came from China and other Southeast Asian countries went through screening procedures with thermal cameras. Soon, this procedure was extended to all passengers. The information about the virus and hygiene rules to combat the virus were distributed to the public through brochures and posters. At the end of February, all flights to and from China, Italy, Iraq, Iran, and South Korea had been suspended.

The first COVID-19 case was reported on March 11. The first virus-related death occurred on March 15. After the virus entered the country, immediate restrictive measures were put in place. In line with the recommendations of the SAB, all incoming passengers were placed in quarantine for two weeks; civil servants were banned from traveling abroad; schools, universities, cafés, restaurants, theaters, and gyms were closed; a partial curfew was first imposed on people who are above 65 and who have chronic diseases and later extended to those under 20 years old; intercity travels were suspended. Furthermore, hospital visits were restricted; court hearings, cultural, and sport activities were postponed; civil servants with chronic diseases were permitted to take administrative leave; flexible working hours were adopted.

Furthermore, a COVID-19 helpline was established; the number of health personnel and diagnosis laboratories was increased; COVID-19 test kits were distributed throughout the country; contract tracing was conducted by health teams working in the field as well as family practitioners. Pandemic boards were gathered in all provinces (Hurriyet 2020). All private hospitals were declared pandemic hospitals that treat COVID-19 patients as well as conduct COVID-19 tests. At the beginning of April, mask-wearing became mandatory in public places such as markets. Masks were distributed by the Ministry of Health free of charge.

A national "stay home campaign" was launched. Policymakers continuously urged citizens to adhere to public health hygiene rules. While policymakers highlighted the gravity of the situation by sharing statistics about cases and deaths, they gave an utmost attention not to create a panic environment, warning citizens about a torrent of disinformation spread in social media. A presidential decree, issued on April 13, stipulated that COVID-19-infected people (irrespective of their health coverage) would have free access to personal protective equipment, diagnostic testing, and medical treatment.

The first general (two-day) curfew was implemented on April 11. Two-day and four-day curfews were intermittently imposed until June 1. Since its establishment, the SAB has conveyed at least two times a week and made recommendations to the Ministry of Health by following closely the current scientific developments about the pandemic. After the meetings, Mr. Koca often appeared on TV, informing the public about the number of infected people, the number of tests conducted, age, and health problems of those who died of COVID-19 and sharing the guidelines laid out by the Board. He also actively used Twitter to keep citizens updated and remind them of social distancing rules. Frequent meetings were held between Mr. Koca and provincial health directorates and head physicians.

The number of infected people reached a peak on April 25 (with 80,808 cases) and then sharply declined until June. President Erdogan announced a normalization plan on May 3 that included the easing of restrictions on those who were above 65 years and below 20 years; the opening of shopping malls, stores, hairdressers, etc. on the condition that they comply with specific conditions such as general hygiene rules, the measurement of customers' temperature, etc.; the beginning of military service procedures; the restart of court hearings, etc. While preparations were made for normalization, two-day and four-day national curfews were imposed until the end of May (Daily Sabah 2020a).

The normalization process gained pace at the beginning of June. Intercity travel restrictions were lifted, and restaurants, cafés, and gyms were reopened. International flight restrictions gradually eased. The easing of some restrictions came at the expense of the introduction of additional measures. A HES code (which reveals information about the COVID-19-related risk status) became mandatory for those who travel by train, bus, or plane. In addition, wearing masks outdoors became mandatory in three major cities in Turkey: Istanbul, Ankara, and Bursa. Monetary fines were imposed on the violators of public health rules. In addition to COVID-19 tests, antibody tests started to be conducted in order to identify asymptomatic people and measure the level of immunity status. Starting from the last week of June, the Ministry of Health published COVID-19-related data that entail information about infected people by age, sex, and region. It also announced algorithms about treatment procedures of COVID-19 patients and contact-tracing (The Ministry of Health 2020a). In August, nationwide inspections regarding COVID-19-related rules were conducted by police officers and other local security forces in work places, parks, restaurants, mass transport vehicles, etc. (Hurriyet Daily News 2020). Provincial and district contract tracing boards were set up as part of efforts to contain the spread of the virus.

In the first week of September, mask-wearing became compulsory in all places except home. With the arrival of the flu season in October, mass inspections were conducted across the country. An economic recovery plan, worth approximately USD15m was introduced that included the postponement of tax payments of 1.9 million citizens; the deferral of more than two million taxpayers' social security contribution payments for six months; financial support to minimum wage workers; an increase in lowest retired pension; the provision of short time working allowance; the recruitment of 32,000 healthcare personnel (KPMG 2020). Yet, the unemployment rate was increasing before 2020, and it increased over the course of the pandemic (OECD 2021).

In October, the police and security forces increased controls with respect to social distancing rules and mask wearing. Through repeated announcements, citizens were warned of the dangers of crowded gatherings and reminded of the necessity of ventilation of indoor areas. Thirty-four locations in 19 provinces were placed under quarantine (Daily Sabah 2020b). In the first week of November, cafés, restaurants, cinemas, and other businesses were ordered to close at 10:00 PM, and a smoking ban was introduced in crowded outdoor spaces. On November 17, Erdogan announced new restrictions that included partial weekend curfew; partial curfew on the elderly and youngsters; the closure of restaurants, cafés, and cinemas. In November, Turkey signed a contract to purchase to 50 million doses of CoronaVac (Reuters 2020a). In the following month, Mr. Koca announced that Turkey would purchase 30 million doses of BioNTech vaccine (Daily Sabah 2020c).

Taken all together, Turkey's crisis management with respect to the COVID-19 can be broken down into three stages. The first stage between January and March 2020 is marked by preemptive measures taken in order to prevent the entrance of the virus into the country. The second stage started with the announcement of the first COVID-19 case in the country on March 11 and lasted until the end of May. This stage is characterized by intermittent lockdowns, the restriction of intercity travels, the closure of schools, stores, restaurants, etc., and the gradual easing of restrictions. The normalization process started in June with the end of lockdowns, restart of intercity travels, the opening of public places, etc. Yet, with the start of flu season in October, inspections were expanded, and a month later, restrictions were reintroduced. Figure 4.1 shows the number of daily cases from March 16, 2020 to January 14, 2021. The first lockdown period (April–June 2020) corresponds to a significant decrease in daily cases. However, November witnessed a significant surge in COVID-19 cases. Cases started to decline in December with slight fluctuations. From December 17 to January 14, there were sharp decreases in COVID-19 cases.

Figure 4.2 shows the number of daily deaths from March 16, 2020 to January 14, 2021. From March 15 to April 22, COVID-19 deaths increased exponentially and then started to decline sharply until June. After fluctuations in June, July, and August, the death toll increased in September. COVID-19 deaths increased severely from November 19 to December 29 and then started to decline until January 14.

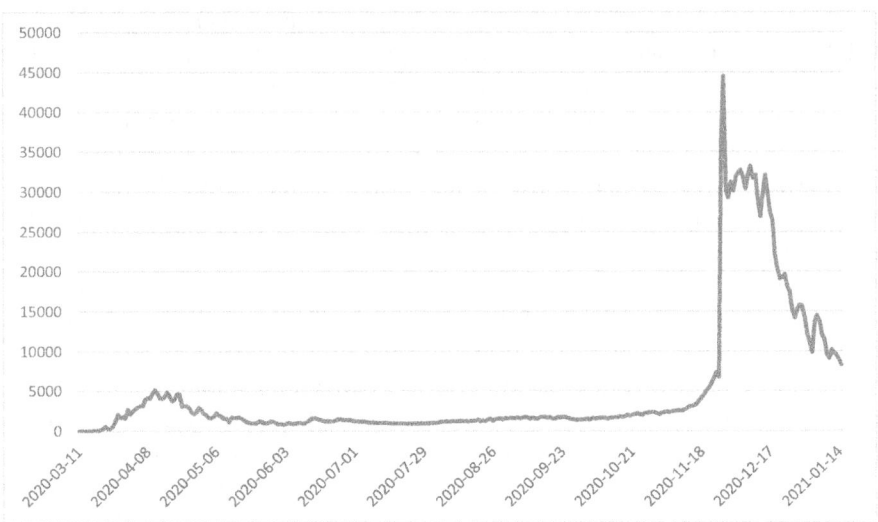

FIGURE 4.1 New Daily Confirmed COVID-19 Cases in Turkey.

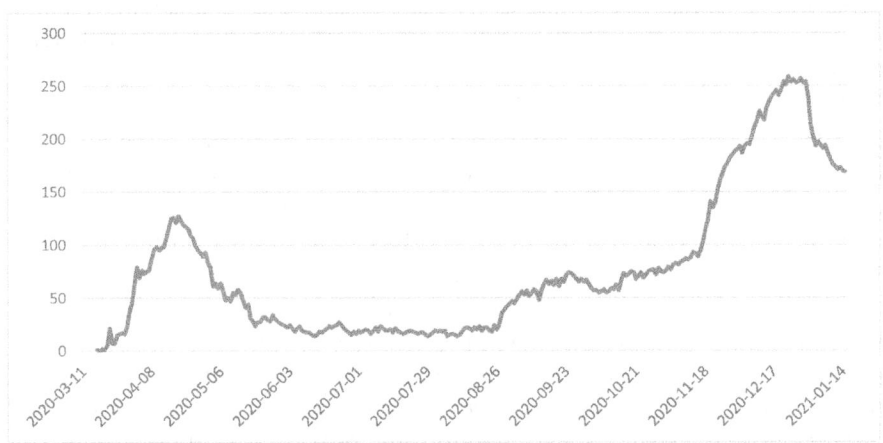

FIGURE 4.2 Daily Deaths from COVID-19 in Turkey.

Discussion and Conclusion

While Turkey has a tradition of top-down policymaking, under the JDP, it has shifted toward "the impositional end of the policy style spectrum" (Richardson 2018) since the political role of citizens, civil society organizations, and bureaucratic actors has been severely reduced. Turkey occupies the low end of the spectrum of policy capacity with its reactive-imposition policy style. Policymaking is not characterized by inclusiveness, as public participation in policymaking is not encouraged, and diverse views are not incorporated in policymaking processes. Overall, with its lower administrative policy capacity, lower inclusiveness, and reactive approach to problem-solving, Turkey fits into administrative policy style.

Turkey's administrative policy style and low trust in government account for why the country adopted a top-down centralized response to the COVID-19 pandemic. The President, the SAB, the Ministry of Interior, and the Ministry of Health have been the central players in the pandemic management. President Erdogan' instructions (informed by the recommendations of the SAB) have determined Turkey's courses of action during the pandemic. Ministries have played important roles in the implementation of COVID-19-related decisions. Erdogan' instructions in presidential cabinet meetings were issued as circulars by the Ministry of Interior. Restrictions to contain COVID-19 such as suspension of flights, lockdowns, mandatory mask wearing, mass inspections, the establishment of provincial, and district filiation boards coupled with easing of restrictions such as were all ordered through circulars and sent to 81 provinces.

These ordered governors and district governors to urgently implement specified measures in accordance with the relevant legislation. Provincial health directorates transformed the actions stipulated by the circulars into their "decisions" (The Human Rights Association 2020). While they are given the leverage to adopt "additional" measures to prevent the spread of the disease, the circulars played a decisive role in their course of action. The Ministry of Health also played a pivotal role in the pandemic management by working in coordination with provincial authorities, assessing provincial plans, training of health care workers, and informing the public (World Health Organization 2020b).

All in all, command and coordination, communication and information management, and resource management took place through hierarchical policy-making processes. Turkey's imposition policy style that characterizes its normal policymaking processes has been reflected in the pandemic management with the concentration of responsibility in the hands of a few executives as well as advisors (health experts) and the exclusion of major health associations (such as the Turkish Medical Association) from policymaking processes.

In view of President Erdogan's instructions that were informed by the recommendations of the SAB, it is safe to argue that Turkey's policymaking during the pandemic is marked by collaboration between policymakers and health experts. Considering high trust in health practitioners, the very establishment of the SAB and the design of policies in line with the recommendations of SAB can be evaluated as a governmental strategy to increase the legitimacy of, and generate maximum compliance to, the restrictive measures. In light of Turkey's low degree of inclusiveness in policymaking and its hierarchical bureaucratic structure, it is reasonable to deduce that the creation of the SAB was not a strategy aimed at increasing *agency autonomy*. Basing their decisions on the advice of the SAB enabled policymakers to ensure citizens' acceptance of restrictive measures against the backdrop of high trust in scientist and doctors in the society. The SAB also enabled Turkish policymakers to depoliticize the issue and avoid blame in an extraordinary situation which necessitated politically costly decisions (Zahari-adis, Petridou, and Oztig 2020).

Yet, despite strategies to generate citizen compliance and repeated warnings by the Health Ministry, crowded gatherings did take place (such as weddings) in which no compliance was observed with respect to social distancing and mask wearing. Trust in government plays a crucial role in the implementation process of public policies, as it lowers social resistance to measures and facilitates coop-eration between policymakers and citizens (Exadaktylos and Zahariadis 2014). In the case of Turkey, lower trust in government explains why the government introduced legal measures and monetary fines for quarantine violators as well as for those who do not abide by mask-wearing and social distancing rules. Viola-tion of public health rules and the enforcement of these rules through monetary fines point out that citizens abide by COVID-19 rules not because they have faith in the system but because they are obliged to do so by the central authority. Furthermore, along with Indonesia, China, and Iran, Turkey has placed charges against people who made comments about the pandemic and criticized the government's response in online platforms under criminal defamation laws (Kisa and Kisa 2020). These measures are indicative of *mutual distrust* between the government and citizens.

Interestingly, Turkey's hierarchical/imposition policymaking style led to the successful management of the health crisis through institutional and legislative agility. More interestingly, Turkey diverged from its reactive approach by having been prepared for a possible pandemic since 2004. Its anticipatory approach resulted in a swift response to the pandemic. Turkey informed the citizens in a timely way and adopted immediate proactive and restrictive measures to prevent the spread of the virus. It quickly increased its daily testing capacity, reaching up to 40,000 per million as of June 30, outpacing many developed countries. It was also successful in quick tracing of close contacts that led to the rapid isolation/quarantine and treatment measures (World Health Organization 2020b). Strict restrictions on the social life along with rapid health measures coincided with a sharp decline in the number of daily cases between April and June 2020. While the number of daily cases ranged between 4000 and 5000 in April, it declined to approximately 900 in June (Worldometer 2020).

As of October, case fatality ratio in Turkey was 2.7%, lower than that of Canada, the United Kingdom, and Sweden (4.7%, 5.6%, 5.5%) (John Hopkins University Coronavirus Research Center 2020). Through strategic stockpiles and local production, it eschewed critical shortages of drugs and medical equipment (World Health Organization 2020b). The strengthening of digital infrastructure throughout 2000s also enabled the country to quickly digitalize COVID-19-related data in the first phase of the pandemic which is of immense importance for the virus research (The Ministry of Health 2020c). Turkey's fight against the virus is not limited to the containment of the virus, but also includes the vaccina-tion research. Currently, 14 centers across the country conduct vaccine research. They gather under Joint Vaccine Study Group under the chairman of Mr. Koca

(The Ministry of Health 2020b). As of October, Mr. Koca announced that three COVID-19 vaccine candidates came to clinical trial phase.

As of November, Turkey ranks 11th in the number of tests conducted nationwide (more than 15 million) (Worldometer 2020). Turkey also provided personal protective equipment and made donations to more than 80 countries. Foreign patients are admitted for treatment (Insight Turkey 2020). There are currently 180 Migrant Health Centers at which COVID-19 temperature screenings are performed, and infected people are referred to hospitals. Undocumented people are also admitted to these centers after they are recorded as "stateless persons" under the Public Health Management System (Heinrich Boll Stiftung 2020).

In its 2020 report, the World Health Organization assessed Turkey's management of the health crisis as successful and effective in consideration of its performance in therapeutic algorithms; preventive measures; case fatality ratios; hospital bed/population ratios; early medication; flexibility in treatment procedures that included the usage of antivirals and even traditional Chinese medicine; local manufacturing of personal protective equipment; the preparation of COVID-19 guidelines that include evidence-based recommendations (World Health Organization 2020b). The World Health Organization's Regional Director for Europe, Dr. Hans Kluge also framed Turkey's response to the pandemic as a success, mentioning the importance of Turkey's vaccine development efforts as well as the provision of healthcare service to asylum seekers (The Ministry of Health 2020c).

On the other hand, Turkey's administrative policy style coupled with lower inclusiveness in policymaking constrained the development of transparent and inclusive policies with respect to the pandemic. Differing from Bakir (2020) who argues that Turkey's pandemic management diverged from its exclusionary policymaking style, this article argues that Turkey's normal governing style has been reflected in the pandemic management albeit in different forms. While collaboration between policymakers and experts determined Turkey's course of action, Turkish Medical Association, the Association of Public Health Experts, and other major health associations were excluded from the SAB and other health policy processes (Kisa and Kisa 2020). The government was criticized by a number of medical associations for the lack of transparency on issues that ranged from medication to access to tests (Hekimlik 2020). Human rights organizations in Turkey (such as Human Rights Foundation of Turkey and Progressive Lawyers Associations) issued a public statement that called the government to share information regularly with respect to the condition of prisons and prisoners' health (Human Rights Foundation of Turkey 2020).

These criticisms have resulted neither in increased transparency nor inclusiveness with respect to COVID-19 policies. Turkey's COVID-19 data do not reveal information about the number of infected children, asylum seekers, and migrants. In September 2020, Mr. Koca's admission that asymptomatic cases are not included in the COVID-19 data sparked backlash from some health workers (Reuters 2020b). In September, Devlet Bahceli, the leader of the Nationalist Movement Party (junior coalition partner of the JDP), went so far to advocate for the closure of the Turkish Medical Association by arguing that it incites panic among the population. Taken all together, especially when compared to many countries, Turkey has effectively handled the pandemic by virtue of its anticipatory approach to the pandemic; timely warnings to the public; immediate preemptive and restrictive measures; early detection of the virus (through large-scale virus-testing and contact-tracing); effective and free treatment of patients. Yet, the deliberation and implementation of COVID-19-related policies as well the enforcement of COVID-19-related rules mirror Turkey's administrative policy style and state-society relations.

Notes

1 There are also private providers in the system. In addition to delivering health care services, the Ministry of Health determines health policies and implements national health strategies. While discussions were made with respect to the decentralization of health services as part of health reforms, it has not been put into practice. Currently, Turkey has a centralized health system in which the Ministry of Health occupies a pivotal place (Tatar et al. 2011).
2 Richardson (2018) and DeLeo (2016) note that electoral concerns prompt many governments (including democratic ones) to choose short-term policymaking over anticipatory policymaking.

References

Ahmad, Feroz. 1993. *The Making of Modern Turkey*. London: Routledge.
Aslan, Imran, Orhan Cinar, and Ustun Ozen. 2014. "Developing Strategies for the Future of Healthcare in Turkey by Benchmarking and SWOT Analysis." *Procedia – Social and Behavioral Sciences* 150: 230–40.
Bakir, Caner. 2020. "The Turkish State's Responses to Existential Covid-19 Crisis." *Policy and Society* 39 (3): 424–41.
Bolukbasi, H. Tolga and Ebru Ertugal. 2019. "Napoleonic Traditions, Majoritarianism, and Turkey's Statist Policy Style." In *Policy Styles and Policymaking Exploring the Linkages*, eds. Michael Howlett and Jale Tosun. New York: Routledge, 351–374.
Burki, Talha. 2017. "Health Care in Turkey in the Erdogan Era." *Lancet* 389 (10081): 1786–87.
Cinar, Menderes. 2006. "Turkey's Transformation under the AKP Rule." *Muslim World* 96: 469–86.
Clemens, Elisabeth S. and James M. Cook. 1999. "Politics and Institutionalism: Explaining Durability and Change." *Annual Review of Sociology* 25: 441–66.
Daily Sabah. 2020a. "One Last Curfew? Turkey Sees Improved Outlook on Pandemic." May 19. At https://www.dailysabah.com/turkey/one-last-curfew-turkey-sees-improved-outlook-on-pandemic/news
Daily Sabah. 2020b. "No Curfews but Tight Measures Remain in Place Amid Pandemic in Turkey." October 19. At https://www.dailysabah.com/turkey/no-curfews-but-tight-measures-remain-in-place-amid-pandemic-in-turkey/news o-curfews-but-tight-measures-remain-in-place-amid-pandemic-in-turkey/new
Daily Sabah. 2020c. "BioNTech Says Turkey to Receive 4.5 Million Coronavirus Vaccine doses by March." December 27. At https://www.dailysabah.com/turkey/

biontech-says-turkey-to-receive-45-million- coronavirus-vaccine-doses-by-march/
news

DeLeo, Rob A. 2016. *Anticipatory Policymaking. When Government Acts to Prevent Problems
and Why It Is So Difficult.* Abingdon: Routledge.

Esen, Berk and Sebnem Gumuscu. 2016. "Rising Competitive Authoritarianism in
Turkey." *Third World Quarterly* 37 (9): 1581–606.

Esen, Berk and Sebnem Gumuscu. 2018. "Building a Competitive Authoritarian
Regime: State–Business Relations in the AKP's Turkey." *Journal of Balkan and Near
Eastern Studies* 20 (4): 349–72.

Eurobarometer. 2005. "Eurobarometer 63: Public Opinion in the European Union." At
https://ec.europa.eu/commfrontoffice/publicopinion/archives/eb/eb63/eb63_exec_
tr.pdf

Eurobarometer. 2009. "Eurobarometer 72: Public Opinion in the European Union." At
https://ec.europa.eu/commfrontoffice/publicopinion/archives/eb/eb72/eb72_tr_tr_
nat.pdf

Eurobarometer. 2010. "Eurobarometer 73: Public Opinion in the European Union." At
https://www.ab.gov.tr/files/BasınMusavirlik/haberler/eb73.pdf

Eurostat. 2018. "Persons Reporting Unmet Needs for Medical Examination or Treatment." At https://ec.europa.eu/eurostat/statistics-explained/index.php?title=Unmet_
health_care_needs_statistics&oldid=461732

Exadaktylos, Theofanis and Nikolaos Zahariadis. 2014. "*Quid pro Quo*: Political Trust
and Policy Implementation in Greece during the Age of Austerity." *Politics & Policy*
42 (1): 160–83.

Freedom House Index. 2020. "Country and Territory Ratings and Statuses, 1973-2020."
At https://freedomhouse.org

Heinrich Boll Stiftung. 2020. "Migrants and Refugees in a Time of Pandemic: Access
to Healthcare Services in Turkey." May 18. At https://eu.boell.org/en/2020/05/18/
migrants-and-refugees-time-pandemic-access-healthcare-services-turkey

Hekimlik. 2020. "Public Statement." At http://www.hekimlik.org/koronavirus/
merhaba/

Heper, Metin. 1985. *The State Tradition in Turkey.* Walkington: The Eothen Press.

Howlett, Michael and Jale Tosun. 2019. (eds.) *Policy Styles and Policymaking Exploring the
Linkages.* New York: Routledge.

Human Rights Foundation of Turkey. 2020. "COVID-19 Salgını ve Hapishanelerde Ac-
ilen Alınması Gereken Onlemler." [COVID-19 Pandemic and Immediate Measures
that should be taken in Prisons] March 20. At https://tihv.org.tr/basin-aciklamalari/
covid-19-salgini-ve-hapishanelerde-acilen-alinmasi-gereken-onlemler/

Hurriyet. 2020. "Tüm valiliklerde Pandemi Kurulları toplandı." [Pandemic boards were
gathered in all governates] March 28. At https://www.hurriyet.com.tr/gundem/
son-dakika-haberi-icisleri-bakanligindan-koronavirus-aciklamasi-tum-valiliklerde-
pandemi-kurullari-toplanacak-41480076

Hurriyet Daily News. 2020. "Turkey Performs Nationwide Inspections against Outbreak."
August 10. At https://www.hurriyetdailynews.com/turkey-to-perform-nationwide-
inspections-against-outbreak-157291

Insight Turkey. 2020. "Turkey's Management of COVID-19 Measures and Strategies
of Health Policies." September 22. At https://www.insightturkey.com/commentary/
turkeys-management-of-covid-19-measures-and-strategies-of-health-policies

John Hopkins University Coronavirus Research Center. 2020. "Mortality Analyses."
October 22. At https://coronavirus.jhu.edu/data/mortality

Keyder, Çaglar. 1997. "Whither the Project of Modernity." In *Rethinking Modernity and National Identity in Turkey*, eds. Sibel Bozdogan and Resat Kasaba. Seattle: The University of Washington Press, 37–51.

Kirişci, Kemal and Amanda Sloat. 2019. "The Rise and Fall of Liberal Democracy in Turkey: Implications for the West." *Brookings Institute, Policy Brief.* At https://www.brookings.edu/research/the-rise-and-fall-of-liberal-democracy-in-turkey-implications-for-the-west/

Kisa, Sezer and Adnan Kisa. 2020. "Under-reporting of COVID-19 cases in Turkey." *The International Journal of Health Planning and Management.* DOI: 10.1002/hpm.3031

Kisa, Adnan, Mustafa Z. Younis and Sezen Kisa. 2007. "A Comparative Analysis of the European Union's and Turkey's Health Status: How Health-care Services Might Affect Turkey's Accession to the EU." *Public Health Reports* 122 (5): 693–701.

Koker, Levent. 1995. "Local Politics and Democracy in Turkey: An Appraisal." *Annals of the American Academy of Political and Social Science* 540 (1): 51–62.

KPMG. 2020. "Turkey: Government and Institution Measures in Response to COVID-19." September 30. At https://home.kpmg/xx/en/home/insights/2020/04/turkey-government-and institution-measures-in-response-to-covid.html

Lijphart, Arend. 2012. *Patterns of Democracy: Government Forms and Performance in Thirty-Six Countries.* 2nd ed. New Haven: Yale University Press.

Lord, Ceren. 2012. "The Persistence of Turkey's Majoritarian System of Government." *Government and Opposition* 47 (2): 228–55.

OECD. 2017. "Government at Glance 2017." At https://www.oecd-ilibrary.org/governance/government-at-a-glance-2017_gov_glance-2017-en

OECD. 2019a. "OECD Statistics." At https://stats.oecd.org/index.aspx?queryid=24879

OECD. 2019b. "Country Fact Sheet: Turkey." At https://www.oecd.org/gov/gov-at-a-glance-2019-turkey.pdf

OECD. 2021. "OECD Economic Surveys. Turkey: Executive Summary." At https://www.oecd.org/economy/surveys/TURKEY-2021-OECD-economic-survey-executive-summary.pdf

Okem, Zeynep Güldem and Mehmet C. Akar. 2015. "What Have Health Care Reforms Achieved in Turkey? An Appraisal of the 'Health Transformation Programme'." *Health Policy* 199 (9): 1153–63.

Oniş, Ziya. 2012. "The Triumph of Conservative Globalism: The Political Economy of the AKP Era." *Turkish Studies* 13 (2): 135–52.

Oniş, Ziya. 2015. "Monopolising the Centre: The AKP and the Uncertain Path of Turkish Democracy." *The International Spectator* 50 (2): 22–41.

Our World in Data. 2021. "Turkey: Coronavirus Pandemic Country Profile." At https://ourworldindata.org/coronavirus/country/turkey

Ozbudun, Ergun. 2011. *The Constitutional System of Turkey: 1876 to the Present.* New York: Palgrave Macmillan.

Ozbudun, Ergun. 2014. "AKP at the Crossroads: Erdoğan's Majoritarian Drift." *South European Society and Politics* 19 (2): 155–67.

Ozen, Hayriye. 2013. "Informal Politics in Turkey during the Ozal Era (1983-1989)." *Alternatives Turkish Journal of International Relations* 12 (4): 77–91.

Peters, B. Guy. 2008. "The Napoleonic Tradition." *International Journal of Public Sector Management* 21 (2): 118–32.

Peters, B. Guy. 2015. "Policy Capacity in Public Administration." *Policy and Society* 34 (3–4): 219–28.

Peters, B. Guy and Jon Pierre. 2002. *Bureaucrats, Politicians and Administrative Reform.* London: Routledge.

Poushter, Jacob. 2015. "Deep Divisions in Turkey as Elections Nears." *Pew Research*. October 15. At https://www.pewresearch.org/global/2015/10/15/deep-divisions-in-turkey-as-election-nears/

Reuters. 2020a. "Turkey could Start Chinese COVID Vaccination this Month." December 11. At https://www.reuters.com/business/healthcare-pharmaceuticals/turkey-could-start-chinese-covid-vaccination-this-month-sozcu-newspaper-2020-12-10/

Reuters. 2020b. "Turkey Has Only Been Publishing Symptomatic Coronavirus Cases – Minister." September 30. At https://www.reuters.com/article/health-coronavirus-turkey-int-idUSKBN26L3HG

Reporters without Borders. 2020. "World Press Freedom." At https://rsf.org/en/ranking

Richardson, Jeremy, ed. 1982. *Policy Styles in Western Europe*. London: Allen & Unwin.

Richardson, Jeremy. 2018. *British Policymaking and the Need for a Post-Brexit Policy Style*. New York: Palgrave, Macmillan.

Şahin, Haluk. 2008. *Liberaller, Ulusalcılar, Islamcılar ve Otekiler* [Liberals, Nationalists, Islamists and Others] Istanbul: Say Yayınları.

Şahiner, Duygu D. and Lacin Ozer. 2020. "Digitalisation of the Health Services in Turkey." *Lexology*. July 2. At https://www.lexology.com/library/detail.aspx?g=02970f1d-2f88-4936-a958-d3e8fa8576f5

Statista. 2021. "Institutions that Citizens Lack Confidence in Turkey 2018." At https://www.statista.com/statistics/932664/confidence-in-institutions-in-turkey/

Tan, Evrim. 2014. *Towards a Managerial State: Turkey's Decentralization Reforms under the AKP Government. In Public Sector Reforms in Developing Countries Paradoxes and Practices*, eds. Charles Conteh and Ahmed Shafiqul Huque. New York: Routledge.

Tatar, Mehtap et al. 2011. "Turkey: Health System Review." *Health Systems in Transition* 13 (6): 1–186.

The Corruption Perception Index. 2019. "World Map." At https://www.transparency.org/en/cpi/2019/results/tur

The Human Rights Association. 2020. "COVID-19 ile Mücadele Kapsaminda Alinan Tedbirlerin Yasalliği Ve İdari Para Cezalari." [Legality of Measures taken to Combat COVID-19 and Administrative Monetary Fines] August 12. At https://www.ihd.org.tr/wp-content/uploads/2020/08/20200811_IHD-Kovid19TedbirleriRaporu.pdf.

The Ministry of Health. 2019. "Pandemik Influenza Ulusal Hazirlik Plani." [Pandemic Influenza National Preparedness Plan. At https://grip.gov.tr/depo/saglik-calisanlari/ulusal_pandemi_plani.pdf

The Ministry of Health. 2020a. "COVID-19 Algorithms." At https://covid19.saglik.gov.tr/TR-66303/covid-19-algoritmalar.html

The Ministry of Health. 2020b. "Minister Koca Chairs Joint Vaccine Study Group." October 14. At https://www.saglik.gov.tr/EN,75089/minister-koca-chairs-joint-vaccine-study-group.html

The Ministry of Health. 2020c. "Minister Koca Meets WHO Regional Director for Europe." June 11. At https://www.saglik.gov.tr/EN,65967/minister-koca-meets-who-regional-director-for-europe.html

Tosun, Tanju. 2015. "Electoral Systems in Turkey and Their Impact on Elections. Freedom Research Association." No. 3. At https://oad.org.tr/en/report/electoral-systems-in-turkey-and-their-impact-on-elections114

Trustworthiness Index. 2019. "Global Trust in Professions: Who Do Global Citizens Trust?" At https://www.ipsos.com/sites/default/files/ct/news/documents/2019-09/global-trust-in-professions-ipsos-trustworthiness-index.pdf

Üstüner, Yılmaz and Nilay Yavuz. 2017. "Turkey's Public Administration Today: An Overview and Appraisal." *International Journal of Public Administration* 41 (10): 820–31.

World Bank. 2018. "Government Effectiveness Index." At https://govdata360. worldbank.org/indicators/h1c9d2797?country=TUR&indicator=388&viz=line_ chart&years=1996,2018

World Health Organization. 2020a. "Hospital Beds (per 10 000 Population)." At https://www.who.int/data/gho/data/indicators/indicator-details/GHO/hospital-beds-(per-10-000-population)

World Health Organization. 2020b. "Turkey's Response to COVID-19: First Impressions." July 11. At https://www.euro.who.int/en/countries/turkey/publications/turkeys-response-to-covid-19-first-impressions-ankara,-turkey,-11-july-2020

World Justice Project. 2020. "The Rule of Law Index." At https://worldjusticeproject. org/sites/default/files/documents/WJP-ROLI-2020-Online_0.pdf

Worldometer. 2020. "Turkey." At https://www.worldometers.info/coronavirus/country/turkey/

Yalçın-Riollet, Melike. 2019. "Coproduction of Participation Policies in Turkey: The Making of City Councils." *Mediterranean Politics* 24 (3): 338–55.

Yaman, Hakan and Evrim D. Güneş. 2016. "Family Practice in Turkey: Observations from a Pilot Implementation." *Scandinavian Journal of Primary Health Care* 34 (1): 81–82.

Yılmaz Zafer. 2020. "Erdoğan's Presidential Regime and Strategic Legalism: Turkish Democracy in the Twilight Zone." *Southeast European and Black Sea Studies* 20 (2): 265–87.

Zahariadis, Nikolaos, Evangelia Petridou, and Lacin Idil Oztig. 2020. "Claiming Credit and Avoiding Blame: Political Accountability in Greek and Turkish Responses to the COVID-19 Crisis." *European Policy Analysis* 6 (2): 159–60.

5

CENTRALIZATION AND LOCKDOWN

The Greek Response

Nikolaos Zahariadis and Vassilis Karokis-Mavrikos

We are at war with an enemy who is invisible but not unbeatable.
(Prime Minister Kyriakos Mitsotakis, March 17, 2020)

I am more afraid of our own mistakes than of our enemies' designs.
(Pericles in Thucydides, *The Peloponesian War 1.144*)

When the COVID-19 pandemic hit the world in January 2020, Greece, like many other countries, was caught unaware and unprepared. Barely out of ten years of austerity and still in the middle of a devastating migrant crisis, the country was resource-poor and politically polarized. Nevertheless, because of its administrative policy style—low policy capacity and low inclusiveness—as well as the low trust that Greek citizens have toward public institutions, the country's response followed the hypothesized trajectory specified in Chapter 2: high centralization. However, deep problems emanating from the illusion of total success during the first wave of the crisis (February–May 2020) exposed institutional deficiencies and generated social discontent and political distrust, leading to centrifugal tendencies during the second wave (September 2020–January 2021). The country's response has subsequently shifted to a more regionally nuanced approach, changing the dynamics of crisis management and partially amending our original centralization hypothesis.

The chapter first describes Greece's policy capacity and trust and then explores how they shaped the national response. The analysis of the response strategy is informed by 20 interviews with Greek policymakers and academics conducted over two waves (July–August 2020 and December 2020–February 2021). The selection of respondents was based on relevant scientific expertise as well as

DOI: 10.4324/9781003137399-7

experience in formal positions during the current or a previous pandemic. The interviews were semi-structured, guided by the analytical axes of the policy styles framework. The names and affiliations of all respondents are listed in the appendix. Comparing the insights collected through the interviews between the two waves, we note the factors that pressed for a shift away from centralization. Still heavily centralized, national response has begun to acquire more centrifugal elements as the Greek government has shifted priorities to a more carefully calibrated public health-economy trade-off. We conclude with observations about our case and identify theoretical gaps in the argument.

An Administrative Policy Style in the Making

Greece has an administrative policy style. In terms of policy capacity, the country exhibits top-heavy concentration of powers, a hierarchical mode of decision-making and implementation, and a high degree of constant institutional change and jurisdictional ambiguity. Similar to other South European countries, it has a profoundly politicized bureaucracy, steeped in formalism and heavily influenced by political patronage (Sotiropoulos 2004). Reasons for these pathologies include historical legacy, partisanship, clientelism, nepotism, and widespread corruption in the transition to democracy (since the fall of the military dictatorship in 1974) as well as a culture of perennial reforms and implementation gaps.

Owing to its legacy in the Napoleonic tradition (Spanou 2008), the Greek administrative system has followed the path of heavy statism. Because the system proved economically very successful following World War II (Pagoulatos 2003), public organizations became deeply entrenched and centralized, functioning on the basis of formal rules and procedures and subjected to direct political control. The fall of the military dictatorship added new issues in terms of partisan politics, democratization, and state-society relations (e.g., Lyrintzis 1984). The arrival of the populist left in power in 1981 saw the dramatic expansion of state bureaucracy through increases in public employment in the name of democracy and modernity (Sotiropoulos 1996). Following the path of least resistance, the ruling Socialists (and their conservative successors) chose to add layers of more state bureaucrats rather than eliminate agencies which were no longer needed. The tendency was perpetuated and propagated by the introduction of temporary general and special secretariats in various ministries, usually abolished by the next administration in power, clogging the already crowded bureaucracy and producing implementation gaps (Makrydemetres 1999). The end result was a huge increase in patronage as a source and consequence of political power (Spanou 1996), clientelism and a labyrinth of agencies, and rules that were often in conflict with one another.

Institutional ambiguity, widened through jurisdictional overlap, produced endemic conflict. As Hajer (2003) reminds, the multiplicity of meanings embedded in ambiguity empowers public agencies to continually (re)interpret institutional opportunities and constraints. (Re)interpretation generates instability and political tension (Zahariadis 2016). In this environment, political patronage becomes the main vehicle to cement benefits and ensure survival. The high politicization that continues to characterize the Greek political system and public bureaucracy, including health care, has tended to overshadow the economic-cum-managerial dimension of operating hospitals, favoring political criteria of organizational and individual performance (Ballas and Tsoukas 2004). Modernizing hospital management "has been in the agenda for years, but staffing has been inconsistent and practices remain outdated" (interview with Emeritus Professor of Management Aris Sissouras).

Minimal Inclusiveness, Perennial Reforms, and Low Trust

What is more, laws have often been adopted by the legislature with minimal consultation with social actors (low inclusiveness). Despite legal obligations in years past to consult with affected social actors, usually meaning labor unions, successive governments have done so in politically expedient ways due to centralized powers. Consultation and inclusiveness were often attempted in form than in substance. Governments have used party-affiliated experts not to meaningfully inform but to legitimize decisions, usually for the benefit of a partisan network of actors in each policy sector (Kalyvas et al. 2012). Austerity and creditor demands since 2010 have strengthened political expediency and reduced inclusiveness (Ladi 2014). Laws are now passed with dizzying speed, hardly any inclusiveness of social actors, and under emergency procedures in the name of obligations to meet creditor targets.

The situation is exemplified by the perennial state of reform that Greek bureaucracy finds itself. In addition to the flux encountered in the 1980s, major reforms to streamline administration have been attempted throughout the 1990s and 2000s including, most recently, capacity-building reforms encouraged by the bailout packages. With the exception of tax collection tools to help balance public books, reforms have mostly failed to take hold (Lampropoulou and Oikonomou 2018). Obstacles have included lack of preparation and cohesion, lack of political will, weak social support and input, and a general political environment that rewards most of the spoils to the electoral winners (Spanou and Sotiropoulos 2011). To this list, we may add suspicion by affected (health) professionals of a biased state; reforms are met with selective consent and dissent (Bolton et al. 2018). In this case, trust in the system and in reforms evaporates. Perennial and unsuccessful reforms increase ambiguity, further feeding low capacity and trust and cementing the downward spiral.

Trust in Greek political institutions is generally low. The perceived lack of transparency, corruption, and widespread nepotism have made Greeks expect less from their government. As Norris (2011) argues, in countries where democratic performance fails, citizen expectations plummet and distrust increases. Successive European Social Surveys show that Greeks have less trust in their government and political institutions than most of their European allies. The rate of decline accelerated once the economic crisis hit, just like it did in other South European countries hit hard by the economic crisis (e.g., Torcal 2017). As Ervasti et al. (2019, 1222) categorically assert, the Greek "people have been repeatedly disappointed with the attempts of politicians of various persuasions to implement policies guiding the nation out of the crisis." By 2018, the country had been hit hard by perceptions of declining quality of governance, lack of accountability, and political transparency, all leading to confidence and trust levels in government and public health services hovering around an abysmal 16% and 42% relative to the OECD average of 42% and 70%, respectively (OECD 2019).

The Greek Health Care System

Such dysfunction and public sector pathologies have long manifested in the Greek health policy sector. Beginning with the establishment of the Greek National Health System (GNHS), in 1983, the sector has been defined by immense centralization, jurisdictional conflict, narrowness in policy outputs, and continuous formal and informal rapport between the government and a highly integrated policy community (Sissouras 2012). The sector has exhibited a clear orientation toward hospital care, encouraged by the hegemonic Ministry of Health (MoH) and the powerful doctor guild (Kyriopoulos and Telloglou 2019). Reform design has been delegated to a small community of health experts with close ties to the government (Petridou et al. 1999) who undertook an array of formal and informal positions and engaged in constant role switching. They undermined inclusiveness from within, legitimizing the institutional configurations in place and maintaining the prevailing balance of interests.

Efforts to introduce decentralized instruments, although legislated on multiple occasions, have largely proven futile during implementation (Athanasiadis et al. 2015). Professor Christos Zilidis categorically states:

> the regional pillars of the system never really functioned effectively and, despite provisions in the health bills of 2001, 2003 and 2005, power remained concentrated in the hands of central political and administrative instruments; specifically, the MoH and the Greek Center for Disease Control (CDC).

Moreover, as Professor Christos Lionis asserts:

> the integral parts of the Greek health services system – hospital, primary and social care – lack integration. Social care services are supervised by the Ministry of Labor, local public health is under the auspices of the Ministry of Interior and primary health care lies with the MoH.

The resultant jurisdictional ambiguity has exposed deficiencies in health monitoring capacity and the absence of updated vaccination and disease registries, inform Professors Dimopoulos and Tsouros. These are key elements of any strategy to effectively combat a pandemic. Missing clear division of labor, consistent co-operation across levels and sectors, and long-term coordination, Greek health care lacks administrative instruments, funding, and the legal infrastructure to adequately address issues at the regional and local levels. Research on public health systems and services and in public health law concludes that creating such instruments is pivotal to policy innovation, infrastructure development, and effective implementation (Burris et al. 2012).

The decade-long financial crisis (2010–2020) only made things worse. Hospitals were one of the main contributors to the ballooning public deficit, the other being the railroad company (Zahariadis 2013). Public funding was unavoidably slashed, supplies were cut back as part of the broader government initiative since 2015 to generate large primary budget surpluses, and staff was decimated in terms of numbers, salary, and morale (Bolton et al. 2018). The GNHS continued to be viewed as highly problematic, inefficient, and corrupt (Sissouras 2012). Following ten years of economic austerity and five years of a concurrent migration crisis, the GNHS found its budget cut by three-quarters in 2020 and the number of Intensive Care Unit (ICU) beds standing at a mere 560 beds (Psaropoulos 2020). To put it into context, this number represents 5.2 beds per 100,000 population (Greece's population in 2019 was 10.72 million according to data from Eurostat) as opposed to the OECD-22 average of 12 beds per 100,000 (OECD 2020).

The COVID-19 Response

A centralized top-down approach emerged as the only course of action for Greece against the COVID-19 threat, especially during the first wave. Despite belated pushback from businesses, some civilians, the Church, and political opposition parties, the Greek government used scientific advice and symbolic politics to legitimize a very stringent lockdown. The pandemic hit the country in two waves. The first lasted from late February to early May 2020. After hesitant measures designed to help the economy recover from the blow caused by the pandemic, the country experienced a second wave of cases and consequent deaths that was far worse than the first. We first track the Greek response during the first wave, then briefly discuss the summer interlude, and finally focus on the second wave from late September 2020 to January 2021.

Centralization and Success during the First Wave

Closely tracking Italy's predicament at the time, Greece realized that it could not afford an epidemic of a similar magnitude to neighboring Italy. "There was opposition [to a general lockdown], mainly from our unit on the economy, but it was quickly overcome, with the images that were starting to come from Italy definitely playing a part," stated Prime Minister Kyriakos Mitsotakis (interview on August 5, 2020). The country's deficiencies in resources and health services capacity precluded any prospect of managing large numbers of patients from the start. Systemic public sector dysfunction forced a proactive response, focusing on prevention, not treatment. "Our single immediate priority was protecting the GNHS from overloading by any means necessary. We shifted all of our attention on how to contain the spread of a threat we knew nothing about," stressed Deputy Minister of Health Vassilis Kontozamanis. "We wanted to make sure we would never reach a state where people would die because we would be incapable of offering care," admitted the Prime Minister.

Action was swift, turning weakness into strength. "Other countries, with much better hospital infrastructure and more ICU units per population, maintained an illusion that their systems would be able to cope, so they delayed [countermeasures]," informs Ioannis Tountas, head of Greece's Institute for Social and Preventive Medicine (in Labropoulou 2020). On February 23, 2020, the Prime Minister set up an 11-man National Committee for the Protection of Public Health against COVID-19, composed of the MoH's general secretaries and directors for public health services and emergencies, the presidents of the national agencies for public health, medicines, and emergency services and four experts specializing in microbiology and infectious diseases. While the international community failed to settle on common guidelines, the Greek Prime Minister prepared to introduce strict measures.

> The international scientific community did not provide clear directions at the start. Let me remind you that the WHO has made quite a few U-Turns so far. It was late to declare a state of world pandemic, it did not advise on using masks in the beginning etc. I spent time educating myself on what this new threat was. I spoke directly with people on the frontlines – people offering care at ICUs – and realized quickly this is and can be ugly. And this led me to the quick personal decision to proceed with a lockdown.

In the low-trust, adversarial Greek polity, he knew that fingers would soon be pointed and blame games were sure to follow.

During the first wave (Figure 5.1) and consistent with our hypothesis, the government drafted a concentrated command-and-control plan with very stringent measures. On February 27, as a result of three confirmed cases, the government canceled carnival events throughout the country, leading to significant political pushback. Social disruption increased resistance from political opposition and individual voters. However, as the number of confirmed cases continued to climb, all educational institutions across the country were closed on March 10. A new Committee of 26 scientists "for the Response to Emergency Public Health Threats from Infectious Causes," which became known as the COVID-19 Specialists Committee, was created on March 11. On March 12, movie theaters, gyms, and courtrooms were closed. On March 13, with 190 confirmed cases and one death, malls, cafés, restaurants, beauty parlors, museums, and archaeological sites were ordered shut followed by beaches and ski resorts the next day, including banning flights to/from Italy. The most impactful

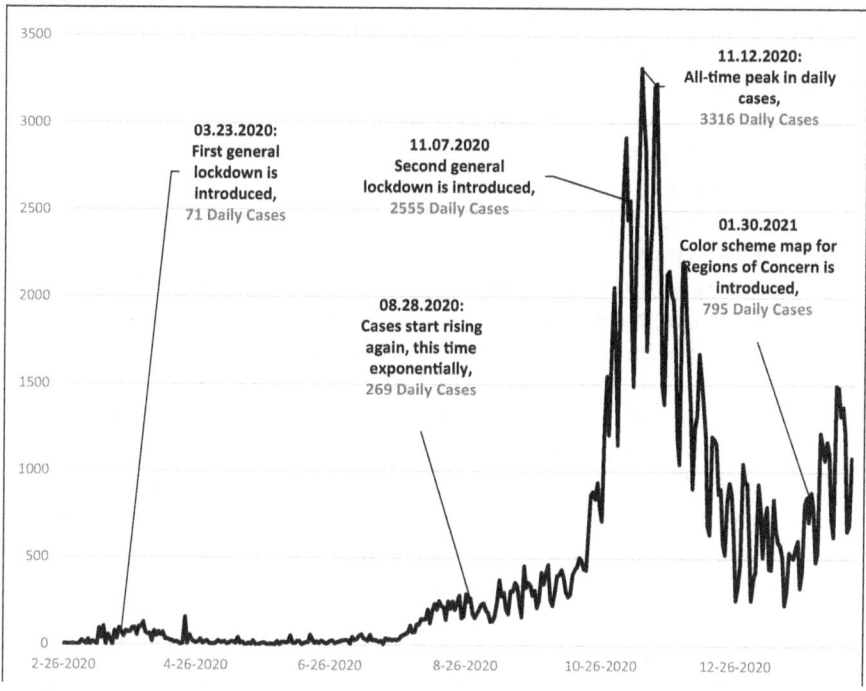

FIGURE 5.1 New Daily Confirmed COVID-19 Cases in Greece.

measures came on March 23, when, following examples by other EU countries, the government banned all non-essential travel and imposed restriction of movement nationwide. Subject to heavy fines, citizens could leave their homes only with special permits and for specific reasons.

With no prospect of making structural changes to the process of policymaking during an emergency, decision-making and coordination were handled by a handful of politicians and bureaucrats, with the Prime Minister undertaking the leading role. As Mahoney and Thelen (2010) predict, Greeks engaged in some institutional change, especially in the form of layering or bricolage (addition or *ad hoc* recombination of capacity). But, unlike their argument, they did not need to overcome political friction. Three new instruments emerged as vital sources of input, prompting a higher-than-expected degree of inclusiveness, albeit in a clearly centralized mode. First, the National Public Health Organization (NPHO), founded by the preceding radical left–right (SYRIZA-Independent Greeks) government to replace the Greek CDC, acted on its mandate as "Greece's designated authority on infectious diseases and public health emergencies." It started issuing directives as early as of February 9, 2020, published a provisional Pandemic Response Plan, had some of its proposals acted upon immediately (e.g., setting up the national COVID-19 case registry hosted by the NPHO website), and undertook all digital communication with the public. Second, the COVID-19 Specialists Committee "met daily" since its establishment at the MoH and "saw most of its proposals accepted by the leadership" (interview with Panagiotis Gargalianos, member of the COVID-19 Specialists Committee). Blamed by many for its narrow composition—by Greek standards—the COVID-19 Specialists Committee did not have the "interdisciplinary and intersectoral character" of similar committees established during the 2009 H1N1 pandemic or the 2002 Sars-Cov-1 epidemic (interview with Emeritus Professor Ioannis Kyriopoulos). Nevertheless, unlike its predecessors, it undertook a more meaningful role, serving as the central advisory body rather than the usual symbolic recognition mechanism as had been the case in the past. Third, the General Secretary of Civil Protection and Crisis Management, Nikos Hardalias, was upgraded to Deputy Minister, within the Ministry of Citizen Protection. Minister Hardalias notes that

> following the Prime Minister's decision in February [2020], Civil Protection undertook the central coordinating role in the fight against Covid-19. Additionally, in close cooperation with police units, fire departments, the coast guard, the MoH and the NPHO, it developed and carried out all contact tracing as well as data processing, in the new National Data Analysis Centre hosted in the new Civil Protection headquarters.

In line with the government's broader agenda of a more meritocratic and efficient state apparatus, efforts were made to increase inclusiveness and enhance administrative capacity from the start while maintaining concentration of powers at the highest level. "Acting early bought us time to prepare for what will come because the pandemic is far from over," stresses Deputy Minister Kontozamanis.

Coordination was exemplified by a consistent message delivered in daily briefings by the spokesperson of the MoH and member of the COVID-19 Specialists Committee, Dr. Sotirios Tsiodras, a professor of infectious diseases at the University of Athens. He was often accompanied by Minister Hardalias. This is a coup for the Greek civil service because it combines transparency and expertise. This did not go unnoticed neither by the public nor by the political opposition. "It gave legitimacy to the measures and support to the socially costly decisions. It was hard to refute through political debate a set of measures so strongly grounded on science" (Professor Zilidis). The scientific legitimation of the strict lockdown policies added to the "initial terror widely publicized in the media from deaths in Italy and Spain" (interview with Associate Professor Effie Simou) in achieving compliance. The government managed to induce higher trust, turning "the traditionally reactionary Greek public to an obedient one" (interview with Professor John Yfantopoulos). The Prime Minister categorically declares:

> I think we found a great balance between the fear and strictness that Nikos Hardalias inspired and the expertise and sweet voice that Sotiris Tsiodras brought. This was not explicitly planned from the start, but when we saw it was working, we heavily invested in it.

Decision-making seemed particularly responsive to feedback.

Frustration and Concern Grow Exponentially during the Summer Interlude

Greece's early response with horizontal measures of strict social distancing introduced through a centralized mode of policymaking catapulted the country to a success story and cultivated citizen trust in government (Petridou and Zahariadis 2021). The number of cases, and more importantly deaths, were kept to a minimum. Key social alliances were formed "in fronts that could threaten trust and compliance, such as with the Greek Orthodox Church," as Professor Zilidis informed. Public funds as well as considerable private donations increased the number of ICU beds to 1,017 in May 2020, close to the threshold of 1,200 that would put the country on par with the EU average of ICU beds per 100,000 people (Athens News Agency 2020). With the risk of a GNHS collapse significantly minimized and with less than 10 daily cases, lockdown measures started being lifted on May 4. The hospitality sector was allowed to resume operations on May 25, and international travel restarted on June 15, in an effort to deliver a much-needed boost to the economy through Greek tourism. Greece relies on tourism for a fifth of its income and a quarter of jobs, making it the single most important economic sector (Tugwell and Nikas 2020). Showing awareness of the long-term persistence of the COVID-19 threat, the government created the Governmental Committee of Coordination for the COVID-19 response at the end of June to collect information and propose or amend government programs under consideration during the pandemic.

Nevertheless, despite the seeming goodwill and increasing trust in government, preparedness for a second wave proved lackluster, and the country was soon plagued by policy capacity deficiencies. Three factors during the crucial summer months generated frustration and concern causing trust to plummet again. Declining levels of trust shaped the Greek response during the second wave of the pandemic (September 2020–January 2021). First, the trade-off between public health and economic objectives made prolonged lockdown measures very difficult to implement. The COVID-19 crisis came on the heels of a 10-year economic recession, devastating a fragile and hesitant economic recovery. Professor Kyriopoulos stressed this point: "The trade-off between public health and the economy was very pertinent in the Greek case. Capitalizing on the early success and opening up following the example of other EU success stories was way too appealing for the government." In fact, in a public opinion poll in early June, more worried about their financial situation (32%) as opposed to those worrying about their health (23%)—42% were concerned about both (ekathimerini.com 2020). As a result, the number of cases began to rise (Figure 5.1). Whether cases were the result of infected tourists coming through land borders in Macedonia and Thrace, where initially no tests were administered in contrast to air travel, or of more tests, the fact is that the government lost a major tool in its successful response against COVID-19: contact-tracing. As the World Health Organization (WHO) makes abundantly clear, "contact tracing ... is a key strategy for interrupting chains of transmission" (WHO 2021, 1). However, because it requires abundant manpower, sensitivity to local context, close engagement with communities, relevant and continuing training, and exhaustive investigation (WHO 2021, 2–4), effective contact-tracing is difficult to perform beyond a certain threshold of cases.

Second, the success generated by responses to the first wave created a false sense of security. Because the general lockdown was so effective, it was thought that the country's authorities could implement the same policy response with similarly successful results. But the centralized response meant that all regions were treated equally without regard to the nuances of local context. Precisely because regional health authorities were underdeveloped and understaffed, the country lost precious time in both monitoring and responding in a timely manner. In other words, centralization's success became its own weakness during the second wave (interview with Marios Themistokleous, General Secretary for Primary Health Care). The signs had been there since the first wave, but were masked underneath the nationwide mobility restrictions. "When spikes in cases would emerge in Northern Greece, the response was always to send NPHO personnel, or Tsiodras and Hardalias in a helicopter, to go check the situation" stresses Professor Zilidis. "During the daily briefings there were no qualitative indices and no information on the geographical spread of the cases. Local communities never understood whether the danger levels were increasing or falling in their area," suggests former Minister of Health Andreas Xanthos. And the Prime Minister adds: "I wish municipalities and administrative regions took greater initiative. Since that was rarely the case, I was forced to intervene." For as long as the only priority was containing the spread of the virus, problems with policy capacity lay dormant underneath the luster of self-congratulations.

Sustainable economic performance demanded learning to live with the virus and delaying a second nationwide lockdown as much as possible. Most of the summer was spent managing the rapid lift of all mobility restrictions. People understood the need for the protection of public health, but as early as June 2020, 65% favored restrictions only in places experiencing spikes in cases and only 21% of those surveyed in a public opinion poll favored horizontal measures similar to those imposed in the spring of 2020 (ekathimerini.com 2020). Early attempts at regional lockdowns came with significant delay and little or no planning. On July 14, then Minister of Health, Vassilis Kikilias, spoke on national TV about the "Plan B of regional lockdowns." But the country did not acquire the monitoring and implementation capacity to take such regionally nuanced measures until November.

Third, the duration of the pandemic took a toll on trust and consequently compliance. New daily cases crept up during the summer, surpassing 200 on August 9 for the first time (Figure 5.1). The March lockdown had been introduced with less, although daily testing had increased since. On August 17, the Prime Minister announced lockdowns in areas with high numbers of cases, which included curfews, restrictions to gatherings, and mandatory mask-wearing. The August local lockdowns did not envision business closures. Tsiodras and Hardalias returned to television for bi-weekly briefings. "Now we need to kick the population's caution back up again, and we are bringing them back" stated the Prime Minister during our interview. However, despite bringing back the proven-worthy messengers, the message was no longer as powerful or even appropriate in some cases. Local lockdowns caused political and popular pushback, and with more relaxed measures than the ones employed during the first wave, they were very often breached. The lack of capacity at the local level meant that centrally taken decisions could not be effectively implemented. "If you do not take into account the diverse needs of the different population groups and do not deliver tailor-made messages involving local authorities, the communication strategy cannot be effective" stresses Christos Lionis sharing first-hand experience from mass non-compliance in Crete. The high trust in the government's successful response to the first wave began to erode. One study, conducted between March and August 2020, reported that levels of high trust resulting from initial successes by the Greek government and health authorities decreased by 31 and 21 percentage points, respectively, during that period (Kanellopoulou et al. 2020).

As the initial approach to local lockdowns seemed to be failing and while cases continued to rise, low monitoring capacity further delayed meaningful interventions. Nightclubs and bars were secretly breaking curfew in rural areas (Skai Online Newsroom 2020). Many nursing homes, "most being private institutions without proper quality and legal auditing," informs Professor Lionis, "lacked the capacity to stop the spread among the elderly." Despite great effort by Civil Protection to cooperate with local and regional authorities in containing the disease and implementing measures, the government could never stay "a step ahead of the disease" (Prime Minister). Aware of institutional deficiencies, the government also knew that it could not engage in wholesale change during the crisis.

Chronic deficiencies in developing regional administrative capacity in public health rendered this feat impossible. Greece's seven Health Regional Authorities are understaffed, uneven in size, and with unclear jurisdiction over public health matters, cooperating uncomfortably with the 13 Administrative Regions and the NPHO. Figure 5.2 provides a map showing the different administrative regions. "The Sixth Health Regional Authority is managed only by a chief administrator and two deputies and covers [an area of] nearly one-fourth of the country" (Minister Xanthos). "The Regional Public Health Labs – created in 2003 for disease monitoring – were never staffed and the one in Thessaloniki has remained locked up," asserts Professor Zilidis. The head of Attica's Administrative Region, in collaboration with the Union of Athens Doctors, voluntarily donated 10 mobile care units to government, to be used for testing in Attica in cooperation with the NPHO. While trying to improve the country's monitoring capacity, these acts rendered the massive institutional gaps more visible at the same time. "The Attica Regional Authority, when activated, proved more effective than the NPHO in identifying needs and intervening" comments Professor Yfantopoulos. Regional instruments performed as well as they could but chronic understaffing and jurisdictional ambiguity did not optimize results. The policy context required upgrading of infrastructure, but the legal foundations, let alone administrative expertise and funding, were simply not there.

Highly centralized monitoring and tracing could not contain the rise in cases. Low capacity and trust prompted a centralized response, but when trust began to rise, low capacity produced centrifugal pressures. In the beginning of fall, daily cases increased exponentially (Figure 5.1). Committed to avoiding a second nationwide lockdown, the government opted to continue with regional measures, in combination with some nationwide tightening up. But during September 2020, trust levels in both the government and the scientific community deteriorated. Measures seemed to change daily, as did the recommendations of the COVID-19 Specialists Committee. Schools opened with mandatory mask-wearing on September 11, following long discussions on classroom size. A 12–5-am curfew was introduced for mini-markets following a record-high (at the time) 453 cases on September 21, according to data from the Johns Hopkins University. Professor Simou states categorically: "Decisions were viewed as contradictory and untimely by citizens." Meanwhile, the blame shifting harmed politicians and experts alike. The second wave of the Dianeosis (2020) survey on COVID-19 showed "high trust on scientists" dropping from 85% to 65.6% and "high trust on the welfare state" dropping from 56.7% to 42% between April and September 2020.

Delaying a second lockdown and maintaining an open economy eventually forced treatment, not just prevention, to become a priority. Low policy capacity

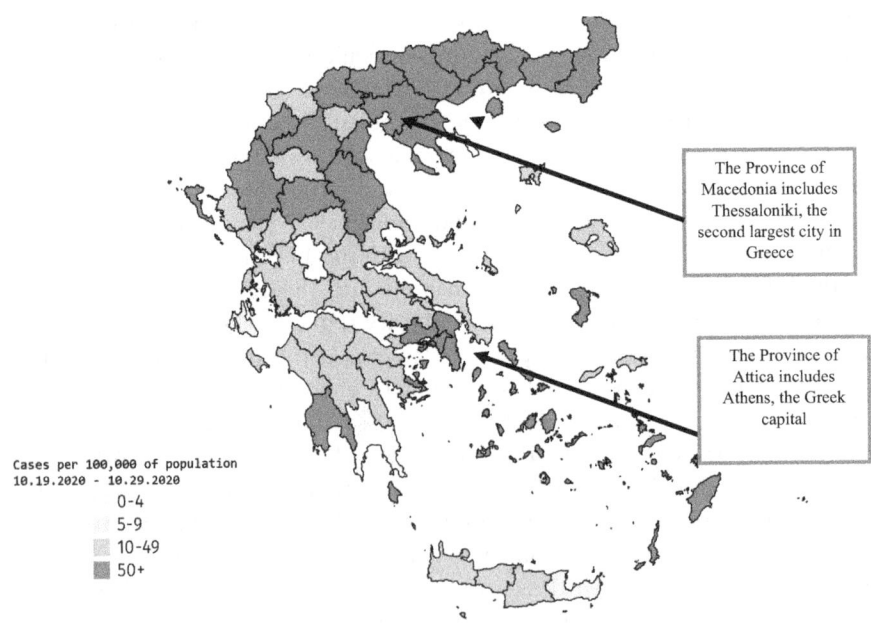

The Province of Macedonia includes Thessaloniki, the second largest city in Greece

The Province of Attica includes Athens, the Greek capital

Cases per 100,000 of population
10.19.2020 - 10.29.2020
0-4
5-9
10-49
50+

FIGURE 5.2 Regional Map of COVID-19 Cases per 100,000 of Population in Greece (October 19, 2020–October 29, 2020).

tested the GNHS, pressuring it to the verge of collapse. Primary care services in the country have been rudimentary and unembedded in the public culture. "Eighty percent of cases exhibit symptoms which can be dealt at the primary care level but only 15% of Greeks are registered to their dedicated family doctor," claims Minister Xanthos. Home care for people unable to visit hospitals or in high danger of infection "is non-existent," added Professor Kyriopoulos. At the end of the day, the chronic problems of the health sector made matters worse. "An integrated system of healthcare services was never achieved in Greece," said Professor Sissouras, forcing all patients to hospital care. During October, daily cases started surpassing 2,000, while daily ICU patients moved past 100. The designated COVID-19 hospitals established during the first wave—predominantly in urban centers—reached capacity limits while hospitals in rural areas faced a lack of equipment and specially trained personnel. The GNHS's durability was questioned daily. It became clear that the country lacked the structural foundations to handle a nationally open economy with only regional measures in place. Neither ensuring compliance nor monitoring and tracing cases, let alone treatment, were feasible.

General Measures and Regional Lockdowns during the Second Wave

Political pushback and plummeting trust led to the worst of both worlds: rising cases and failing measures. During the national holiday weekend of October 26–28, no further restrictions were imposed although celebrations were canceled. The holiday is a double celebration for the city of Thessaloniki, the capital of the Province of Macedonia, where most cases were traced during the fall (Figure 5.2). As the Minister of Development Adonis Georgiadis stated on Skai TV (January 5, 2021): "Not imposing stricter restrictions on Thessaloniki was the biggest mistake we made. The Covid-19 Specialists Committee made recommendations for a lockdown, but we wanted to show respect to the Orthodox Church." Daily cases jumped by more than 1,000 in the following week, continuously reaching new record numbers. "We (the Committee) were blamed for failing to contain the epidemic in Northern Greece. If you have three cities acting as super-spreaders it only takes a day or two for a whole region to come under siege," underlines Professor Gargalianos. The delay had reached the breaking point. On November 3, 2020, the government announced a lockdown in Northern Greece, and on November 7, 2020, a general lockdown was introduced across the country. The centralized mode of response that proved so effective in the spring returned "with a vengeance" in late fall. Swift, centrally made decisions and public health priorities over the economy prevented the catastrophe that Greece's neighbors had faced in the course of the pandemic.

The task of maintaining "normal" life without complete lockdown demanded a more centrifugal response—that is, with higher trust. Because Greece structurally lacks the institutions for higher administrative capacity—and little was done to build it because of lackluster preparedness during the summer and insurmountable problems in making deep structural changes during the crisis— it could not achieve the needed response flexibility. Maintaining a centralized response, because again, this is what the country could do, created problems mainly driven by low trust (in compliance), low administrative capacity (in treatment and monitoring), and low inclusiveness (in monitoring, communication, and enforcement regarding local measures). When things reached the breaking point in November, a couple of quick decisions managed to get the situation back on track (for the most part). But, when the aim shifted to also addressing economic problems, the centralized response was slow, rigid, overwhelmed, and ultimately ineffective. The government did not act in time, made costly mistakes, lost the public's trust, and finally brought the GNHS back to the brink. Only during and after the second nationwide lockdown did things begin to change, and a more appropriate, regionally nuanced—centrifugal in this book's terms—response has hesitantly begun to be implemented.

To mitigate the public health toll and economic cost that were by now decimating voter goodwill, the national government finally mustered the resources to create better regional monitoring capacity. An initiative by Professor of Chemistry Nikos Thomaidis to test waste water for COVID tracing—identifying viral loads at the regional and local levels three–four days before symptoms are expressed in the population—was enthusiastically adopted by the government, providing a costless solution to the lackluster regional monitoring capacity. With an effective tool for regional intervention in hand, the government introduced a color scheme map on January 30, 2021 to designate Regions of Concern, making them subject to significant mobility restrictions. There are three levels of measure stringency:

- Horizontal measures in the entire country such as mandatory use of masks in all public areas inside and outside, restrictions of movement within regions and prohibition of movement across regions, prohibition of private congregations, and others.
- Measures in specific areas under scrutiny, that is, areas where COVID-19 cases are on the rise, such as a curfew from 9 pm to 5 am, one person per 25 square meters in retail stores, and others.
- Measures in high-risk regions—that is, areas where the number of cases exceeds a threshold level—such as a curfew from 6 pm to 5 am, church service with up to nine individuals present, and click away service, that is, pre-ordering goods and picking up only by appointment (GSCP 2021).

More recent examples of centrifugal response tendencies involve the government's plan to achieve vaccination coverage of at least 70% of the population by actively engaging local primary care facilities (historically underutilized services for vaccination), pharmacists, and regional mobile units (interviews with General Secretary Marios Themistokleous and Pharmacist Evie Papathanasiou). As the past summer's experience demonstrates, decentralized response and inclusiveness of social actors require timely and meticulous planning.

It is evident that monitoring capacity, and to a lesser extent the message, is devolving to a more regional approach that is targeted and specific to the particular local context. Institutional capacity has been built but mostly *ad hoc* through bricolage and some layering (Mahoney and Thelen 2010). The message has also had to change from almost exclusively safeguarding public health to a more balanced health-economy calibration. While a centralized response formed the essence of the Greek response to the first wave of the pandemic, the crisis that ensued has prompted more centrifugal tendencies during the second wave.

Conclusion

In this chapter, we have argued that policy style interacted with political trust to shape the Greek response to the crisis created by the COVID-19 pandemic. We showed that when the pandemic hit the country in February 2020, Greece exhibited an administrative style coupled with low trust in government and other relevant public institutions. Focusing on measures taken during the response phase, that is, reaction to the pandemic, we have confirmed our hypothesis. However, we have also uncovered a certain dynamism driven by feedback from earlier response measures. While we anticipated a more-or-less "fixed," that is, centralized response, we also uncovered centrifugal tendencies during the second wave. Command and coordination remained firmly in central–national hands throughout the two waves. But the message changed as the trade-off between public health and economic performance became more visible, and politically pressing, while there were attempts at more regionally nuanced outcomes. To be sure, centralization is still the norm—after all, policy styles cast a long shadow onto the future—but trust and the direction of response appear to wax and wane, further buttressing our argument for an interactive effect of style and trust on national crisis response. Figure 5.3 summarizes the findings.

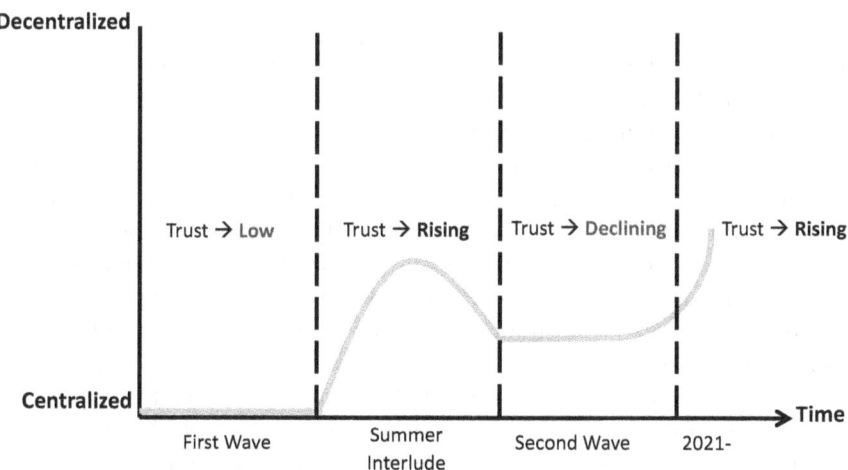

FIGURE 5.3 Greece's Response as a Function of Administrative Style and Fluctuating Political Trust.

As predicted, Greece initially adopted a highly centralized response. Low administrative capacity interacting with low trust prompted a coordinated and clear response. Action was swift largely driven by weakness. Ten years of austerity and a gargantuan migrant crisis left health care understaffed and severely underfunded. Precisely because the Greek leadership knew that capacity in the health care sector was too low to withstand high numbers of cases, it decided to focus on prevention. Weakness turned to strength. The success of the first wave hid structural capacity deficiencies that were highlighted during the interlude. Affecting trust levels (Cairney and Wellstead 2020), they shaped the centrifugal response during the second wave. A change in aims as well as lapses in monitoring, staffing, and more importantly, poor regional infrastructure created huge problems that could not be overcome. Institutional inertia created friction that generated political tension in addition to centrifugal tendencies.

While the argument appears to explain the actual response quite well, it leaves important questions unanswered. Why was the response so well coordinated and implemented in a country better known recently for chaos and paralysis? Is it because "Greece has shown a tendency to create alarm reflexes during crises, exhibiting much more effective management than in normal times" (Professor Kyriopoulos)? Or is the answer found in political leadership (Rhodes and 't Hart 2014)? Our analysis cannot but commend the current leadership for insight and forethought, at least relative to past governments' performance, as stressed by most of our interviewees. Whatever the answer, these are interesting questions that await further research.

Three theoretical implications should be emphasized. First, the argument has to incorporate the notion of feedback (e.g., Béland 2010; Mettler and Sorelle 2018). The Greek response was shaped by interactions of policy style and trust, but changes in trust (and to a lesser degree capacity) altered the effects over time. Positive and negative effects were felt within a very short period of time, leading to contradictory pathways: the need to change course but still experience the same results (Daugbjerg and Kay 2020). And all that without much capacity or trust to do it. The argument on policy styles needs to conceptualize feedback.

Second, confirming the literature's expectations (e.g., Lavazza and Farina 2020), experts played a significant but secondary role. The response was shaped by experts, but decisions were fundamentally political. Experts framed, communicated, and legitimated the message of essentially political decisions: whether, where, and when to implement a lockdown, compliance issues, and the like. The key command-and-coordination unit was Civil Protection, which is located within the Ministry of Citizen Protection, that is, the police. It further buttresses our argument regarding the essence of administrative style: crisis response focuses attention and resources on units with administrative, not substantive expertise.

Third, the findings partially support Mahoney and Thelen's (2010) institutional change argument but also extend it. Compliance is not just a variable affecting institutional change, and therefore policy capacity, but also crisis management. While they hypothesize gradual institutional change, we find more abrupt changes under crisis conditions. The changes observed in Greece fit Mahoney and Thelen's institutional outcomes: bricolage, that is, mostly *ad hoc* recombination and expansion of capacity, and layering, that is, the addition of capacity to address new purposes. Amending their argument, the changes were affected by policy context but not by political friction, that is, overcoming veto players. This makes sense as crisis conditions temporarily mute opposition. The mechanism linking compliance to change is trust. Policy styles cast long shadows into public policymaking under extraordinary conditions. Interacting with political trust, both variables affect compliance rates, which, in turn, open power-distributional opportunities to bring changes that affect policy style and trust. Such interactive loops over iterations in a short period of time go a long way toward explaining the Greek response to the crisis caused by the COVID-19 pandemic.

APPENDIX

Interviewee Name	Description	Date
Kyriakos Mitsotakis	Prime Minister of Greece (2019–)	August 5, 2020
Vassilis Kontozamanis	Deputy Minister of Health (2019–) President of the National Organization for Medicines (2008–2009)	August 5, 2020
Ioannis Kyriopoulos	Emeritus Professor of Health Economics— National School of Public Health, Athens Member of the 2009 Pandemic Response Committee as Dean of the National School of Public Health	July 27, 2020 and January 27, 2021
Effie Simou	Associate Professor of Mass Media and Health Communication, Department of Public Health Policy—University of West Attica Coordinator and author of the "National Action Plan for Public Health 2008–2012" (Ministry of Health)	August 3, 2020
Christos Zilidis	Professor of Social Medicine and Epidemiology, University of Thessaly Leading Member of the Design Committee for Greece's first Public Health Law (2003)	July 28, 2020 and December 15, 2020
Aris Sissouras	Emeritus Professor of Management, University of Patras Leading Member of the Committee for the Design of the Greek NHS (1981–1982)	July 26, 2020
Ioannis Tountas	Professor of Social and Preventive Medicine, National and Kapodistrian University of Athens Greece's National Representative for Health at the OECD (2009)	July 29, 2020 and December 18, 2020

Christos Lionis	Professor of General Practice and Primary Health Care, University of Crete Deputy General Director of the Regional Health and Welfare system of Crete (2001–2004)	August 1, 2020
Meletios- Athanasios Dimopoulos	Professor of Haematology/Oncology, National and Kapodistrian University of Athens Rector of the National and Kapodistrian University of Athens (2015–)	August 18, 2020 and January 28, 2021
Agis Tsouros	Emeritus Professor of Epidemiology and Public Health—University College London Former Director of the Division of Policy and Governance for Health and Wellbeing, WHO, Regional Office for Europe	August 7, 2020
Nikos Hardalias	Deputy Minister for Civil Protection and Crisis Management (2019–)	February 5, 2021
Panagiotis Gargalianos	Pathologist, Infectious Disease Specialist, Athens Medical Center President of the Hellenic Society of Infectious Disease Specialists and Member of the COVID-19 Specialists Committee	January 23, 2021
Marios Themistokleous	General Secretary for Primary Health Care, Ministry of Health (2019–)	February 3, 2021
John Yfantopoulos	Professor of Health Economics and Social Policy, National and Kapodistrian University of Athens President of the National Council for Public Health (2014–2016)	January 21, 2021
Andreas Xanthos	Minister of Health (2015–2019)	January 27, 2020
Evie Papathanasiou	Pharmacist General Coordinator of Eastern and Northern Attica Party Staff Registry (New Democracy)	January 21, 2021

References

Athanasiadis, Athanasios, Stella Kostopoulou, and Anastas Philalithis A. 2015. "Regional Decentralisation in the Greek Health Care System: Rhetoric and Reality." *Global Journal of Health Science* 7 (6): 55–67.

Athens News Agency-Macedonian Press Agency. 2020. "Health Minister Kikilias: Our Aim is 1,200 Beds in ICUs." May 3. https://www.amna.gr/en/article/454434/Health-Minister-Kikilias-Our-aim-is-1-200-beds-in-ICUs.

Ballas, Apostolos A., and Haridimos Tsoukas. 2004. "Measuring Nothing: The Case of the Greek National Health System." *Human Relations* 57 (6): 661–90.

Beland, Daniel. 2010. "Reconsidering Policy Feedback: How Policies Affect Politics." *Administration & Society* 42 (5): 568–90.

Bolton, Sharon C., Vasilis Charalampopoulos, and Lila Skountridaki. 2018. "Selective Consent and Dissent: Professional Response to Reform in the Post-crisis Greek NHS." *Work, Employment and Society* 33 (2): 262–79.

Burris, S. et al. 2012. "Moving from Intersection to Integration: Public Health Law Research and Public Health Systems and Services Research." *The Milibank Quarterly* 90 (2): 375–408.

Cairney, Paul and Adam Wellstead. 2020. "COVID-19: Effective Policymaking Depends on Trust in Experts, Politicians, and the Public." *Policy Design and Practice*, DOI: 10.1080/25741292.2020.1837466.

Daugbjerg, Carsten and Adrian Kay. 2020. "Policy Feedback and Pathways: When Change Leads to Endurance and Continuity to Change." *Policy Sciences* 53: 253–68.

Dianeosis. 2020. "Panhellenic Dianeosis Survey on Covid-19" (in Greek). https://www.dianeosis.org/research/covid-19/.

Ekathimerini.com. 2020. "Greeks against Second Lockdown, Survey Finds." June 15. https://www.ekathimerini.com/news/253643/greeks-against-second-lockdown-survey-finds/.

EODY. 2020. "Daily Epidemiological Monitoring Report of Infections from the New Coronavirous (Covid-19)" (in Greek). https://eody.gov.gr/wp-content/uploads/2020/10/covid-gr-daily-report-20201029.pdf.

Ervasti, Heikki, Antti Kouvo, and Takis Venetoklis. 2019. "Social and Institutional Trust in Times of Crisis: Greece, 2002–2011." *Social Indicators Research* 141: 1207–31.

General Secretariat of Civil Protection (GSCP). 2021. "Map of Health Safety and Protection Measures against Covid-19" (in Greek). January 29. https://www.civilprotection.gr/el/simantika-themata/hartis-metron-ygeionomikis-asfaleias-kai-prostasias-apo-ti-loimoxi-covid-19.

Hajer, Maarten. 2003. "Policy without Polity? Policy Analysis and the Institutional Void." *Policy Sciences* 36: 175–95.

Kalyvas, Stathis, George Pagoulatos, and Haridimos Tsoukas, eds. 2012. *From Stagnation to Forced Adjustment: Reforms in Greece 1974–2010*. New York: Columbia University Press.

Kanellopoulou, Afroditi et al. 2020. "Awareness, Knowledge and Trust in the Greek Authorities Towards COVID-19 Pandemic: Results from the Epirus Health Study Cohort." University of Ioannina. November 17. https://www.medrxiv.org/content/10.1101/2020.11.10.20229146v2.full.pdf.

Kyriopoulos, John and Tasos Telloglou. 2019. *The Adventure of Reform in Health and Care* (in Greek). Athens: Papazisis

Labropoulou, Elinda. 2020. "Greece Has Been a Coronavirus Success, But it Will Be Hit Economically Anyway." *Washington Post*. April 22. https://www.washingtonpost.com/world/europe/greece-coronavirus-success/2020/04/22/47e018ee-7f38-11ea-84c2-0792d8591911_story.html.

Ladi, Stella. 2014. "Austerity Politics and Administrative Reform: The Eurozone Crisis and Its Impact Upon Greek Public Administration." *Comparative European Politics* 12 (2): 184–208.

Lampropoulou, Manto and Giorgio Oikonomou. 2018. "Theoretical Models of Public Administration and Patterns of State Reform in Greece." *International Review of Administrative Sciences* 84 (1): 101–21.

Lavazza, Andrea and Mirko Farina. 2020. "The Role of Experts in the Covid-19 Pandemic and the Limits of Their Epistemic Authority in Democracy." *Frontiers in Public Health* 8: 356.

Lyrintzis, Christos. 1984. "Political parties in Post-Junta Greece: A Case of 'Bureaucrartic Clientelism'?" *West European Politics* 7 (2): 99–118.

Mahoney, James and Kathleen Thelen, eds. 2010. *Explaining Institutional Change: Ambiguity, Agency, and Power.* Cambridge: Cambridge University Press.

Makrydemetres, Anthony. 1999. *Administration and Society* (in Greek). Athens: Themelio.

Mettler, Suzanne and Mallory Sorelle. 2018. "Policy Feedback Theory." In *Theories of the Policy Process*, 4th edition, eds. Christopher M. Weible and Paul A. Sabatier, 103–34. New York and London: Routledge.

Norris, Pippa. 2011. *Democratic Deficit: Critical Citizens Revisited.* Cambridge: Cambridge University Press.

OECD. 2019. *Government at a Glance: Greece.* At http://www.oecd.org/gov/gov-at-a-glance-2019-greece.pdf. Accessed on February 21, 2021.

Organization for Economic Cooperation and Development (OECD). 2020. *Intensive Care Beds Capacity.* At https://www.oecd.org/coronavirus/en/data-insights/intensive-care-beds-capacity. Accessed on May 5, 2021.

Pagoulatos, George. 2003. *Greece's New Political Economy.* London: Palgrave.

Petridou, Evangelia et al. 1999. "Public Health Policies and Priorities in Greece." In *Public Health Policies in the Europe Union*, eds. Walter Holland, Elias Mossialos, Paul Belcher and Bernarnd Merkel, 127–48. London: Routledge.

Petridou, Evangelia and Nikolaos Zahariadis. 2021. "Staying at Home or Going Out? Leadership Response to the COVID-19 Crisis in Greece and Sweden." *Journal of Contingencies and Crisis Management*, DOI: 10.1111/1468–5973.12344.

Psaropoulos, John. 2020. "How Greece Flattened the Coronavirus Curve." *Al Jazeera.* April 7. https://www.aljazeera.com/news/2020/04/greece-flattened-coronavirus-curve-200407191043404.html.

Rhodes, R. A. W. and Paul 't Hart. 2014. *The Oxford Handbook on Political Leadership.* Oxford Handbooks Online. https://www.oxfordhandbooks.com/view/10.1093/oxfordhb/9780199653881.001.0001/oxfordhb-9780199653881.

Sissouras, Aris. 2012. *The Suspended Step of the Greek NHS* (in Greek). Athens: Kastaniotis.

Skai Online Newsroom. 2020. "Patrols in the Islands: 10,000 Euro Fines in Nightclubs in Syros." August 5. https://www.skai.gr/news/greece/elegxoi-se-nisia-prostimo-10000-eyro-se-mpar-sti-syro.

Sotiropoulos, Dimitri A. 2004. "Southern European Public Bureaucracies in Comparative Persepctive." *West European Politics* 27 (3): 405–22.

Sotiropoulos, Dimitri A. 1996. *Populism and Bureaucracy.* Notre Dame, IN: University of Notre Dame Press.

Spanou, Calliope. 2008. "State Reform in Greece: Responding to Old and New Challenges." *International Journal of Public Sector Management* 21 (2): 150–73.

Spanou, Calliope. 1996. "Penelope's Suitors: Administrative Modernization and Party Competition in Greece." *West European Politics* 19 (1): 97–124.

Spanou, Calliope and Dimitri A. Sotiropoulos. 2011. "The Odyssey of Administrative Reforms in Greece, 1981–2009: A Tale of Two Reform Paths." *Public Administration* 89 (3): 723–37.

Torcal, Mariano. 2017. "Political Trust in Western and Southern Europe." In *Handbook on Political Trust*, eds. Sonja Zmerli & Tom W. G. van der Meer, 418–39. Cheltenham: Edward Elgar.

Tugwell, Paul and Sotiris Nikas. 2020. "Greece's Reliance on Tourism is a Weakness in the Corona Age." Bloomberg.com. March 17. https://www.bloomberg.com/news/articles/2020-03-17/greece-s-reliance-on-tourism-is-a-weakness-in-the-age-of-corona.

World Health Organization (WHO). 2021. "Contact Tracing in the Context of Covid-19." February 1. https://www.who.int/publications/i/item/contact-tracing-in-the-context-of-covid-19.

Zahariadis, Nikolaos. 2016. "Delphic Oracles: Ambiguity, Institutions, and Multiple Streams." *Policy Sciences* 49 (1): 3–12.

Zahariadis, Nikolaos. 2013. "National Fiscal Profligacy and European Institutional Adolescence: The Greek Trigger to Europe's Sovereign Debt Crisis." *Government & Opposition* 48 (1): 33–54.

6

KENYA'S RESPONSE TO COVID-19

Lockdown and Stringent Enforcement

Shadrack W. Nasong'o

Reports of the outbreak of the Coronavirus in Wuhan, Hubei Province of China, hit the international media headlines in January 2020. Despite the reported deadly nature of the novel Coronavirus, the Kenyan government seems to have not taken the outbreak seriously enough at the beginning. Whereas the country's national airline, Kenya Airways, ceased its flights to China for fear of importing the virus, the government continued to allow flights from China to land in Nairobi, including one in late February 2020 carrying 236 passengers from China. The arriving passengers were simply advised to "self-quarantine" (Achuka & Kabale 2020). Kenya recorded its first case of the Coronavirus on March 12, 2020, presumably brought in from the US as the patient had arrived from the US via London seven days earlier (Aluga 2020). Two days later, two more cases were confirmed by the National Influenza Centre Laboratory at the National Public Health Laboratories. The government was thus forced to craft a response strategy to mitigate the deleterious implications of the spread of the deadly Coronavirus.

This chapter examines the nature of Kenya's response to the COVID-19 pandemic. It utilizes data collected from official policy pronouncements by Kenya's president; official pandemic briefings by the president and his minister of health; reports of the National Coordination Committee on the Response to the Coronavirus Pandemic (NCCRCP) as well as the response to the pandemic mitigation measures by Kenyans as reported by the country's mass media. The chapter seeks to demonstrate that Kenya's response to the pandemic, centered on lockdown and stringent enforcement, was a function of the centralized and personalistic nature of the country's policy style coupled with exclusivist policymaking processes and high levels of citizen distrust of the country's public institutions and its political leaders. The chapter concludes that the nature of the pandemic response, particularly the manner in which the resources mobilized

DOI: 10.4324/9781003137399-8

for mitigating the pandemic were (mis)used, only helped to heighten the level of government mistrust on the part of the ordinary citizens. In other words, the case of Kenya illustrates with particular clarity the argument that, whereas the response to the pandemic was aimed at saving lives, it simultaneously served the purpose of projecting power and enhancing the benefits of those who preside over the status quo.

Kenya as an Administrative State: Centralization, Exclusion, and Mistrust

Kenya's statehood is rooted in its British colonial legacy. The state was established through violence and maintained by the same through an elaborate administrative apparatus from the center down to the localities (Oyugi 1994). The administrative apparatus established under colonialism in the form of the provincial administration remained in place post-independence. The essential role of the provincial administration is one of penetration and control (Oyugi 1994). The country has undergone a significant process of democratization since the 1990s and is now in its second republic with the promulgation of a new liberal democratic constitution in August 2010. One major administrative novelty of the new constitutional dispensation is the devolution of power on local issues to 47 county governments, first elected in 2013. Nevertheless, the centrally determined administrative attributes of the state remain in place, and the country remains a unitary state. The provincial administration was simply transformed into regional administration co-existing with county governments but answerable to the central government. The legislature and the judiciary, though afforded autonomy by the current constitution, remain dominated by the presidency, which enjoys overwhelming executive power.

Against the foregoing, policymaking in Kenya has remained an overly centralized and personalistic affair dominated by the presidency and a few bureaucratic agencies closely tied to the executive branch. For instance, Jomo Kenyatta, the founding president, ruled much like a monarch between the time of independence in 1963 and 1978 when he passed on. His presidency, according to Anyang' Nyong'o (1989), was marked by the disintegration of the nationalist coalitions and the emergence of "presidential authoritarianism." Kenyatta's successor, Daniel arap Moi (1978–2002) presided over an even more centralized state apparatus in a dispensation that some scholars have characterized as a dictatorship (Adar & Munyae 2001; Ajulu 2021; Kariuki 1996). This was particularly so in the period 1982–1992, which can be said to have been the high noon of authoritarianism in Kenya wherein policy was largely dictated by the president.

The third president of Kenya, Mwai Kibaki (2003–2013) came to power in a context of democratization and seems to have been much less inclined to authoritarian tendencies. His policymaking style comes closest to what Guy Peters (2015) describes as the New Public Management, which emphasizes the autonomy of public sector organizations with the assumption that "managers in the public sector could, if permitted the autonomy and given the resources, do a better job of providing services than could their political leadership" (Guy 2015, 222–223). Kibaki, a London School of Economics-trained economist, attempted to staff state bureaucracies with competent managers and granted them autonomy to manage their agencies and make policy with minimal political interference from the presidency. Furthermore, Kibaki's government made efforts to consult relevant stakeholders and social actors whenever major policies were being considered as a way of involving them in shaping policies that had a direct effect on them. Interestingly, critics, so used to a historically robust presidency that dominated policymaking, viewed Kibaki's leadership as somewhat weak, describing it as "hands off," "aloof," or "absentee leadership" (Jopson & Wallis 2007). Nevertheless, Kibaki's leadership style led to economic revival and sustained economic growth throughout his decade in power.

Instead of building on the legacy of his predecessor in terms of leadership style, the current president of Kenya, Uhuru Kenyatta (2013–present), has been keen on replicating the authoritarian style of the Moi days in spite of the remarkable achievements of the process of democratization and institutional reform in the country. Uhuru Kenyatta and his deputy, William Ruto, assumed power in 2013 under the new constitution that provided for a presidential candidate and a running mate as the deputy president-to-be. In functional terms, the deputy president played a more active role in appointment powers post-2013 elections than previous vice presidents. It turns out, however, that the alliance between the president and the deputy president has been simply another coalition for managing the already entrenched spoils system at the national level. Strategic cabinet positions were shared, for the most part, among members of two ethnic groups, the president's Kikuyu, and the deputy president's Kalenjin. According to Eric Otenyo (forthcoming), each of the dominant players maintains their own gatekeepers and negotiates national issues in a give-and-take manner. Policymaking is centered in the hands of the president and his deputy, though the two have recently fallen out owing to the politics of succession in the run-up to 2022 when the president's second and final term comes to an end. In this context, bureaucratic and political corruption has been perpetrated to levels never seen before. Public institutions are largely treated as havens for self-aggrandizement rather than arenas of policymaking and implementation for the benefit of the country and its citizens.

Against the foregoing, policymaking in Kenya tends to be exclusivist and personalistic rather than inclusive and consultative. It is dominated by the top political actors in the executive branch of government with very little if any consultation with sectors within civil society. Even in a context in which parliament has been legally afforded autonomy under the 2010 constitution, legislation is still influenced by the executive to a great extent. On account of the fact that Kenyan legislators are among the best paid in the world (their individual annual pay is 76 times the country's GDP per capita), they tend to identify more with the political system and its interests than with their constituents and their representational needs (*Business Day*, July 23, 2013). The legislators are thus always inclined to serve the interests of the president and 'the system' more generally than those of their own constituents and the citizens at large. Sometimes, they are cajoled to do so by their party leaders; at other times, they are financially induced depending on the political premium of the stakes involved (Akech 2011; Nyamori 2018).

The level of mistrust of government, political leaders, and public institutions on the part of Kenyans is very high on account of the foregoing, especially the scourge of corruption. As pointed out above, corruption in Kenya has reached epidemic proportions. In the 1960s and 1970s, bureaucratic corruption manifested itself in bureaucrats' demands for kickbacks valued at around 10% of the total cost of a public tender, development project, or whatever goods or services were under procurement. By the 1980s and 1990s, the rates had escalated to around 40%. In the current dispensation in Kenya, the rates have maxed out to 100%! This is the situation where, for instance, a development project is conjured up, it is costed, awarded, and paid for, but nothing is done (Nasong'o 2020a). The exemplification of this is the Kimwarer and Arror Dams project scandal in which billions were paid out for nothing (Kahura 2019). Alternatively, public funds are simply withdrawn from institutional bank accounts and directly pocketed by public officers in charge of such institutions. This is a most brazen form of corruption that was amplified by the investigative report on the financial shenanigans at Maasai Mara University (Kigotho 2020). The healthcare system in Kenya suffers from this same scourge of corruption and the concomitant mistrust of the general population. The frequent strikes by doctors, nurses, and other healthcare workers in the country are a function of this reality.

The Healthcare System in Kenya

In an institutional arrangement that mirrors the centralized administrative nature of the Kenyan state, the country's healthcare system is hierarchically structured into six levels as shown in Table 6.1. Kenya's public healthcare system is presently undergoing transformation, resulting from the constitutionally mandated devolution of health services delivery to county governments. The country is in the process of implementing relatively new and untested mechanisms ranging from policy and regulatory interventions to health care financing models (WHO 207: 8).

TABLE 6.1 Hierarchy of Kenya's Health Institutions

Level	Type of Institution
Level 1	Community services
Level 2	Dispensaries and clinics
Level 3	Health centers and maternity and nursing homes
Level 4	Sub-County hospitals and medium-sized private hospitals
Level 5	County referral hospitals and large private hospitals
Level 6	National referral hospitals and large private teaching hospitals

Source: Compiled from WHO (2017).

Public healthcare facilities are governed by health facility committees, which include the facility in-charge and community representatives. For private healthcare facilities, government oversight is provided by the Ministry of Health (MoH) through regulation, which is implemented through eight regulatory agencies (WHO 2017, 4). Public healthcare services are primarily provided at levels 1–3. The higher up the level you go, the higher the quality and sophistication of the healthcare services and thus the more expensive and less accessible to the general public. To enhance accessibility to healthcare by Kenyans, the government, through an Act of Parliament, set up the National Hospital Insurance Fund (NHIF) in 1966 as a department under the MoH. The NHIF's core mandate is to provide medical insurance cover to all its members and their dependents. Over the years, the original Act of Parliament that set up the NHIF has been reviewed to accommodate the changing healthcare needs of the Kenyan population, employment, and restructuring in the health sector. In 1998, a new NHIF Act No. 9 transformed the NHIF from a department in the MoH to an autonomous State Corporation. This transformation was aimed at improving effectiveness and efficiency.

As a State Corporation, the NHIF's mission is to contribute toward universal health coverage in the provision of affordable, accessible, sustainable, and quality health insurance through strategic resource pooling and healthcare purchasing in collaboration with stakeholders. NHIF membership is mandatory for those in the formal employment sector whose dues are directly deducted from their payroll and transmitted to the NHIF by their employers. For those in the informal sector and retirees, membership is open and voluntary. As of 2021, the NHIF has over 25 million members including 7.3 million principal contributors. Like other state institutions, the management of the NHIF is centralized at NHIF House in Nairobi, although it has about 95 branches and satellite offices across the country. Awash with liquidity derived from mandatory statutory deductions from all workers in the formal sector, NHIF has been an arena of mega corruption where billions have been stolen through inflated tenders, payment to phantom hospitals, pay-outs to hospitals that do not qualify to receive NHIF funds, and inflation of insurance claims among other avenues (Macharia 2012; Ombati & Obala 2019; Wasuna 2018).

Despite scandal after scandal at NHIF, efforts at reforming the Fund and the healthcare system in general are reserved for the same top bureaucrats and political operatives at the national center to the exclusion of other stakeholders. Even the reforms alluded to at the beginning of this section related to implementing relatively new and untested mechanisms ranging from policy and regulatory interventions to healthcare financing models are decided exclusively by the same policy circles that oversee the perpetration of theft and pilfering of public resources. It thus is no wonder that public trust in the healthcare system, its institutions, and its capacity to deliver is very low.

Overall, at the outbreak of the COVID-19 pandemic in early 2020, Kenya's healthcare system, plagued by corruption, exclusivist centralized management, and low public trust, was ill-equipped to handle the crisis. With a population of 52 million, the country had a total capacity of 64,181 hospital beds across all sectors (public, faith based/NGO, private for profit). Of these beds, 37,216 (58%) were in hospitals that have oxygen supply. Even worse, the country had only 537 ICU beds and a total of 256 ventilators. Therefore, 281 (52%) of existing ICU beds did not have the accompanying equipment to provide care for COVID-19 critically ill patients (Barasa et al. 2020). This dire situation is compounded by geographical disparities in the distribution of ICU units across the country. Barasa et al. (2020) note that only 22 (47%) of the country's 47 counties have at least one ICU unit. In comparative terms, Kenya's critical care capacity is below the continental average. For instance, the 537 ICU beds translate to one ICU bed for every 100,000 Kenyans compared to the continental average of three ICU beds for every 100,000 persons. Similarly, whereas Kenya's capacity of roughly 0.5 ventilators per 100,000 is higher than the East African regional average of 0.23 ventilators per 100,000, it is lower than the continental average of 0.97 ventilators per 100,000. Even the sheer hospital bed capacity of 123 beds for every 100,000 Kenyans (64,181 for 52 million) is lower than the continental average of 135 beds per 100,000 (Craig et al. 2020).

Kenya's Response to COVID-19

Kenya recorded the first case of Coronavirus on March 12, 2020, and on March 14, two more cases were recorded. Following these developments, President Uhuru Kenyatta took a number of measures in response. In his first briefing on the pandemic on March 15, 2020, the president suspended travel by air into Kenya from any country that had recorded COVID-19 cases. Kenyan citizens and foreigners with valid residence permit were allowed to travel to Kenya and self-quarantine for 14 days. Learning was suspended in all educational institutions, which were ordered closed. With an emphasis on minimizing social gatherings, employers were encouraged to allow their employees to work from home in order to reduce congestion in public transport. Businesses were encouraged to use cashless transactions in order to reduce contact and thereby minimize the possibilities of infection (GoK March 15, 2020).

One of the most stringent measures taken was imposition of a daily curfew countrywide from 7:00 PM to 5:00 AM with the exemption of essential service providers, especially medical professionals. By the first week of April 2020, it was noted that Nairobi and the Coast Counties of Kilifi and Mombasa were COVID-19 hotspots in the country. Consequently, in his third briefing on the pandemic on April 6, the president ordered a 21-day lockdown of Nairobi including cessation of movement by road, rail, and air in and out of Nairobi. The Coast Counties of Mombasa, Kilifi, and Kwale were put under partial lockdown, and security services were directed to upgrade their alert and response measures in border areas. The 21-day dusk-to-dawn curfew and Nairobi lockdown were extended several times as the Coronavirus cases continued to grow. By May 16, 2020, Kenya had a record of

830 cases and 50 deaths. Of these cases, 43 were cross-border transmissions. Based on the rise in imported cases, the president, in his 6th briefing on the pandemic, directed cessation of movement in and out of Kenya through the Kenya–Tanzania and Kenya–Somalia borders except for cargo vehicles, whose drivers were required to undergo mandatory COVID-19 testing before entering Kenya.

The government adopted further containment measures at the social and health levels. These include social distancing; heightened restriction on gatherings in most non-essential social spaces; encouragement of teleworking where possible; establishment of isolation facilities; limitations on public transportation passenger capacity; and mandatory mask-wearing in public spaces. These policy decisions were reported as a collaborative activity among various stake holders and state agencies. However, these efforts to contain the spread of Coronavirus were led by the National Coordination Committee on the Response to the Coronavirus Pandemic (NCCRCP. The committee, chaired by the Cabinet Secretary for the Ministry of Interior and Coordination of National Government, was tasked with coordinating actions undertaken by various state agencies. Decision-making on all pandemic issues was concentrated in the hands of the top political leaders and a few of their political appointees.

The task of communication fell on President Uhuru Kenyatta and his Cabinet Secretary for Health, Mutahi Kagwe. Between March and end of July 2020, the president made a total of ten briefings to the country. These focused on the impact of the pandemic and what the government was doing to combat the same. It is at these briefings that the president communicated his policy directives and extended curfews and lockdowns as well as announced relief measures to mitigate the pandemic's deleterious effects on the economy and on livelihoods. For his part, the Cabinet Secretary for Health, who held more frequent press briefings than the president, focused his communication on updating the public on the extent of infections in the country, emphasizing what the public needed to do to stem the tide of infection, and what his ministry was doing in conjunction with County governments to enhance preparedness for COVID-19.

The messaging on the pandemic was thus dominated by politicians to the exclusion of health experts who were the source of the statistics and the pandemic mitigation recommendations that political leaders communicated to the public. In fact, power games were on display with the whole pandemic communication issue. In late April 2020, the Cabinet Secretary for Health, Mutahi Kagwe, was delayed in his scheduled press briefing on account of late delivery of COVID-19 sample testing results from the Kenya Medical Research Institute (KEMRI), an autonomous State Corporation under the Cabinet Secretary's docket. Without bothering to establish the cause of the diagnostic delay, Kagwe instructed KEMRI's Director-General, Yeri Kombe, to demote the Director of KEMRI's Center for Virus Research, Dr. Joel Lutomiah with immediate effect. Dr. Lutomiah, with decades of experience in entomology, parasitology, pandemic influenza, and arbovirology, was thus demoted for "failing in his duty to honor a matter that is of very serious national importance" (Shimanyula 2020).

In a nutshell, in response to the first confirmed cases of Coronavirus in Kenya in March 2020, the government closed all learning institutions, imposed a curfew, banned public gatherings, required burial of COVID-19 victims within 48 hours of death with only five relatives in attendance, closed houses of worship, and at various times, imposed a lockdown and restricted movement in and out of the most-affected regions. These staggered measures clearly slowed the spread of the virus, while threading the difficult balance between protecting lives and protecting livelihoods. By the end of 2020, the country had recorded a total of 96,802 cases of Coronavirus and 1,685 deaths according to MoH statistics (Obulutsa 2021).

Stringent Enforcement of Mitigation Measures

The manner in which the pandemic containment measures were enforced demonstrated the centralized command-and-control orientation of Kenya's policy style. The police were deployed to enforce the dusk-to-dawn curfew and mask-wearing throughout the country. Those found outside their homes during the curfew hours—including those in transit from their workplaces—were brutally assaulted by the police, and some actually lost their lives. For instance, following the March 25 announcement of the dusk-to-dawn curfew, police across Kenya used excessive force, including beating and tear gassing crowds on their way home in an effort to enforce the curfew. On March 31, a 13-year-old boy was shot and killed on his balcony in Nairobi as police moved through the neighborhood, enforcing the Coronavirus curfew. In Mombasa, media reported that police descended on people who were queuing to board the ferry after work and mercilessly beat them for "violating the curfew hours" (HRW 2020; Wasike 2020a).

Police brutality sparked protests and led to demonstrations, particularly in Nairobi where marchers hit the streets on June 8 to demonstrate against police brutality, with marchers lamenting that the "police have killed us more than Corona" (*The Guardian* 2020; BBC 2020). Indeed, as Andrew Wasike (2020b) reports, as of April 16, 2020, 12 Kenyans were confirmed to have been killed by the police in their overzealous attempt to enforce the dusk-to-dawn curfew with many more bruised and badly injured from police beatings. At the same time, the death toll from COVID-19 stood at only 11. By June 2020, the number of casualties from police brutality in the enforcement of pandemic mitigation measures had increased to more than 20 (Wasike 2020a).

Furthermore, the police introduced instant 'fines' for those found in public spaces without wearing masks. The fact that courts of law were suspended in the wake of the pandemic afforded the police a chance to extort Kenyans without fear of being challenged in court. Accordingly, as one civil society activist put it, "the people fear the police more than Covid-19, people are putting on masks not because they fear Covid-19, they fear that they would be arrested and extorted" (Wasike 2020b). In other words, mask-wearing became more of a protection against police brutality and extortion rather than a health measure against the Coronavirus.

The protests and pushback against police brutality yielded some positive outcomes. First, in early June, the Independent Policing Oversight Authority (IPOA)—the agency tasked with holding the police accountable—reported that it had received 87 complaints against the police and documented 21 killings by the police. IPOA proceeded to arraign six police officers on charges of murder and assault. Second, the dusk-to-dawn curfew hours were revised from 7:00 PM to 5:00 AM to 10:00 PM to 4:00 AM (Obulutsa 2021; Wasike 2020a).

Overall, measures put in place by government to contain COVID-19 were met with criticism by Kenyans including street demonstrations as mentioned above because of the stringency of their enforcement and their negative impact on the livelihoods of a majority of Kenyans who depend on face-to-face interactions to earn their living. Some were of the opinion that some measures such as the curfew would make them poorer, and some expressed fear of dying of hunger rather than from COVID-19. The curfew and its stringent enforcement may have helped slow the spread of the virus but at a major cost on livelihoods. For millions, who live in urban slums or in rural poverty, social distancing is not an option. Their livelihoods depend on daily face-to-face interactions. Other measures such as e-learning were met with criticism owing to the fact that for the majority of Kenyans owning a tablet/laptop is a luxury which most students can't afford.

Economic Relief and Recovery Measures

One of the major impacts of the stringently enforced lockdown measures in response to the COVID-19 pandemic was loss of employment and livelihoods for a great proportion of Kenyans. Consequently, the government implemented a number of measures aimed at protecting livelihoods and sources of income and cushioning businesses. At his second briefing on the COVID-19 pandemic on March 27, 2020, President Uhuru Kenyatta directed the National Treasury to offer Kenyans immediate relief and increase their disposable income by effecting 100% tax relief to Kenyans earning Kshs. 24,000 (USD 240) per month and below and by reducing personal and corporation income tax (popularly known as PAYE—pay as you earn) from 30% to 25% for those earning Kshs. 25,000 (USD 250) per month and above. Similarly, value-added tax (VAT) was reduced from 16% to 14%, and the turnover tax rate was reduced from 3% to 1% for all Micro, Small, and Medium Enterprises (MSMEs). Additionally, Kshs. 1 billion (USD 10 million) was released from the Universal Health Coverage Kitty for recruitment of additional health workers. The Central Bank was directed to lower bank interest rates from 8.25% to 7.25% and cash reserve ratio from 5.25% to 4.25% (*Daily Nation* March 27, 2020).

In addition to the above measures, on April 16, 2020, the president directed the MoH to develop a package to cushion front-line health workers and extended to the country's 47 county governments a three-month tax waiver from the Kenya Medical Supplies Agency (KEMSA) for the purchase of masks and personal protective equipment (PPEs). The national government undertook to support county governments with Kshs. 5 billion (USD 5 million) to cushion the vulnerable and protect health workers and rolled out a weekly COVID-19 support stipend for the vulnerable in Nairobi County. A major presidential announcement was the release of Kshs. 8.5 billion (USD 8.5 million) for the elderly and vulnerable across the country (GoK, April 16, 2020). Furthermore, on May 1, the National Treasury created a fund of close to Sh100 billion to cushion distressed MSMEs against the Coronavirus effects. This was designed to ensure that loan rates remain affordable to MSMEs.

Generally, these economic relief and recovery measures were well received. Nevertheless, as Matthew Tyce (2020) notes, the measures were received with some reservations. One major concern was that the relief measures would benefit only the small proportion of Kenya's formally employed population that pays taxes and do little for the vast informal and agricultural sectors that Kenyan policymakers and others across Africa have long ignored (Tyce 2020). Khadiagala (2020) adds that "the pandemic and its economic fallout have disproportionately affected disadvantaged groups within Kenyan society, heightening the class, ethnic, and regional inequalities that have driven polarization [in the country]." Accordingly, Kenyans were not so positive about their government's COVID-19 mitigation efforts. A poll conducted by GeoPoll in Benin, Cote d'Ivoire, Democratic Republic of Congo, Ghana, Kenya, Mozambique, Nigeria, Rwanda, South Africa, Tanzania, Uganda, and Zambia established that of the 12 countries, Kenyans were the least impressed by their government's efforts to stop the spread of Coronavirus, rating the effort an average 2.9 out of 5. Kenya was followed by Nigeria (3.0) and Zambia (3.0). The most positive were Rwandans who rated their government's effort an average 4.4 out of 5 followed by Uganda at 4.0 and Ghana at 3.8 (Tyce 2020).

Indeed, there is no evidence that the funds earmarked for the elderly and other vulnerable groups in Kenya were ever disbursed to them. Designation of funds for helping the vulnerable seems to have been designed as a conduit for the well-connected to siphon public resources as detailed in the section below. Many Kenyans who lost their sources of income due to COVID-19 became highly frustrated by the government misuse of the aid given for mitigating the COVID-19 pandemic. Most claimed not to have received any sort of help from the government. A quick, unscientific survey conducted on people living in Kawangware, a large informal settlement in Nairobi, established that none of the people, who had either been laid off or had to close down their small businesses, had ever received any payment from the government fund designated for this purpose (Warah 2020).

In his frequent addresses to the country on the pandemic, President Kenyatta exhorted Kenyans to channel their innovative spirit toward combating the Coronavirus. Kenyans seem to have responded positively with some innovative measures that contributed immensely to mitigating the spread of the Coronavirus. The country's tech community developed a software to assist laboratory testing and a digital dashboard to monitor supplies. This development enhanced existing HIV testing infrastructure capacity to a point where it could test upward of 37,000 Coronavirus samples in 12 hours. Additionally, some county governments such as Kitui and Mombasa worked with garment manufacturers to re-orient production toward PPE equipment like face masks. Toward this end, the national government provided support by suspending restrictions on firms within Export Processing Zones, where most manufacturers are located from selling their products in the domestic market (Tyce 2020).

Power Politics, Opportunism, and COVID-19 Millionaires

The Kenya government's response to the COVID-19 pandemic was characterized by power politics, opportunism, corruption, and a personalistic policy style. COVID-19 corruption led to what Kenyans on social media have dubbed 'COVID-19 millionaires.' With the incumbent president's second and final term coming to an end in 2022, succession politics had heated up by the time COVID-19 hit. Accordingly, the country's top political leaders did not direct all of their energies toward the pandemic, prompting growing accusations of ineffective leadership. Focused on the 2022 succession politics, the president was not fully focused on protecting lives and livelihoods. Instead of placing toxic politics into suspension, to ensure that all the state's energies and resources were directed into the war against the virus, the president "joined other leaders around the world in using the crisis to bolster his position and marginalize opponents" (Tyce 2020; Khadiagala 2020). Tyce (2020) notes that President Kenyatta's allies were given 'presidential blessings' to flout travel restrictions and attend political meetings on succession issues and how to undermine perceived opponents (*The Standard*, Nairobi: April 19, 2020).

Political opportunism was manifested in the parliamentary enactment of the tax relief measures mentioned above. As Tyce (2020) writes, by the time Kenya's draft Tax Laws (Amendment) Bill (to help cushion Kenyans) was tabled in parliament, it had become "a 97-page tome of deletion after deletion and insert after insert," leading to accusations of measures being introduced by 'stealth.' Tyce cites Professor Attiya Waris, a fiscal policy expert at the University of Nairobi, who identified various proposed measures that seemed to represent "opportunistic funding of lobby groups … and the loudest voices in government and those connected to them." These criticisms and pushbacks, inside and outside of parliament, led to some measures being dropped, notably increased taxes on certain staple food items. Nevertheless, others remained including tax exemptions on helicopters that politicians are so fond of using (Tyce 2020; Kabaara 2020). In other words, politicians took advantage of the pandemic to selfishly help themselves even as they purported to be protecting the public's lives and livelihoods. Indeed, there is no evidence that monies set aside for the elderly across the country and for the vulnerable in Nairobi were ever dispersed to the intended recipients.

Perhaps, the ugliest part of the whole pandemic saga was the manner in which political leaders and their close associates misappropriated funds meant to fight the pandemic. Two major scandals help illustrate this—one at the MoH and one at the KEMSA. In May 2020, Kenya's Catholic Bishops raised concerns over the alleged misappropriation of the over Kshs. 1.3 billion (US$10.3 million) COVID-19 Emergency Fund. A leaked memo on the breakdown of Kshs. 1.3 billion spent in the first month of the fight against COVID-19 showed that Kshs. 42 million (USD 420,000) had been spent on leasing 15 ambulances (at the cost Kshs. 2.8 million (US$28,000) per ambulance), Kshs. 4 million (USD 40,000) for tea and snacks, and Kshs. 2 million (USD 20,000) on airtime! The expenditure was part of the Kshs. 1 billion (USD 10 million) donated by the World Bank for an emergency response that was to cater for the procurement of PPE, medicines, and the setting up of isolation facilities. Naturally, these revelations attracted angry reactions from a section of Kenyans who, through online forums, condemned the opportunism of implicated government officials. In response during his Labor Day address on May 1, 2020, President Uhuru Kenyatta dismissed the claims of misappropriation of COVID-19 emergency kitty, assuring Kenyans that the money will be audited "to the last cent" (Maina 2020; Nasong'o 2020c). Such an audit was never done, and in fact, three months after the president's speech, on August 16, NTV, one of the top TV stations in the country, did an expose on corruption in COVID-19-related matters that indicated about Kshs. 43 billion (USD 430 million) COVID-19 funds were missing (Maina 2020).

The second scandal involved the KEMSA, the state agency tasked with supplying hospitals and health institutions with medical equipment. In the face of funds pouring into the country in response to the Coronavirus pandemic, companies that had previously done business with KEMSA were abandoned, and newly formed, politically connected ones were contracted to make COVID-19-related supplies including PPEs and infections prevention consumables (IPCs). These companies, all incorporated in the aftermath of the pandemic and all with links to top political leaders and their associates, were given no-bid tenders by KEMSA and paid in millions and billions of Kenya Shillings to supply PPEs and IPCs at inflated prices. Kilig Ltd. is an illustrative example from more than a dozen of such companies. Kilig Ltd., a briefcase company with no capacity to supply anything, was awarded a tender and paid Kshs. 4 billion (USD 40 million) to supply PPEs and IPCs to KEMSA. Kilig owners simply pocketed Kshs. 1 billion (USD 10 million) and used Kshs. 3 billion (USD 30 million) to subcontract the tender to Entec Technology Co. Ltd. Through these shenanigans, USD 400 million of the COVID funds is said to have been pilfered from KEMSA by August 2020 (Maina 2020; Mboga 2020; Nasong'o 2020c). Meanwhile, as this was going on, scores of healthcare providers were dying on account of lack of PPEs and IPCs in public health institutions.

Conclusion

By the end of the first week of July 2020, a consensus emerged among Kenya's health experts that the country had reached a reasonable level for re-opening. Accordingly, President Uhuru Kenyatta issued directives that lifted the cessation of movement in and out of the counties of Nairobi, Mombasa, and Wajir; allowed domestic and international air travel to resume on July 15 and August 1, respectively; allowed the phased opening of houses of worship with restrictions on maximum numbers and ages 13–58; and required the Ministry of Transport to ensure public transport operators complied with MoH guidelines on COVID-19 mitigation. In addition, students in grades 4, 8, and 12 were allowed to resume school in October 2020. This was for the purpose of facilitating them to take examinations required for them to transition to middle school, high school, and university, respectively. Schools across the country did not resume in full until the first week of January 2021, nine months since they were closed down in March 2020. Nevertheless, the 10:00 PM to 4:00 AM curfew remained in place across the country well into 2021.

The import of this chapter is confirmation of the hypothesis about policy style impacting response to crisis situations as much as it does impact routine policymaking in non-crisis situations. The chapter has demonstrated that Kenya's response to the COVID-19 pandemic was highly centralized, personalistic, and exclusive, mirroring the policy style of the country's leadership even in non-emergency situations. The stringent measures employed by the government and the forceful and violent manner in which they were enforced reflected not only the country's authoritarian style and high levels of mistrust of government on the part of the citizens, but actually helped reinforce the same mistrust. The political maneuverings and general non-compliance of elites with COVID-19 countermeasures, particularly those aligned to the president, coupled with the violence inflicted on citizens by police in the name of enforcing curfews and lockdowns, had the effect of exacerbating the pre-existing lack of trust in Kenya's political leadership and its institutions. They also served to erode the social capital required to combat the pandemic. This was particularly accentuated by perceptions on the part of the general public that COVID-19 affected the elite more than ordinary citizens. Indeed, perceptive Kenyans were quick to note that whereas Malaria affects the lower classes the most, when HIV/AIDS struck, it hit the middle classes the hardest; while COVID-19 appeared to be the disease of the elite!

The exclusivist nature of the Kenyan policy style was also evident in the manner in which decision-making on issues pandemic was centralized at the top of the political system. Even the messaging on the matter remained the preserve of the president and his appointee, the Cabinet Secretary for Health. Medical and public health experts were side-lined and, though they were consulted, were never made the face of the pandemic messaging, but were subordinated to the dictates of the political leaders. As indicated above in the case of Dr. Joel Lutomia, some were even victimized and unceremoniously dismissed "for delay in sending testing results to the political leaders" so the latter could communicate the same to the public. The case of Kenya's response to the COVID-19 pandemic thus illustrates the argument that policy styles cast long shadows and, ipso facto, help explain policymaking under normal and extraordinary circumstances when the policy terrain is punctuated by a major crisis situation.

References

Academia Kenya Team. 2020. "Uhuru Kenyatta 10th Presidential Address on COVID 19." Nairobi: July 27. Retrieved from: http://academia-ke.org/library/download/uhuru-kenyatta-10th-presidential-address-on-covid-19/.

Achuka, Vincent & Nasibo Kabale. 2020. "Coronavirus: China Flight in Drama at JKIA." *East African*, Nairobi: February 27.

Adar, Korwa G. & Isaac M. Munyae. 2001. "Human Rights Abuse in Kenya under Daniel arap Moi, 1978–2001." *African Studies Quarterly*, 5(1): 1–17.

Ajulu, Rok. 2021. *Postcolonial Kenya: The Rise of an Authoritarian and Predatory State.* London: Routledge.

Akech, Migai. 2011. "Abuse of Power and Corruption in Kenya: Will the New Constitution Enhance Government Accountability?" *Indian Journal of Global Legal Studies*, 18(1): 341–394.

Aluga, Martin A. 2020. "Coronavirus Disease 2019 (Covid-19) in Kenya: Preparedness, Response and Transmissibility." *Journal of Microbiology, Immunology and Infection*, 53(5): 671–673.

Barasa, Edwine W., Paul O. Ouma, & Emelda A. Okiro. 2020. "Assessing the Hospital Surge Capacity of the Kenyan Health System in the face of the Covid-19 Pandemic." *Plos One*, 15(7), July 20: DOI: 10.1371/journal.pone.0236308.

British Broadcasting Corporation. 2020. "Kenya: Police Brutality in the Battle against Coronavirus in Mathare." June 15: https://www.bbc.com/news/av/world-africa-53025934.

Business Daily. 2013. "Kenyan Legislators Emerge Second in Global Pay Ranking." Nairobi: July 23, 2013. https://www.businessdailyafrica.com/bd/economy/kenyan-legislators-emerge-second-in-global-pay-ranking-2037344.

Cheeseman, Nick. 2013. "The Lack of Trust at the Heart of Kenya's Democracy." *Daily Nation*, Nairobi: September 22.

Craig, Jessica, Erta Kalanxhi, & Stephanie Hauck. 2020. "National Estimates of Critical Care Capacity in 54 African Countries." Washington, DC: Center for Disease Dynamics, Economics, and Policy, https://cddep.org/wp-content/uploads/2020/05/National-estimates-of-critical-care-capacity-in-54-African-countries.pdf. DOI:10.1101/2020.05.13.20100727.

Daily Nation. 2020. "Uhuru's Speech in Full as more Covid-19 Measures are Announced." Nairobi: March 27.

Government of Kenya. 2020. "The 4th Presidential Address on the Coronavirus Pandemic, Nairobi: State House." April 16. Retrieved from: https://www.president.go.ke/2020/04/16/the-fourth-presidential-address-on-the-coronavirus-pandemic-16th-april-2020-at-state-house-nairobi/.

Government of Kenya. 2021. "Review of the Covid-19 Containment Measures." Nairobi: Executive Office of the President Press Release, January 2. https://www.nation.co.ke/kenya/news/uhuru-s-speech-in-full-as-more-covid-19-measures-announced-281796.

Hanson, Stephanie. 2008. "Understanding Kenya's Politics." Washington, DC: Council on Foreign Affairs Backgrounder, January 25: https://www.cfr.org/backgrounder/understanding-kenyas-politics.

Hope, Kempe R. 2013. "Tackling the Corruption Epidemic in Kenya: Toward a Policy of more Effective Control." *Journal of Social, Political, and Economic Studies*, 38(3): 287–316.

Human Rights Watch. 2020. "Kenya: Police Brutality during Curfew." Washington, DC: HRW Report, April 22: https://www.hrw.org/news/2020/04/22/kenya-police-brutality-during-curfew.

IPSOS, 2020. Responding to COVID-19: Highlights of a Survey in KENYA. https://www.ipsos.com/sites/default/files/ct/publication/documents/2020-05/kenya_report_0.pdf.

Jopson, Barney & William Wallis. 2007. "Spotlight: Mwai Kibaki – Absentee Leader Seeking Reelection." *Financial Times*, December 23.

Kabaara, Dennis. 2020. "Tax Amendment Bill Not Quite what we Expected." *Business Daily*, Nairobi: April 9: https://www.businessdailyafrica.com/analysis/ideas/Tax-amendment-Bill-not-quite-what-was-expected/4259414-5519480-naenna/index.html.

Kabia, Evelyn, R. Mbau, R. Oyando, C. Oduor, G. Bigogo, S. Khagayi, & E. Barasa 2019. "We are called the et cetera: Experiences of the Poor with Health Financing Reforms that Target them in Kenya." *International Journal for Equity in Health*, 18(1): 98.

Kahura, Dauti. 2019. "Lies, Dam Lies and Intrigues: The Arror and Kimwarer Dams Saga." *The Elephant*, Nairobi: April 11: https://www.theelephant.info/features/2019/04/11/lies-dam-lies-and-intrigues-the-arror-and-kimwarer-dams-saga/.

Kang'ethe, G. T. 1994. "Policy Analysis in Eastern Africa, Especially Kenya." In *African Development and Public Policy*, ed. Stuart S. Nagel. London: St. Martin's Press, 3–20.

Kariuki, James. 1996. "'Paramoia': Anatomy of a Dictatorship in Kenya." *Journal of Contemporary African Studies*, 14(1): 69–86: DOI: 10.1080/02589009608729582.

Khadiagala, Gilbert M. 2020. "Kenya: Elite Clashes and Coronavirus Quarrels." *Carnegie Endowment for International Peace*, April 28: https://carnegieendowment.org/2020/04/28/kenya-elite-clashes-and-coronavirus-quarrels-pub-.

Kigotho, Wachira. 2020. "Vice-Chancellor and Staff Charged with Embezzlement." *University World News*, August 27: https://www.universityworldnews.com/post.php?story=20200827090219221.

Macharia, James. 2012. "Kenyan Minister Urged to Resign over Medical Scam." *Reuters*, May 8: https://www.reuters.com/article/ozatp-kenya-corruption-20120508-idAFJOE84709Z20120508.

Maina, Mercy. 2020. "'We are Concerned': Bishops in Kenya Over Alleged Misuse of Covid-19 Emergency Fund." *Association for Catholic Information in Africa (ACI Africa)*, Nairobi: May 5: https://www.aciafrica.org/news/1277/we-are-concerned-bishops-in-kenya-over-alleged-misuse-of-covid-19-emergency-fund.

Masenge, D. O., & B. K. Kimolo. 2019. "Integration of University Research Uptake on Public Policy Development Practice in Kenya: A Case of University-Stakeholders Research Partnerships." *American Journal of Public Policy and Administration*, 4(2): 1–15.

Mauti, Joy, L. Gautier, J. W. De Neve, C. Beiersmann, J. Tosun, & A. Jahn 2019. "Kenya's Health in All Policies Strategy: A Policy Analysis Using Kingdon's Multiple Streams." *Health Research Policy and Systems*, 17(1): 15.

Mboga, Jael. 2020. "Uhuru dismisses Report that Covid-19 Misappropriated." *The Saturday Standard*, Nairobi: May 1: https://www.standardmedia.co.ke/nairobi/article/2001369790/covid-19-funds-not-misused-uhuru.

Nasong'o, W. S. 2020a. "The War on Corruption: What Singapore Got Right." *The Elephant*, Nairobi: January 16: https://www.theelephant.info/features/2020/01/16/the-war-on-corruption-what-singapore-got-right/.

Nasong'o, W. S. 2020b. "Disaster Capitalism in the Age of Covid-19." *The Elephant*, Nairobi: April 17: https://www.theelephant.info/ideas/2020/04/17/disaster-capitalism-in-the-age-of-covid-19/.

Nasong'o, W. S. 2020c. "Covid-19 and the Specter of Disaster Capitalism: Fragments of Evidence from Kenya." In the 63rd Annual Meeting of the African Studies Association, Online: November 19–21.

Nyamori, Moses. 2018. "Muturi Team Told MPs were Bribed in Toilets." *The Standard*, Nairobi: September 26: https://www.standardmedia.co.ke/kenya/article/2001296895/mps-our-colleagues-were-bribed-in-the-toilets.

Nyong'o, Anyang' P. 1989. "State and Society in Kenya: The Disintegration of a Nationalist Coalitions and the Rise of Presidential Authoritarianism, 1963–78." *African Affairs*, 88(351): 229–251.

Obulutsa, George. 2021. "Kenya extends Night Curfew to March to Curb Covid-19 Spread." *Reuters*, January 3: https://www.reuters.com/article/health-coronavirus-kenya/kenya-extends-night-curfew-to-march-to-curb-covid-19-spread-idINKBN2980DJ.

Ombati, Cyrus & Roselyne Obala. 2019. "Over 10 Billion Feared Lost in New NHIF Pay Scandal." *The Standard*, Nairobi: February 25: https://www.standardmedia.co.ke/business-news/article/2001314296/over-sh10b-feared-lost-in-new-nhif-pay-scandal.

Otenyo, Eric E. (forthcoming). "Presidential Leadership Styles from Jomo to Uhuru." In *Palgrave Handbook of Kenya and its History*, ed. Wanjala S. Nasong'o, Maurice Amutabi & Toyin Falola. New York: Palgrave Macmillan.

Oyugi, Walter O. 1994. *Politics and Administration in East Africa*. Nairobi: East African Educational Publishers.

Peters, B. Guy. 2015. "Policy Capacity in Public Administration." *Policy and Society* 34 (3–4): 219–28.

Shimanyula, Andrew W. 2020. "Kenya Sacks top Covid-19 Scientist over Delayed Results." Anadolu Agency, Ankara: https://www.aa.com.tr/en/africa/kenya-sacks-top-covid-19-scientist-over-delayed-results/1819508.

The Conversation. 2020. "COVID-19 Exposes Weaknesses in Kenya's Healthcare System. And What Can Be Done." https://theconversation.com/covid-19-exposes-weaknesses-in-kenyas-healthcare-system-and-what-can-be-done-143356.

The Guardian. 2020. "'They have Killed us more than Corona': Kenyans Protest against Police Brutality." *The Guardian*, June 9: https://www.theguardian.com/global-development/2020/jun/09/they-have-killed-us-more-than-corona-kenyans-protest-against-police-brutality.

Tyce, Matthew. 2020. "Kenya's Response to Covid-19." *Effective States and Inclusive Development*, April 29: https://www.effective-states.org/kenyas-response-to-covid-19/.

"Uhuru's Triple Headache." *The Standard*, Nairobi: April 19: https://www.standardmedia.co.ke/mobile/amp/article/2001368471/uhuru-s-triple-headache-pandemic-economy-and-2022-succession-wars.

Wakaya, Jeremiah. 2017. "Kenya's Politicians Least Trusted in Society, Survey Indicates." https://www.capitalfm.co.ke/news/2017/06/kenyas-politicians-least-trusted-society-survey-indicates/.

Warah, Rasna. 2020. "What Covid-19 has Revealed about our Callous and Clueless Leaders." *The Elephant*, Nairobi: May 15: https://www.theelephant.info/op-eds/2020/05/15/what-covid-19-has-revealed-about-our-callous-and-clueless-leaders/.

Wasike, Andrew. 2020a. "Hundreds Protest Police Killings in Kenya during Curfew." Anadolu Agency, Ankara: June 8: https://www.aa.com.tr/en/africa/hundreds-protest-police-killings-in-kenya-during-curfew/1869419.

Wasike, Andrew. 2020b. "Kenya Police Kill more during Curfew than Covid-19." Anadolu Agency, Ankara: April 16: https://www.aa.com.tr/en/africa/kenya-police-kill-more-during-curfew-than-covid-19/1807930.

Wasuna, Brian. 2018. "NHIF Scandal – How Theft of Billions Unfolded from 2014." *Daily Nation*, Nairobi: December 12.

World Health Organization. 2017. *Primary Healthcare Systems: Case Study from Kenya*. Geneva: World Health Organization.

3

Centripetal Responses

7

NORWEGIAN CORPORATISM

A Centripetal National Response to the Pandemic

Jörgen Sparf

Introduction: An Overview of Policy Styles in Norway

Norway is an advanced welfare state characterized by a robust political system with high levels of trust and legitimacy, competent politicians, reliable bureaucracy, and a strong state (Christensen and Lægreid 2020; Sverdrup, Ringen, and Jahn 2020). Policy change is the result of routinized interactions between the government and institutionalized interest groups, whose role extends beyond policy advocacy to policy planning and policy administration (Einhorn and Logue 2003; Rust 1990). Ascribing a policy style to Norway is perhaps a less straightforward proposition than one might expect from a small Northern European country that shares a considerable number of features with its neighbors. We often speak of a Nordic model, but this tends to gloss over the differences between Danish, Norwegian, and Swedish policymaking, not to mention Finland and Iceland. A Nordic model of politics and administration is broadly characterized by many and de-politicized commissions of inquiry and evaluations feeding into the policymaking cycle; the connection between the articulated policy goals at the central level and the implementation at the local level is fairly loose, while governance is generally polycentric. Even though governance and administration have been underpinned by democratic ideals and striving toward equity, in practice, administration runs based on cost-effectiveness (Petersson 2005). Having said this, scholarship has nuanced the administrative heritage of the Nordic countries through the development of the *East–West* model (Greve, Lægreid, and Rykkja 2016; Petersson 2005). The East Nordic (Swedish) administrative model privileges collegial governmental decision-making in the sense that individual ministers lack the type of individual ministerial power and responsibilities that are associated with the ministerial model of administration and is the norm in most European administrative systems. The ministries are small scale, and state

DOI: 10.4324/9781003137399-10

agencies are independent part of the Swedish dualism of the executive (Hall 2016). Finland oscillates toward the East Nordic model to a certain extent, while Norway, Denmark, and Iceland follow the West Nordic model that "entails significant ministerial administration (the 'ministerial model') that allows for a high degree of spontaneous, individual ministerial steering of state authorities" (Greve and Ejersbo 2016: 85).

Writing about policy styles in Norway in 1982, Olsen, Roness, and Sætren paint an image of a modern welfare state based on order, incrementalism, and compromise underpinned by problem-solving, bargaining, and self-governance. The authors go on to note that there are deviations from this business-as-usual mode of policymaking involving many and perhaps unexpected participants, different frames of goals, problems, and solutions to these problems, disagreement, lack of legitimacy, and sometimes dynamic change. More recently, scholars have noted a move toward increased central control of the state vis-à-vis the local authorities belying the image of compromise and self-governance (Sverdrup, Ringen, and Jahn 2020; Tranvik and Fimreite 2006; see also Olsen 2019).

In this chapter, I argue that despite the large degree of autonomy of public agencies and local authorities as well as inclusion of a number of actors in the policymaking process, the Norwegian policy style is more accommodative than managerial due to its pronounced (for the Nordic context) centralized character. This has resulted in a centripetal policy response to the pandemic, with the state taking control of the national response quite early in the process. I support this argument in the remainder of the chapter, which is structured as follows: in the section that follows, I further outline the Norwegian policy style, followed by a brief note on method and data. I then present the Norwegian response to the pandemic, followed by an analysis and concluding remarks.

Policymaking in Norway: Processes and Institutions

Norway is a constitutional monarchy, led by a parliament [*Storting*] and a government with a prime minister. The government consists of 16 ministries (also called departments), including the office of the prime minister (Greve and Ejersbo 2016; Government of Norway n.d.a). The ministries employ about 4,600 people, while about 7,800 are employed in government agencies, 1,600 of whom are employed at the central level (Greve and Ejersbo 2016). Lægreid (2016) notes that the number of ministries has remained fairly constant, but the number of state-owned companies has increased vis-à-vis civil society organizations outside the ministries (Greve and Ejersbo 2016).

Traditionally, Norwegian cabinets are cohesive, underpinned by close ministerial cooperation, strong identification with the government, and presenting a united front with team work (Sverdrup, Ringen, and Janh 2020). The government derives its power by the control it asserts on political initiatives and by being the head of the bureaucracy. Constitutionally, the government is the more active party compared to the parliament in the sense that it submits the annual budget every October, and when it deems it appropriate, it prepares policy proposals to submit to the parliament. It has the power to appoint top personnel in the civil service and to set up commissions of inquiry to evaluate existing policies and measures in any policy sector. Commonly, these commissions result in proposals for new policies or policy amendments. The parliament cannot initiate a policy proposal—it can only vote for or against a proposal submitted by the government (Heidar 2001).

Administration and public services are planned and provided at different levels. At the national level, departments are the secretariats consisting of staff supporting the ministers and the government. The minister is simultaneously the head of the department, a part of the government, and accountable to the parliament for the actions (and inactions) of the department. It is a powerful position, though bureaucracy (the public agencies or directorates) can resist new policies, and thus, ministers must have experience in navigating politically motivated obstruction of policy implementation. Generally, ministers in charge of recently established departments are more likely to face resistance from directorates than some of the legacy departments such as foreign affairs or justice. The mandate of the directorates is to carry out the policies decided by the department to which they belong (Heidar 2001).

Norway's extensive welfare system necessitates an administration that is close to its citizens and thus results in a large degree of decentralization where municipalities are in charge of practically all welfare services. Even though Norway is not a federal state, the local level has considerable autonomy, funded by income and wealth taxes as well as intergovernmental transfers in the form of block grants and earmarked grants (Heidar 2004). The Local Government Act of 1992 [1992:107] was the result of reforms that intended to increase local autonomy, while a 2017 reform taking effect in 2020 puts the number of municipalities to 365 and the regions at 11 (OECD 2019a).

Actors in Scandinavian politics opt for compromise and consensus as well as inclusion of all possible organized interests rather than open conflict and exclusion (Goodin 2003). Drafting legislation at the national level requires systematic consultation of a multitude of groups—all major interest groups involved, mainly through the process of remiss. This is an extensive process during which the proposal is sent out to all relevant organizations for feedback, encouraging a rational debate about the merits of the proposal and finding points of consensus among major parties and interest organizations (Einhorn and Logue, 2003). Public servants are expected to provide expertise and policy guidance, while the role of elected officials is to provide legitimacy, political know-how, and guidance (Peters and Pierre 2003).

When it comes to health care, the municipalities have the responsibility to provide most of primary health care, while public hospitals and specialist health care are administered by four special jurisdictions: North, Mid-Norway, West, and South-East (Helsenorge.no n.d.; Norwegian Ministry of Health and Care Services n.d.). Further structural reforms enacted in 2002 saw the ownership of public hospitals transferred to the national government. This means that the special jurisdictions above manage and are responsible for the delivery of health care services, but without ownership rights (OECD 2019b; Sverdrup, Ringen, and Jahn 2020). The OECD reports that "Norwegians lead longer and healthier lives than most other Europeans" (OECD 2019b n.p). Indeed, health care spending, which has grown steadily recently, is a full two-thirds higher than the EU average accounting for 10.4% of GDP, also above EU average, which is 9.8%. Public funding accounts for 84% for health care spending, while the remainder is out-of-pocket expenses by health care recipients (OECD 2019b). In 2018, the country reported 3.5 hospital beds and 2.9 physicians per 1,000 people, while public spending on health care per person for that year was USD8,293 (World Bank 2018a; 2018b; World Health Organization 2018). Norway entered the pandemic crisis with favorable conditions in the health care sector in terms of capacity and public spending.

At the national level, the Norwegian Directorate of Health is the public agency tasked with analyzing conditions that may affect public health and is the entity responsible for compiling knowledge regarding health and health care services. It also has the mandate to implement the policies of the Ministry of Health and Care Services. The directorate is also thus a regulatory professional agency that is both an administrator and an "interpreter of legislation" (Norwegian Directorate of Health n.d. n.p.). Ministers, who are members of the cabinet and head governmental departments, have slightly different roles when considered comparatively in Nordic countries. Norway, Denmark, and Iceland, which follow the West Nordic administrative model (as mentioned earlier in this chapter), are allowed greater intervention in the day-to-day work of public agencies (Greve and Ejersbo 2016). This results in comparatively less autonomy of public agencies compared to their Swedish counterparts (see Petridou, this volume). Indeed, public agencies have autonomy when it comes to their area of expertise, in that they are advisory bodies consulting the government. In practice, they rarely take a difference stance going against the directive of the ministries (Sverdrup, Ringen, and Jahn 2020).

In summary, Norwegian policymaking is characterized by stability, continuity, and incrementalism (Sverdrup, Ringen, and Jahn 2020). Its economic policies earn Norway a top spot internationally despite the country's dependence on oil revenues. In fact, the Norwegian economy is aimed at reducing that dependence, boasting robust growth and sound public finances. Norway occupies the top spot for 2020 Sustainable Governance Indicators (SGI) ranking, with very high educational attainment, generous social insurance programs, low crime rates, and universal health care (Bertelsmann Stiftung 2020). Policymaking has become increasingly centralized, and there is some tension regarding the (decreasing) autonomy of local authorities. What is more, the state is the largest owner of capital, holding about 40% of equity traded at the Oslo stock exchange. Indeed, in practice, the state solely funds areas such as culture, education, and research, as well as health (Sverdrup, Ringen, and Jahn 2020).

Note on Data and Method

The data used for this study mainly consist of governmental documents relevant to the response to the pandemic. Governmental documents include press releases, legislative documents, decrees, and other crisis communication documents that outline contagion mitigation and economic relief measures, mainly at the national level. The character of this crisis has, to some degree, determined the data sources for this study. This has also been the case for a number of COVID-19-related recently published studies (see, e.g. Capano, 2020; Capano et al., 2020; Christensen and Lægreid, 2020; Petridou 2020; Petridou and Zahariadis 2021; Petridou, Zahariadis, and Ceccoli 2020; Pierre, 2020; Zahariadis, Petridou, and Oztig 2020). The timeframe under research includes the entire 2020, including the first phase lasting until approximately mid-May, the lull in the summer, and the subsequent waves in the fall and winter of 2020.

Pandemic Response

Christensen and Lægreid (2020: 775) describe the Norwegian response as "a suppression strategy followed by economic measures," including the harshest restrictions imposed on the Norwegian population since World War II. The national response privileged health over economic concerns and a fairly centralized national strategy over flexibility of the local level featuring a set of mandatory regulations combined with softer guidelines (Christensen and Lægreid 2020). In this section, I outline the Norwegian response to the pandemic, starting with the preparedness plans that were in place at the onset of the crisis. I then discuss the measures aimed at mitigating contagion as well as the ones providing financial relief to households and businesses.

Preparedness

The pandemic's character renders it, of course, a public health issue. However, its consequences are far-reading, multi-sectoral, and cast long shadows on the whole of society, and in that respect, it is relevant to understand preparedness when it comes to crisis management in general. I will begin with the country's preparedness in terms of public health and the contagious diseases and continue with the institutional and procedural landscape regarding crisis management.

The comprehensive and multi-sectoral *National Health Preparedness Plan* provides the basis for health preparedness in Norway. It is a document outlining not only a series of statutes relevant to health-related incidents but it also provides guidance when it comes to relations of institutions in multi-level governance, the role of expert scientific knowledge and resources, and coordination and crisis management. The plan is meant to be used as a guide for the subnational entities when they draw up their own contingency plans. Specific to communicable diseases is the *Act Relating to Control of Communicable Diseases*. In the interest of protecting the Norwegian population from communicable diseases, the act states that health and other authorities will implement the measures necessary to control contagion, providing for the imposition of measures such as quarantine, movement, and travel restrictions (Norwegian Ministry of Health and Care Services 2014).

Four fundamental principles underpin crisis management in Norway: (i) the principle of responsibility; (ii) the principle of subsidiarity; (iii) the principle of equivalency; and (iv) the principle of cooperation. The principle of responsibility conveys the idea that the entity responsible for service of public interest or empirical field during normal times retains that responsibility during extraordinary events, including emergency preparations and management of such events. The principle of subsidiarity states that crises must be handled at the lowest possible level of government, while the principle of equivalency (following the principle of responsibility) requires that any organization established to handle a crisis to be as equivalent as possible to the corresponding organization during normal times. Finally, according to the principle of cooperation, entities are mandated to ensure coordination and collaboration with other relevant entities in preventing, preparing for, and managing crises (Lovdata 2017).

The following organizational chart describes the landscape of collaboration in implementation activities among the institutions in Norwegian multi-level governance (Norwegian Ministry of Health and Care Services 2014). Decisions originate at the ministry level, while the public agencies (the Directorate of Health and the Directorate for Civil Protection and Emergency Planning as well as more public agencies if needed) push these further down to the subnational levels. The county governors act as the representative of the state to the

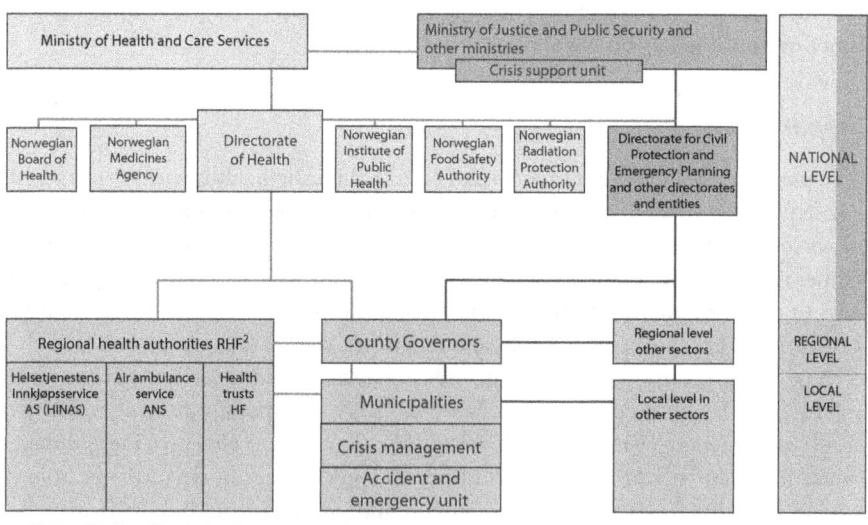

— Ministry of Health and Care Services' line　— Line to other sectors

FIGURE 7.1 Notification and reporting lines in the health sector in the event of crises.
Source: Norwegian Ministry of Health and Care Services 2014.

municipalities, thus playing the role of the intermediary facilitating relations and cooperation between the state and municipalities.

Contagion Mitigation Measures

The Norwegian Directorate of Health (NDH) and the Norwegian Institute of Public Health (NIPH—under the Ministry of Health and Care Services) were important actors in the government's response, with the NDH being assigned extended powers in late February and early March for the protection of the population from the virus (Government of Norway n.d.b). The Ministry of Health was initially the lead agency, but as the scope of the crisis expanded, the Ministry of Justice and Public Security was assigned the leading role instead (Christensen and Lægreid 2020). In addition to soft measures and guidelines such as a ban on large gatherings or broad guidelines about working from home, restricting travel, and online teaching at universities and high schools, Norway imposed highly stringent measures aimed at containing the spread. The Government's timeline of corona measures (Government of Norway 2020b) accounts that: Norway closed down schools and imposed a lockdown on March 12; on March 17, the Ministry of Health and Care Services issued the decision that local (municipal) rules to stop contagion may not be such that they hinder important societal functions; on March 18, the government proposed a six-month extraordinary legislation due to the coronavirus to ensure that society functions smoothly and negative consequences are mitigated; on March 19, a ban on spending the night in one's second home [*hytte*] (an activity which is part of Norwegian identity) was enforced. The ban concerned second homes that were in a different municipality than someone's first residence. Schools started opening from April 20 to May 11, while on May 7, the government announced that the goal was to resume activities by June 15 (Christensen and Lægreid 2020).

Norway's Prime Minister, Erna Solberg, was prominent in communicating the measures and became the public face of the government's response. The timeline of measures was listed on the official government website while politicians generally engaged in public debate. What is more, the emergency legislation in practice concentrated power at the national level and away from the municipalities for a six-month period. Finally, closing the schools at the national level had followed the closing of schools in the municipalities of Oslo and Bergen, the two most populous municipalities in the country (Helljesen et al. 2020).

The complete lock down lasted 26 days. At the end of April, the government relaxed the stringency of measures but still recommending keeping a two-meter distance among people in public places, frequent hand-washing, working from home, avoiding public transportation, and staying home if exhibiting any symptoms at all. In May 2020, national measures allowed the gathering of 20 people along as a one-meter distance between individuals could be maintained, while sport halls could open. Travel abroad remained discouraged. National guidelines stayed in place for the remainder of 2020. The central government was able to avoid further 'hard' lockdown orders, while local governments were permitted more leeway in their handling of the pandemic. In September 2020, after an upsurge of cases, local measures included avoiding public transportation, caping the maximum people in gatherings to 50, while recommending that private gatherings not exceed 10 individuals. Restaurant operations were curtailed (with the option of mandated closure open), mask-use was recommended when maintaining physical distance was not an option, while university teaching was recommended to take place online. In the latter part of the year, several local governments enforced stricter measures for a time if the number of cases rose. The national response in December 2020 included cancelation of flights to and from the UK due to the most recent mutation discovered in that country and a recommendation to download and use a phone application "intended to help prevent coronavirus from spreading among the population" (Helsenorge.no n.d: n.p.). An earlier version of that application, also launched by the NIPH, received harsh criticism by Amnesty International and was taken down due to the centralized collection of personal information (Finell and Carlsson 2020).

The stringency of the national response, *inter alia*, was presented as one of the reasons behind the 'Corona Commission,' convened in April 2020. Commissions of inquiry are fairly common policymaking tools at the national level in the Nordic context. They are set up by the government, but they are independent in the sense that they are led by experts, though politicians participate. Commission members normally represent a variety of interests (Rust 1990). Their role is to gather information in a specific area and submit recommendations to the government, often resulting in legislative change. The goals of this commission, scheduled to submit its findings in March 2021, were to evaluate the governmental response as well as the preparedness in place prior to the outbreak of the pandemic for the purpose of learning when it comes to crisis management of the next pandemic or the next extraordinary event (Government of Norway 2020).

Financial Support to Business and Households

Norway's labor market policy has traditionally been proactive, aiming at retaining long-term unemployed workers. Unemployment benefits are generous, and labor laws limit dismissal procedures, though layoff costs are low for companies that want to downsize (Sverdrup, Ringen, and Jahn 2020). The pandemic had almost immediate consequences in the labor market evidenced in unemployment rates, shooting up from 2.3% to 10.4% in the month of March. This prompted a swift reaction by the national government in enacting financial relief measures. Indicatively, on March 13, measures were introduced to help viable businesses avoid layoffs and bankruptcies as well as support jobs. Just three days later, on March 16, 100b NOK were allocated in the form of guarantees as loans to businesses as crisis support (Christensen and Lægreid 2020). Lockdown measures hit the cultural and volunteer sectors as well as sports quite hard, so throughout 2020 and into 2021, the national government introduced several financial support packages (Government of Norway n.d.b). By April 3, additional measures supporting businesses had added up to 241b NOK taken from the petroleum fund. Compared to the previous year's budget, public spending had increased by 17% (Christensen and Lægreid 2020). The Norwegian Labor and Welfare Administration (NAV) implemented a series of temporary measures aimed at addressing the negative consequences of the contagion mitigation measures on households and individuals. These included sickness benefits, unemployment benefits to those that had been laid off or filed for bankruptcy, as well as support to self-employed individuals (Norwegian Labour and Welfare Administration n.d.). As Christensen and Lægreid (2020) note, the government paid most of the unemployment benefits as the main measures aimed at supporting businesses with cash and amending layoff rules, which in effect led to more layoffs, than for example in Denmark, where the national government subsidized employers to continue paying their employees at a lower rate.

A Question of Trust

Norway is characterized by high levels of trust in political institutions, transparency, as well as high levels of social capital and high levels of trust in politicians (Bjørnå and Weigård 2020; Pedersen and Kuhnle 2017; Stein, Buck and Bjørnå 2019). High levels of political trust in Norway, in particular, and the Nordic countries, in general, are largely attributed to low levels of corruption and socioeconomic equality (Andersen 2018). The share of people who answered 'a lot' or 'some' when asked if they trust their national government was 89.9% in 2018 (Ortiz-Ospina and Roser 2016; Our World In Data 2020). Norway is a particularly sparsely populated country with a difficult geography, the vicissitudes of which have only relatively recently been alleviated through substantial infrastructure investment, though center–periphery tensions remain with the largest urban centers and the capital region in the south of the country. Stein, Buck, and Bjørnå (2019) add an intriguing dimension in unpacking political trust in Norway: that of space. They find that distance from the (political) center is inversely related to trust in politicians. This spills over even to local politicians. In other words, the farther from the capital, the less trust people place in politicians, both national and local. In a country exhibiting such high levels of political trust, this differentiation is perhaps minor when thinking about trust in a comparative way, but it does serve as a reminder of the center–periphery tensions and the differentiation among regions that exists in Norway.

Having said this, trust in government has increased considerably since 2010. This included trust in government, health authorities, the parliament, local politicians as well as the prime minister. Compared to January 2010, a study conducted in March 2020 reported that citizen satisfaction with the government had increased from 23 to 49%, while satisfaction with politicians in the country had increased from 24 to 43%. The same was true for satisfaction with parliament, which had increased from 41 to 63%. Finally, overall satisfaction with democracy went up from 57 to 63% (Christensen and Lægreid 2020; Medborgerpanelet 2020). Interestingly, the increased levels in citizen satisfaction with the executive and legislative bodies and democracy in Norway in general are registered at the time when the most stringent measures were enacted as part of the national response to the pandemic.

The Corona Commission: Government and Bureaucracy

Indeed, the Corona Commission (an inquiry commissioned by the government in April 2020 to evaluate the pandemic response) credits trust as "one of the factors that made the Norwegian society well equipped to handle the crisis" (Koronakommisjonen 2021: n.p., author's translation). Indirectly, the commission credits the high trust that citizens place on government and bureaucracy for the high compliance rates and, in turn, a successful response. The intrusiveness of the measures was also taken up by the commission, which pointed to the unsustainable character of such measures, including a 26-day hard lockdown, though it credited the public agencies with a swift response based on existing data. Interestingly, for this chapter, the commission argues that the set of measures announced on March 12 (measures that included the lockdown) should have been communicated to the public by the government and not by the directorate. They go on to say that the constitution places the burden on the elected officials and not the public servants to make decisions of such importance as imposing "the strictest measures in peacetime" on the Norwegian population (Koronakommisjonen 2021: n.p.). This is not to say that the commission asserts that the government alone ought to have made such decisions. Rather, it argues that decision-making powers of this magnitude and communication to the public rest with elected officials.

Conclusions

Even though assessing the Norwegian response is beyond the scope of this article, it must be noted that Norway faired quite well in terms of number of cases and deaths. According to data reported by Verdens Gang (2020), at the peak of the first wave, a seven-day average of cases topped 2,089, while deaths registered at 62. During the second wave, the peak case number stood higher at 4,237, while the seven-day average of deaths was lower at 33. As of March 16, Norway had reported a total of 640 deaths compared to 13,146 in Sweden, 2,394 in Denmark, 800 in Finland, and 29 in Iceland (Johns Hopkins 2021). The Norwegian national response result (in terms of people getting sick of dying in relative low numbers) has been deemed paradigmatic by the media as well as academics (see, e.g., Christensen and Lægreid 2020) especially when framed in comparison to its Nordic neighbors and particularly Sweden.

This was not the case during the H1N1 flu pandemic in 2009–2010. Albeit an event of considerably lesser magnitude, Norway fared worse than most European countries and its Nordic neighbors having registered 29 deaths. Evaluations from NIPH and the Norwegian Directorate for Civil Protection (DSB) point to gaps in collaboration, the need for an increase role for the Norwegian Directorate of Health, and the need to revamp the legislative framework governing communicative diseases (Norwegian Directorate of Health 2010; Norwegian Institute of Public Health 2015). The learning process from the previous experience with a pandemic is itself evidence of deliberative policymaking indicating high policy capacity and inclusion through the use of expert evaluations to inform change in legislation and contingency plans.

High level of administrative capacity in Norway and the Nordic countries in general is a well-documented feature of the Scandinavian corporatist political and administrative system, featuring a high status of the bureaucracy, an open recruiting and career system in public service as well as a pronounced accountability of the bureaucracy to the citizens (Kuhlmann and Wollmann 2014). Kuhlmann and Wollmann (2014) go on to note that Scandinavian countries tend to be more centralized than their federalist European countries such as Germany or Switzerland. However, as noted elsewhere in this chapter, there has been tension between increased centralization of decision-making and the autonomy of local authorities to make decisions.

The tendency to curtail the autonomy of subnational levels and centralize decision-making powers may be related to an extraordinary event and the ensuring crisis. Kristinsson and Matthíasson (2016) found some evidence to support this hypothesis when analyzing reforms in Europe after the financial crisis of the late 2000s. Norway, which was affected very little by the economic downturn that devastated countries in the European south and saw banks collapsing in Iceland and Denmark, increased the power of the Ministry of Finance less than other countries, exhibiting less organizational centralization and a very small degree of politicization. Interestingly, Iceland did not increase the power of its Ministry of Finance, also exhibiting comparatively less centralization and politicization of decision-making processes. It is therefore reasonable to expect that the policy style casts a long shadow on policymaking processes and institutions, even during times of crises.

Norway adopted a centralized response to the pandemic and imposed a lockdown with mandatory closures. To do that, Norway's central government assumed decision-making powers which are normally under local level remit including instituting an emergency 'corona law' (albeit with an expiration date) giving it the ability to centralize measure. It is noteworthy, however, that restrictive measures and specifically school and daycare closures were first enacted at the local level (albeit in anticipation of a possible announcement of a national measure), in Oslo and Bergen, the two biggest municipalities in Norway. This, perhaps, all but forced the hand of the national government to impose a nationwide school closure which became part of the national response.

Reflecting the tensions between centralization and decentralization in Norway, I conclude that the policy style may oscillate between managerial and adversarial. Though more research is necessary to confirm this, I put forth that the policy style may partly depend on the policy sector (an early critique of the national policy style argument) and that it may shift over time. For example, in a corporatist system as the Norwegian one, interest groups may become entrenched, rendering the policymaking process less inclusive and more centralized. Olsen, Roness, and Sætren reported this much as early as 1982, referring especially to fiscal policy. They described a political system based on low conflict among cleavage group that found a way to collaborate. Having said that, they found that the general tendency in Norway was that ministries concerned with economic policy tended to coopt the other actors involved in policymaking processes. More recently, we have seen an increased centralization of specialty healthcare with the ownership of the hospitals being transferred to the state, though still run by the subnational health districts. Added to this, the wealth of the Norwegian state and the fact that it contributes considerably more to the health care system in general compared to other European countries essentially holding the purse strings may be indicators pointing inevitability of a tendency to curtail autonomy through increased centralization especially after the perceived failure of the H1N1 pandemic.

An *adversarial* policy style combined with high trust led to a centripetal crisis response, at least during the first phase of the crisis. A few points should be noted here. First, the levels of administrative capacity and inclusiveness are dynamic— on a continuum rather than fixed and better understood when thought of in comparative terms: 'lower' or 'higher,' rather than in the absoluteness that 'low' or 'high' conveys. Indeed, in Norway, the coordination within the executive and between the executive and the parliament was high, and there was coordination between the national and the subnational levels. Public agencies provided input for decision-making; but at the end of the day, the decision rested with the politicians at the state level which made the decisions for the subnational levels in the beginning, and this is what I mean by lower inclusiveness. Particularly, high levels of political trust served as a magnifying glass—citizens trusted the decisions of the central government, even when it impinged on the local jurisdictions. As the year progressed, the national contagion mitigation measures eased, and local measures were foregrounded again. The Corona Commission's results are sure to be part of a larger evaluation of the pandemic response. As Olsen (2019) contends, there are unresolved conflicts in central public administration, conceptual, and otherwise, that Norwegian administration must live with.

References

Andersen, Rasmus Fonnesbaek. 2018. "Trust in Scandinavia: Findings from Moving Borders between Denmark and Germany." *Scandinavian Political Studies* 41: 22–48.

Bertelsmann Stiftung. 2020. "Sustainable Government Indicators: Norway." https://www.sgi-network.org/2020/Norway

Bjørnå, Hilde, and Weigård, Jarle. 2020. "From Public to Private Accountability in Norwegian Local Government." *SAGE Open.* https://doi.org/10.1177/2158244020957042

Capano, Giliberto, Howlett, Michael, Jarvis, Darryl S. L., Ramesh, M., and Goyal, Nihit. 2020. "Mobilizing Policy (in)Capacity to Fight Covid-19: Understanding Variations in State Responses." *Policy and Society* 39: 285–308. https://doi.org/10.1080/14494035. 2020.1787628

Capano, Giliberto. 2020. "Policy Design and State Capacity in the Covid-19 Emergency in Italy: If You Are Not Prepared for the (Un)Expected, You Can Be Only What You Already Are." *Policy and Society* 39: 326–44. https://doi.org/10.1080/14494035.2020. 1783790

Christensen, Tom, and Lægreid, Per. 2020. "Balancing Governance Capacity and Legitimacy - How the Norwegian Government Handled the Covid-19 Crisis as a High Performer." *Public Admnistration Review* n/a. https://doi.org/10.1111/puar.13241

Einhorn, Eric S., and Logue, John. 2003. *Modern Welfare States: Scandinavian Politics and Policy in the Global Age.* 2nd ed. Westport, CT: Praeger.

Finell, Ola, and Carlsson, Sven. 2020. "Stop for app Contagionstop." (16 June). *Swedish Radio.* https://sverigesradio.se/artikel/7496749

Goodin, Robert E. 2003. *Reflective Democracy.* Oxford: Oxford University Press.

Government of Norway. 2020. "The Government Inaugurates the Corona Commission" [Press Release, No70/20]. https://www.regjeringen.no/no/aktuelt/ regjeringen-oppnevner-koronakommisjon/id2699476/

Government of Norway. n.d.a. "Ministries." https://www.regjeringen.no/en/dep/ id933/

Government of Norway. n.d.b. "Timeline: Corona measures under the Department of Culture." https://www.regjeringen.no/no/tema/kultur-idrett-og-frivillighet/ innsiktsartikler/tidslinje-koronatiltak-under-kulturdepartementet/id2828012/

Greve, Carsten, and Ejersbo, Niels. 2016. "Reform Context and Status." In *Nordic Administrative Reforms: Lessons for Public Management*, eds. Carsten Greve, Per Lægreid and Lise H. Rykkja. London: Palgrave Macmillan. 88–126.

Greve, Carsten, Lægreid, Per and Rykkja, Lise H. eds. 2016. *Nordic Administrative Reforms: Public Sector Organizations, Public Sector Organizations.* London: Palgrave Macmillan.

Hall, Patrik. 2016. "The Swedish Administrative Model." In *The Oxford Handbook of Swedish Politics*, ed. Jon Pierre. Oxford: Oxford University Press. 299–314.

Heidar, Knut. (ed.) 2004. *Nordic Politics: Comparative Perspectives.* Oslo: Universitetsforlaget.

Heidar, Knut. 2001. *Norway: Elites on Trial.* Boulder: Westview Press.

Helljesen, Vilde, Svendsen, Roy Hilmar, Mikalsen, Kaja Staude, and Baisotti, Valentina. 2020. "Alle Landets Skoler og Barnehager Stenges." 12 March *NRK.*

Helsenorge.no. n.d. https://www.helsenorge.no

Johns Hopkins University. 2021. "Corona Virus Resource Center." https://coronavirus. jhu.edu/map.html

Koronakommisjonen. 2021. *Kommisjonens hovedbudskap.* [NOU 2021: 6 kapittel 2.2] https://files.nettsteder.regjeringen.no/wpuploads01/blogs.dir/421/files/2021/04/ Kommisjonens-hovedbudskap.pdf

Kristinsson, Gunnar Helgi, and Matthíasson, Pétur Berg. 2016. "Managing the Financial Crisis." In *Nordic Administrative Reforms: Lessons for Public Management*, eds. Carsten Greve, Per Lægreid and Lise H. Rykkja. London: Palgrave Macmillan. 352–93.

Kuhlmann, Sabine, and Wollmann, Hellmut. 2014. *Introduction to Comparative Public Administration.* Cheltenham, UK: Edward Elgar.

Lægreid, Per. 2016. "Nordic Administrative Traditions." In *The Routledge Handbook on Scandinavian Studies*, eds. Peter Nedergaard, and Anders Wivel. London: Routledge. 80–91.

Lovdata. 2017. "Instruks for Departementenes Arbeid med Samfunnssikkerhet (Samfunns- sikkerhetsinstruksen)." https://lovdata.no/dokument/INS/forskrift/2017-09-01-1349

Medborgerpanelet. 2020. Norsk medborgarpanel. March 4. https://www.uib.no/aktuelt/135017/stolar-meir-på-erna-og-mindre-på-naboen

Norwegian Directorate for Civil Protection. 2010. "Rapport. Ny Influensa A (H2N1) 2009. Gjennomgang av Erfaringer in Norge." [Report. New influenza A (H1N1) 2009. Review of experiences from Norway]. https://www.dsbinfo.no/DSBno/2010/Rapport/Pandemirapport/

Norwegian Directorate of Health. n.d. "About the Norwegian Directorate of Health." https://www.helsedirektoratet.no/english/about-the-norwegian-directorate-of-health#publicmandate

Norwegian Institute of Public Health. 2015. "Evalueringer etter influensapandemien 2009 i Norge og internasjonalt." [Evaluations after influenza pandemic 2019 in Norway and internationally]. https://www.fhi.no/sv/influensa/influensapandemier/evalueringer-etter-influensapandemi/

Norwegian Labour and Welfare Administration. n.d. "Corona Virus: What Do I Do?" https://www.nav.no/en/home

Norwegian Ministry of Health and Care Services. 2014. "National Health Preparedness Plan." Version 2.0. https://www.regjeringen.no/en/dokumenter/national-health-preparedness-plan/id761213/

Norwegian Ministry of Health and Care Services. n.d. "The Department of Hospital Ownership." https://www.regjeringen.no/en/dep/hod/organisation-and-management-of-the-ministry-of-health-and-care-services/Departments/the-department-of-hospital-ownership/id1413/

OECD. 2019a. "Country Profiles: Norway." http://www.sng-wofi.org/country-profiles/Fiche%20NORWAY.pdf

OECD. 2019b. "Norway: Country Health Profile 2019." https://read.oecd-ilibrary.org/social-issues-migration-health/norway-country-health-profile-2019_2e821540-en#page3

Olsen, Johan P. 2019. "Sentraladministrasjonen i en utfordrende æra: Tid for ettertanke." *Norsk statsvitenskapelig tidsskrift* 35(01): 4–27.

Olsen, Johan, Roness, Paul, and Sætren, Harald. 1982. "Norway: Still Peaceful Coexistence and Revolution in Slow Motion?" In *Policy Styles in Western Europe* ed. Jeremy Richardson, George Allen & Unwin Ltd [Routlege Revivals 2013]. 47–79.

Ortiz-Ospina, Esteban, and Roser, Max. 2016. "Trust." *Published online at OurWorldInData.org.* https://ourworldindata.org/trust

Our World in Data. 2020. "Trust." https://ourworldindata.org/trust

Pedersen, Axel West, and Kuhnle, Stein. 2017. "The Nordic Welfare State Model." In *The Nordic Models in Political Science. Challenged, but Still Viable?* ed. Oddbjørn Knutsen, Fagbokforlaget. 249–72.

Peters, B. Guy., and Pierre, Jon. 2003. "Introduction: The Role of Public Administration in Governing." In *Handbook of Public Administration*, eds. B. Guy Peters, and Jon Pierre. London: Sage, 1–12.

Petersson, Olof. 2005. *Nordisk Politik.* 5th ed. Stockholm: Norstedts Juridik.

Petridou, Evangelia. 2020. "Politics and Administration in Times of Crisis: Explaining the Swedish Response to the Covid-19 Crisis." *European Policy Analysis* 6: 147–58.

Petridou, Evangelia, and Zahariadis, Nikolaos. 2021. "Staying at Home or Going Out? Leadership Response to the Covid-19 Crisis in Greece and Sweden." *Journal of Contingencies and Crisis Management*, n/a.

Petridou, Evangelia, Zahariadis, Nikolaos, and Ceccoli, Stephen. 2020. "Averting Institutional Disasters? Drawing Lessons from China to Inform the Cypriot Response to the Covid-19 Pandemic." *European Policy Analysis* 6: 318–27.

Pierre, Jon. 2020. "Nudges against Pandemics: Sweden's Covid-19 Containment Strategy in Perspective." *Policy and Society* 39: 478–93.

Rust, Val D. 1990. "The Policy Formation Process and Educational Reform in Norway." *Comparative Education*, 26(1): 13–25, DOI: 10.1080/0305006900260103

Stein, Jonas, Buck, Marcus, and Bjørnå, Hilde. 2019. "The Centre–Periphery Dimension and Trust in Politicians: The Case of Norway." *Territory, Politics, Governance*, 1–19. https://doi.org/10.1080/21622671.2019.1624191

Sverdrup, Ulf, Ringen, Stein, and Jahn, Detlef. 2020. "Norway Report: Sustainable Governance Indicators 2020." Bertelsmann Stiftung.

Tranvik, Tommy, and Fimreite, Anne Lise. 2006. "Reform Failure: The Processes of Devolution and Centralisation in Norway." *Local Government Studies* 32(1): 89–107, DOI: 10.1080/03003930500453609

Verdens, Gang. 2020. Coronaviruset. https://www.vg.no/spesial/corona/?utm_source= coronav-new-front

World Bank. 2018a. Hospital Beds (Per 1,000 People). All Countries and Economies. https://data.worldbank.org/indicator/SH.MED.BEDS.ZS

World Bank Group. 2018. Current Health Expenditure Per Capita (Current US$). All Countries and Economies. https://data.worldbank.org/indicator/SH.XPD.CHEX. PC.CD

World Health Organization. 2018. Medical Doctors (Per 10 000 Population). https://www.who.int/data/gho/data/indicators/indicator-details/GHO/medical-doctors-(per-10-000-population)

Zahariadis, Nikolaos, Petridou, Evangelia, and Oztig, Lacin Idil. 2020. "Claiming Credit and Avoiding Blame: Political Accountability in Greek and Turkish Responses to the Covid-19 Crisis." *European Policy Analysis* 6: 159–69.

8

NEW ZEALAND COVID RESPONSE

Leadership, Communication, and Trust

W. John Hopkins and Annick Masselot

Introduction

The New Zealand government has been rightly lauded for its response to COVID-19 and has been held up as something of a model for future pandemic response. However, the reasons for its success are less obvious than some assume. The New Zealand health sector has suffered from long-term systemic problems stemming from its semi-private model (Health and Disability System Review 2020). In addition, the legal and governance frameworks around pandemic planning are outdated (primarily focused around influenza) and were cruelly exposed in the 2019 measles epidemic, which was tragically exported to Samoa in early 2020 (Hopkins 2021). For this reason, New Zealand ranked a lowly 35th place in terms of preparedness to manage an epidemic outbreak on the 2019 Global Health Security Index (Global Health Security Index 2019). Yet, despite these issues, New Zealand appears to have fared far better in its handling of the COVID-19 pandemic when compared to other, more highly ranked (and thus arguably better-equipped) states. This chapter focuses on why this should be the case.

The first COVID-19 case was diagnosed in New Zealand on 26 February 2020. By the middle of March, community transmission was occurring in New Zealand, and it became clear that the country lacked sufficient testing and contact-tracing capacity to contain the virus (Baker et al. 2020a). In addition, the systemic vulnerabilities within the health system (including a chronic lack of ICU beds), alluded to above, led to the government being presented with modeling which made for sobering reading. This predicted a mortality level of between 12,000 and 36,000 people after six months of uncontrolled transmission. These deaths would disproportionately affect vulnerable and historically disadvantaged populations, including Māori and Pasifika, who represent 16.7% (Statistics NZ 2020) and 7.5% (Statistics NZ 2018) of New Zealand's overall inhabitants.

DOI: 10.4324/9781003137399-11

In response to, and informed by, strong, science-based advocacy, the government adopted a strict countrywide lockdown (styled "Alert Level 4") on March 26, 2020. Cases first increased exponentially but declined rapidly after five weeks, prompting a move to a relaxed lockdown (Alert Level 3) for an additional two weeks.[1] In total, New Zealanders were ordered to stay home, with very limited exceptions, for seven weeks. The last community-transmitted COVID-19 case was detected in early May 2020, which marked the end of identified community spread and the (first) elimination of the virus in New Zealand (Baker, Wilson, and Anglemyer 2020). On June 8, 2020, the government announced a countrywide move to Alert Level 1, thus effectively asserting the end of the domestic pandemic in New Zealand, 103 days following the first identified case. By June 2020, New Zealand had recorded a total of 1,569 cases and 22 deaths.[2] Despite a number of contained community outbreaks, the COVID-related mortality of 4 per 1 million remains the lowest among the 37 OECD countries. The life of most citizens has largely since returned to normality albeit without the option of international travel and with mask requirements on public transport. In addition, although the economic fallout remains a concern, much of the domestic economy has returned to pre-COVID levels, and overall negative economic impacts have been far below than predicted (Smyth 2020).

New COVID-19 cases in the country are exclusively linked to international travelers, who are kept in government-managed quarantine (MIQ) facilities for 14 days after arrival in order to not compromise the country's elimination status.[3] This MIQ system has proved imperfect at times with cases being transmitted through the border by both staff and travelers, but, in most cases, these "leaks" have been contained without community transmission. However, on two occasions, since May 2020, COVID community transmission was detected, prompting a rise to Alert Level 3 in Auckland and Alert Level 2 in the rest of the country for short periods in August 2020 and in February/March 2021. As the entire border workforce is now vaccinated (as of March 2021), the risk of this re-occurring would appear much reduced.

The success of this "elimination" strategy has led to a number of rather simplistic assertions as to why this occurred. Situated in the south-west Pacific Ocean, Aotearoa | New Zealand consists of two main islands as well as some smaller offshore archipelagos. The "tyranny of the distance" (Blainey 1966) appears intuitively as a blessing in the fight against the COVID-19 pandemic. A remote island should be more successful at keeping the virus at bay because it might be better able to manage border crossing than land locked countries. In reality, geographical remoteness was not a decisive factor in successful management of the virus. Indeed, statistics suggest that although geographically isolated, New Zealand receives a high number of visitors; 3.9 million arrivals in 2019 (Dunstan 2020). In addition, New Zealand's close economic relationship with China mean that travel between these countries is relatively common, particularly Wuhan, which was served by direct flights to both Auckland and Christchurch (with which it is a "sister city").

Equally, the relatively small population size of around five million was not critical to managing the crisis. Contrary to popular myth and despite a relative low density,[4] New Zealand is one of the world's most urbanized societies with over 86% of the population living in such environments (United Nations 2018). New Zealand's cities thus represented a fertile ground for the spread of COVID-19 in urban areas.

Geographical isolation (almost all visitors arrive by air) and the delayed arrival of COVID-19 in the South Pacific did play some role in New Zealand's pandemic experience, in particular, in relation to policy learning from the Italian experience. Nevertheless, other factors have been identified as more critical. A 2020 Lancet study (Chaudhry et al. 2020) into the successful management of the pandemic identified three main factors all centered around political leadership; namely the speed of decision-making; the quality of communication, and the compliance of the population. These points were all the more critical when one considers the fragility of New Zealand's legal framework around public health, which was exposed early in the pandemic response. The New Zealand success in managing the COVID-19 pandemic can thus, largely, be attributed to the government's fast and decisive decision-making, its clear, consistent, and efficient communication with the population and the ability to foster a sense of citizenship/team to work together. Prime Minister Jacinda Ardern has, in particular, been a key element in providing leadership during the crisis.

This chapter explores New Zealand policy style and the importance of "public trust" in the state in national response to the COVID-19 pandemic over the period of January–November 2020. In order to do so, the first section provides an outline of New Zealand's legal context and policy style. "Overview of the Country's Policy Style" section considers the level of political trust in the government and health system. The final section aims to link the interactions between policy style and trust in the national response during COVID-19.

Overview of the Country's Policy Style

The policy style of New Zealand can be identified as "accommodative" (based on Chapter 1 in this book) characterized by a combination of moderately low administrative capacity and reasonably high inclusiveness. We illustrate this classification by referring to constitutional as well as disaster management frameworks.

The Legal Context

New Zealand is a democratic constitutional monarchy, based on an uncodified constitutional model. In addition to New Zealand, only the United Kingdom and Israel have a so-called "unwritten constitution." In fact, the term "unwritten" is misleading as the constitution is made of a large number of statutes and other documents providing the framework for New Zealand's map of power. This framework sits upon three constitutional pillars, The Treaty of Waitangi | Te

Tiriti o Waitangi (1840), the Rule of Law, and Parliamentary Sovereignty. Te Tiriti o Waitangi is the founding document of Aotearoa | New Zealand. It establishes the legitimacy and limits of government in New Zealand as well as the relationship with the indigenous Māori population. While it remains, "simply the most important document in New Zealand's history" (Cooke 1990), its role within the constitution remains contentious. In particular, its relationship with Parliamentary Sovereignty, an English constitutional principle, inherited from the United Kingdom's colonial influence, remains problematic. The exact nature and content of the Rule of Law is also open to debate. As a consequence, although the traditional view of the New Zealand constitutional model places Parliament at the apex, more recent academic and judicial development has challenged this orthodoxy, particularly as it is the Executive rather than the Legislature that exercises such authority in practical terms.

For this reason, the judiciary, in particular, has been reluctant to allow legislation to trample upon what are seen as constitutional statutes (e.g., the Constitution Act 1986 or the New Zealand Bill of Rights Act 1990). In addition, courts even considered incorporating supreme constitutional principles in the concept of the Rule of Law, as a means of limiting Parliamentary power (*Taylor v New Zealand Poultry Board* 1984). This has led to courts stretching statutory interpretation to avoid Parliamentary attempts to overrule these "constitutional" statutes (*R v Pora* 2001). Nonetheless, despite these caveats, New Zealand Parliamentary power is atypical, in that it provides the tools for swift legislative change and, in practice, a high degree of discretionary power when an executive wishes to use it. This characteristic is particularly relevant when New Zealand deals with disasters and emergencies.

This extensive power of Parliament needs to be understood in the context of New Zealand's wider constitutional and political framework. New Zealand is a Parliamentary democracy, and all Ministers must be Members of Parliament. The executive and legislature are thus fused. When this is combined with New Zealand's unicameral Parliamentary model and a strong party system, the result is an extremely weak separation of powers where the executive dominates the New Zealand political landscape.

This level of Executive power, once described as "Unbridled Power" (Palmer 1979), was further enhanced by the "First Past the Post" (constituency based) voting system. However, in order to mitigate such excess, a proportional representation system of voting was introduced in 1996, which, in turn, led to coalition government becoming the norm. Nevertheless, the country is characterized by the continued dominance of two major parties (Labour and National), which means that one of them is always the dominant partner in any coalition arrangement. Interestingly, despite the reluctance of the New Zealand electorate to grant majorities to single parties since 1996, Labour achieved this feat in 2020 in the wake of the COVID-19 response.

The ability of the executive to, largely, control Parliament is further strengthened in a time of emergency (or disaster) by the high level of trust most New

Zealanders have in their government in comparison with many overseas examples (Chapple and Pricket 2019). Typically, this means that the opposition finds it politically difficult to challenge the actions of the executive during a disaster. This phenomenon was observed in two recent major (seismic) events. In the wake of the Canterbury earthquake sequence of 2010/2011 and the Hurunui/Kaikoura earthquake of 2016, the opposition Labour Party supported special legislation but voiced concerns over the adoption of extraordinary and wide-ranging executive powers included within it (with only minority parties opposed). It was rewarded by a fall in popularity amongst the electorate (and defeat in the general election of 2011). This occurred again in 2020, when the then leader of the (National Party) opposition, Simon Bridges, adopted a robust critical stance as the lockdown progressed. His behavior was perceived as overly political, ultimately leading to a collapse in public support for his party and an internal party coup resulting in his replacement.

Interestingly, the ability of the government of the day to introduce bespoke legislation to cope with the requirements of any particular disaster is actually baked into the current Disaster Risk Management (DRM) framework. As a consequence of the serial abuse by successive governments of two poorly written generic emergency statutes (the Public Safety Conservation Act 1932 and the Economic Stabilisation Act 1947), a reformist Labour Government was elected to repeal them in 1987. However, rather than replacing them, the government of the time chose instead to rely upon a narrow set of existing sectoral emergency laws to provide for the provision of exceptional powers in "emergency situations." This decision was supported by work undertaken by Law Commission, led by Justice Keith, which advocated for creating additional exceptional legislation when required. Such legislation would require the support of Parliament, which, as already explored, is likely to be provided at a time of crisis. This reliance upon "bespoke" emergency legislation, coupled with a system of Parliamentary Sovereignty, means that their relationship with Human Rights and Constitutional protections is not always harmonious. In addition, connections between the state and local communities are often poor (Hopkins 2016).

Disaster Management in New Zealand

New Zealand is a society which is vulnerable to many hazards and as a result is well attuned to emergencies and disasters. The most common hazard is meteorological, although in terms of economic loss, geological events (both seismic and volcanic) provide the higher risk. As with most developed countries, the hazards posed by human pathogens have not been considered as a particular risk (notwithstanding that Aotearoa | New Zealand experienced a measles epidemic as recently as 2019). For this reason, New Zealand's response mechanisms and legal framework tend to focus on geological hazards, and when health hazards are considered, they are dealt with separately.

The overarching DRM law, which provides for generic emergency powers, is the Civil Defence and Emergency Management Act 2002 (CDEM). This provides for the declaration of a State of Emergency and the provision of executive powers to be exercised by the Director of Civil Defence (or delegate). This act was utilized in the COVID-19 response and the early stages of the recovery process but was largely side-lined as the pandemic progressed. Instead, two sector-specific acts provided the basis for the government's lockdown decisions. These were the Health Act 1956 (HA) and, to a lesser extent, the Epidemic Preparedness Act 2006 (EPA). The Health Act, which dates back to the 1950s, contains sections designed to deal with the control of infectious diseases when an epidemic notice is in force (or a state of emergency).

The Health Act, in particular, empowers the Director of Health to utilize their discretion to control social behaviors as a means of containing a "notifiable disease" (Health Act 1956, Part 3). These powers are extensive but quite narrowly defined and, despite recent amendments, remain focused on measures required to contain known infectious diseases such as measles and influenza. This focus reflects the origin of the act (and the public health system generally) which can be traced back to New Zealand's disastrous handling of the influenza epidemic of 1918/1919.

The EPA by contrast is a modern piece of legislation developed specifically to address the requirements of a modern pandemic and supports the executive with the power to alter primary legislation, in response to such an event. However, the act is primarily limited to the technical and administrative aspects of legislation rather than providing the executive with the ability to undertake major legislative change. Nevertheless, as explored above, New Zealand's constitutional model has allowed a practice of bespoke emergency legislation to develop, introduced to respond to disasters and emergencies in real time. This approach was utilized as part of the COVID-19 response (COVID-19 Public Health Response Act 2020), but importantly, not until after the initial seven-week lockdown had taken place. The pace with which the pandemic unfolded proved too fast even for New Zealand's infamously speedy legislative process.[5]

Within this legal framework, two officials emerge as key to the management of the public health emergencies in New Zealand. These are the Director of Civil Defence (under the CDEM Act) and the Director of Health (under the Health Act). However, emergency response and recovery require more than the narrow exceptional powers provided to these individuals. For this reason, they sit as part of a wider political National Security System. The key national coordination mechanism is the Officials Committee for Domestic and External Security Coordination (ODESC). As the name suggests, this system is heavily "security" influenced with a role for intelligence services. In practice, the small size of the National Emergency Management Agency means that there is no emergency management administrative infrastructure, with individual agencies being coordinated only at the Chief Executive level under ODESC. ODESC itself sits within the Department of Prime Minister and Cabinet (DPMC) and is chaired by its CEO. This coordinating body (which does not exercise decision-making authority) advises the Cabinet (and the External Relations and Security Committee when activated) and, most importantly, the Prime Minister. Importantly, for the discussion that follows, in the absence of systematic coordination and control mechanisms in the New Zealand model, the role of the Prime Minister is crucial to effective emergency management outside the limited framework envisaged by the current emergency and disaster law framework. Overall, the New Zealand model relies heavily on cooperation between political and administrative agents. Political leaders appear to be respectful and reliant upon the expertise of the civil service administration.

The result of this legislative and policy framework is a centralized policy framework around the management of emergencies and a fragmented legal framework around emergencies and disasters. This has consequences for the management of nationally significant disasters as consistently, the New Zealand government has struggled to manage within the existing legal framework (Kipp 2016). This has been evident particularly during the recovery stage of previous geological events, but in the COVID crisis example, the problems became evident much earlier. This weakness of the formal legal framework requires *ad hoc* management of disasters and the creation of new legal frameworks. Such models utilize the high administrative capacity of the New Zealand state but also often lack the enforcement or delivery mechanisms required to ensure policy delivery. In the COVID example, this created the impression of an "adversarial" model (with a strong role for the police), which, in reality, relied upon high levels of population compliance. The model also relied upon effective communication to ensure that the centrally driven policy of lockdown was policed by the population.

A High Level of Political Trust in Government and Health System

Governance in Aotearoa | New Zealand enjoys comparatively high levels of trust amongst the population, as reflected in a number of international comparator indicators. The Rule of Law index, for example, places New Zealand at seventh (out of 113 states surveyed) and first in the Asia-Pacific Region (World Justice Project 2020). This ranking is driven, at least partially, by the confidence shown in the restraints upon government recognized by the survey. In addition, New Zealand jealously guards its position at the top of the Corruption Perceptions Index (CPI) (Transparency International 2020). It is important to note that the CPI is a perception-based index, not a measure of actual corruption and thus reflects the generally positive way that governance is perceived in New Zealand. Domestic indicators tell a similar tale. Longitudinal research by Chapple and Prickett (2020) has shown consistently high (and increasing) levels of trust in New Zealand toward the government, particularly around its ability to deal with national problems (Chapple and Prickett 2020, 10). This latter indicator seems to be the most connected to emergency and disaster management and is perhaps the key to how the New Zealand government was able to navigate an effective COVID-19 response in the context of a problematic legal framework.

The role of such trust should not be underestimated in the context of long-term disaster management. The COVID crisis reflects a very different type of disaster event from that which Aotearoa | New Zealand has traditionally addressed, with an extremely long response phase, unlike that seen with recent volcanic, meteorological, or seismic events. In the latter example, the long process of recovery from the Canterbury earthquakes, undertaken with strong central direction and "bespoke" recovery legislation, saw a loss of trust in government institutions and eventual hostility toward the Canterbury Earthquake Recovery Authority (CERA). In contrast, the long response phase of the COVID crisis has not seen significant falls in government support and, in fact, led to the landslide victory of the Labour party in the 2020 election. The ability of this government to retain trust during this period has been key to the ongoing success of New Zealand's COVID response. Although starting from a high threshold, it would have been easy for poor decision-making to erode confidence in the government's competence and strategy. In fact, although a number of missteps did occur, the leadership of the Prime Minister, Jacinda Ardern, played a large role in retaining the trust needed to maintain the elimination policy during the whole of the pandemic.

Interactions between Policy Style and Trust in Implementing the National COVID-19 Response

High levels of trust in political leadership together with the ability to make quick, decisive, and bespoke decisions have undoubtedly contributed to the successful response in fighting the COVID-19 pandemic on the New Zealand territory. But it was the excellent communication skills from the political leadership that really made all the difference.

Communication

From a political point of view, New Zealand's success can be directly linked to Prime Minister Jacinda Ardern's handling of the pandemic, which has been considered a "masterclass in crisis leadership" (Wilson 2020; Gilby 2021). Ardern's excellent communication skills represent one of the most compelling elements of the New Zealand government's elimination strategy. Such communications were done often personally by the Prime Minister, during a daily briefing which occurred during the lockdown and until the alert level returned to Alert Level 1. This provided clear instructions on expected community behaviors; instructions that were followed by the vast majority of the population.

New Zealand and the rest of the world had previously taken notice of Ardern's communication skills. Prime Minister Jacinda Ardern has arguably disrupted traditional leadership and communication standards by firmly placing human values at the center of the decision-making process in times of crises. Ardern's governing style domestically and on the international scene have fed into global media attention on New Zealand; when she, for example, wore the Kahu huruhuru (Māori cloak) whilst pregnant at Buckingham Palace or when she brought her baby Neve to the United Nations. But, it was her ability to communicate with compassion with the victims of the terrorist attack on the Christchurch mosques, a year before the start of the pandemic, that was remarked as a strikingly different style of leadership. During that crisis, and in response to unimaginable horror, she has deliberately employed language of empathy instead of hate and messages of togetherness rather than the traditional reference to power, retribution, and division between "us and them." Kindness in this context has become a politically radical act, which has been replicated in the environment of the pandemic. Accordingly, communication during the COVID pandemic underscored the importance of the human values underpinning the government decisions and reminded the population to be kind and to act with humanity towards one another. In doing so, political leadership fostered a sense of togetherness and identity building for the population.

The government identified early the need for clear and effective communication with everyone. It required the country's entire population to understand the risk that the virus posed, as well as to prepare each individual to contribute to the response. An easy-to-understand and actionable strategy was therefore necessary. On March 21, 2020, days into the COVID crisis, the government designed and released a clear four-Alert Level system.[6] This provided people with a relatively clear sense of the urgency of the crisis as well as enabling a flexible, swift response to localized outbreaks.

In addition, communication was coordinated between political, administrative, and scientific agents. The substance of the government communication with the New Zealand population regarding COVID appeared to be in harmony with the scientific community and the civil service. In addition, communication was overall clear, consistent, and regular. The government quickly established a "Unite against COVID-19" website. During lockdown, Prime Minister Jacinda Ardern and Director General of Health Ashley Bloomfield held daily 1-pm press briefings, which the population followed assiduously, even receiving an IMDb page, with viewers rating it as their "favourite show of 2020" (Franks 2020). This far-reaching and comprehensive communication strategy drove strong public acceptance of the government response to the COVID pandemic.

National Response Plan

New Zealand's structural ability to respond to a crisis of this scale and type was always limited. In contrast to the political system, the New Zealand health system is highly decentralized. The role of the Ministry of Health is to oversee and to primarily act as a purchaser of services. The "system" is thus fractured and operates along classic New Public Management lines. It also suffers from a legacy of underfunding. As a result, the Ministry of Health faces significant and frequent challenges in providing effective oversight, something that makes it unsuitable for the management of operational matters such as emergency response. In addition, the operational backbone of the health-care system is highly decentralized. It is divided into 20 (partially elected) District Health

Boards (DHB) which deliver health services for their specific geographic area. Public Health is managed through 12 regional public health units charged with the regulation of communicable diseases. The units are owned by the DHBs, but many of their functions are undertaken under the direction of the Director General, particularly under the Health Act. This decentralization is a feature not only in the Health system but across government as a whole, and during a time of national crisis, it has resulted in significant communication and logistics problems (Cameron 2020) requiring the government to find an effective way to coordinate across its own agencies and departments. The disparate nature of New Zealand government, particularly in the field of health, is compounded by serious deficiencies in intensive care capacity driven by chronic underfunding. The result is a system incapable of coping with the requirements of a pandemic and which, according to the modeling discussed above, would soon become overwhelmed with severely ill patients.

In contrast to the administrative executive and specifically the health system, the political executive is relatively centralized in Aotearoa I New Zealand. This allows for swift, bespoke decision-making in emergency situations. The role of the Prime Minister is thus central to crisis response. Such a role for the central government, and particularly the Prime Minister, is thus baked into the New Zealand model. In this particular crisis, faced with a weakened and decentralized health system unsuited to emergency response, this political centralization became crucial. However, this level of centralized executive power and ease of decision-making does not always lead to positive outcomes, although it is an inevitable feature of New Zealand emergency and disaster response (Kipp 2016). In the COVID-19 example, the deficiencies of the health system placed the Prime Minister (and the wider coalition government) in the crucial position of managing a successful response. Poor decision-making at this level would not have been ameliorated by the administrative state, given its inherent weakness, particularly in the field of health. The ability of New Zealand to cope with the COVID-19 emergency (and ensuing disaster) would likely depend upon the decisions of the Prime Minister.

Ardern's response, and that of the government as a whole, proved successful, but it is important to note that in the early days of the pandemic, the approach taken did not have universal support. However, the coalition government (led personally by the Prime Minister) developed a policy response driven by three key principles, which have been enduring throughout the crisis. First and very importantly, New Zealand's response has, uncompromisingly, been based on the importance of community and the value of human life. No life has been seen to be expendable, and there has been little discussion of "cost benefit" analysis around lives and health. Second, while the decision-making has been politically centralized, it has largely followed the advice of the scientific community (at least at the political level), something that has clearly been assisted in Director of Health at the time of the crisis being a globally acknowledged Public Health expert. Finally, citizens have been considered to be an integral part of the response, and the messaging has consistently emphasized that the political leadership is merely an extension of New Zealand's community response. We are the team of "5 million."

Decisions Laden with Human Values Which Ultimately Benefits the Economy

Faced with the fast spreading of the COVID-19 virus in January 2020, New Zealand's early response first followed its existing national pandemic plan, which was primarily based upon influenza. However, informed by strong, science-based advocacy,[7] national leaders decisively switched from a mitigation strategy ("flatten the curve") (Backer, Wilson, and Blakely 2020) to an elimination strategy in the early part of 2020. From the beginning of the pandemic, governments around the world considered two main policy options: a hard, lockdown strategy which appeared to be successful in China and Taiwan (O'Connor et al. 2021) or a "softer" epidemic suppression approach. The "hard" approach had significant impacts upon individual freedoms and economic activity (at least in the short term), while the "softer" approach, although appearing to limit the impact upon economic and personal lives, came with the risk of higher loss of life and greater health impacts. In effect, the latter claimed to find a "balance" between health, economics, and personal liberty. However, the decision was made very early by Prime Minister Ardern (and her coalition government) that New Zealand would not be going down the management route. "That was a values-based decision … [Ardern] made it very clear that we would be protecting the lives and health of New Zealanders from the get-go, and that was non-negotiable" (Ian Town, Chief Science Adviser at the Ministry of Health cited in Cameron 2020, 9).

The elimination strategy raised economic concerns. It was argued that lockdowns would have an intolerable economic impact that would dwarf any positive impact on citizens' health. This argument was based upon a misconception of the nature of the economy and the market. This failed to appreciate their socially constructed nature and the impact that social dislocation would have upon them (Masselot 2019). Because of this, many believed that an elimination strategy would sacrifice the economy and result in longer-term hardship and even higher negative health impacts. In hindsight, this proved to be fundamentally wrong and the countries which have applied elimination strategies have suffered lower economic impacts than those that undertook a policy of suppression (Baker, Wilson, and Blakely 2020).

In addition, elimination strategies based upon the value of human life not only avoid overwhelming hospitals (and thus keep the wider health system functioning) but also prevent the long-term effects of the virus even after mild infections (Lancet 2020). The reality is that public health, care, and the economy are intrinsically linked (Caracciolo di Torella and Masselot 2020), which has been confirmed by the early recovery of the New Zealand economy (Smyth 2020).

Moreover, lockdowns around the world have contributed to a rise in gender-based violence (Ince Yenilmez 2020) and negatively impacted individuals' mental health and wellbeing (Collinson 2020). The New Zealand's hard but short lockdown, focused upon the value of human life, compared to other countries, which have used milder and multiple lockdowns, has meant that these additional social effects have been limited.

Stringency of Measures based on Science and Administrative Capability

Measures taken by the New Zealand government in response to COVID-19 have been stringent but generally time-limited. Importantly, the measures have been based on the recommendation of the scientific community and a reflection of New Zealand's capacity to manage epidemics.

Lockdown

In sharp contrast to other Western countries, the New Zealand government decided to "go hard and early" (Jamieson 2020) once the consequences of uncontained spread were understood. Amid increasing concerns that the virus would spread quickly at large events, the government banned all gatherings of 500 or more people on 16 March and showed the seriousness of the situation by canceling the national remembrance service scheduled for the first anniversary of the mosque attacks in Christchurch. This measure was the first real signal from the government of the gravity of the COVID-19 threat.

The government's decision to move rapidly from "Alert Level 2" to "Alert Level 4" saw the sharp establishment of an extreme level of restriction, unmatched in New Zealand's history (the level of restrictions imposed exceeded even the polio restrictions of the 1940s). The decision to enter into an unprecedented national quarantine, which was amongst the tightest in the world, was crucial to the level of success that New Zealand has achieved. This makes it all the more surprising that the weaknesses that the legal framework suffered from did not impede the policy's ultimate success. Instead, a combination of excellent leadership and a degree of good fortune assisted New Zealand's efforts.

The measures required New Zealanders to be confined to their homes or to short walks in their neighborhood and for shops or businesses to open only with specific authorization. In the main, this was not granted. Only truly essential suppliers (specified supermarkets, fuel outlets, and medical services) were allowed to remain open, under restrictions. These measures represented one of the most restrictive lockdowns seen in the democratic world.

Robust Test and Contact-Tracing System

Following the recommendations of the WHO to test, trace, and isolate, the government began to establish a robust test and contact-tracing system, which utilized relatively traditional techniques. Technology was not a major feature of the system, with tracers instead conducting interviews with the person to identify where they had been and with whom they had been in contact. All these individuals were then contacted and tested, with further places of interest identified. This labor-intensive model was quickly overwhelmed as the number of cases rose during the first week of lockdown. As a result, the Ministry of Health recruited over 200 new staff to work in a new contact-tracing center and centralize the data. Despite the additional resources, the system continued to struggle. As a consequence, the ministry commissioned Dr. Ayesha Verall, an infectious-diseases physician and researcher with expertise in tuberculosis and international health to review the process. The conclusions of her review were adopted by the end of May 2020. However, although the Ministry of Health released a mobile App, the NZ COVID tracer which users could use as a digital diary, as recommended by Dr. Verall, the New Zealand response has remained rather "low tech." This has had consequences for the continued approach to the pandemic, explored below (O'Connor et al. 2021).

Quarantine at the Border

Alongside the hard and short lockdown, New Zealand adopted early and strict border control measures, which have largely prevented the unrestrained re-entry of the virus into the community. As the COVID-19 pandemic emerged overseas, and with only 20 cases confirmed in the country, the New Zealand government implemented strict travel restrictions. After the failure of the attempt to require travelers to self-quarantine, the government closed the border to non-residents on March 18, effective within a two-day window. A compulsory two-week quarantine requirement was established at managed isolation facilities[8] to ensure that there were no further community outbreaks. Although this has not been 100% effective, the quarantine system has remained the cornerstone of the ongoing New Zealand response. As New Zealand continues to rely upon a low-tech model of contact-tracing, should a community outbreak occur, the only response is for citywide lockdowns and nationwide restrictions. These measures reduce the risk of wider spread and allow the contact-tracing system time to isolate the outbreak. Such a model, while effective, requires community acceptance of its necessity. It is this ability to keep the "team of 5 million" together that has been crucial in retaining community acceptance of the legal framework. Without this acceptance, the legal framework underpinning the continued successful New Zealand response to COVID-19 would fail.

Inclusivity of Citizens: Rallying the "Team of 5 Million"

Prime Minister Ardern has fostered the idea of togetherness and unity crystallized in the idea of the "team of 5 million" (Ardern 2020) who were urged to make short-term sacrifice of personal freedoms for the long-term good of their country. The government's far-reaching, regular, and consistent messaging has encouraged citizens to work collectively, fostering national unity and pride around a common goal of defeating the virus. Clear, consistent information ensured that everyone was informed about what needed to be done to save lives and ultimately to eliminate the virus on the territory. This has contributed to a strong public acceptance of the government strategy and overall general compliance with control measures (Cameron 2020).

Although, the virus was first eliminated in May 2020, resurgence has occurred several times and has led to frustration amongst the community around breaches in the MIQ model. Despite this, the response of the community has generally been compliant when such outbreaks have occurred. This messaging of "the team" has been crucial to ensuring such compliance and ensuring that the lockdowns end swiftly. However, "the team" messaging has been notably less successful outside of outbreaks with widespread complacency around the use of the App and mask-wearing requirements (on public transport) are regularly ignored. It has also led to personal attacks on individuals and communities perceived not to be supporting the rest of "the team" (Weekes 2021).

As a consequence of this approach and the community acceptance of the need for lockdowns, challenges to government decisions have been limited. Most have been carefully couched to not undermine the overall effort of the "team of 5 million." A few critical voices were raised but, at least in the early part of the lockdown, most remained constructive. This acceptance has translated into self-policing of the lockdown measures and other restrictions. During the Alert Level 4 lockdown, very few outlets opened without permission and those that did received criticism online and suffered reputational damage. The Police had to establish dedicated procedures for those reporting breaches of the lockdown to avoid their 111 emergency lines being overwhelmed.

Inclusion and legitimacy are key to effective law, particularly in liberal democracies. The lockdown gained legitimacy because of the trust that New Zealanders have in their public authorities and the actions of a Prime Minister and Director General of Health who were able to build upon it. Such trust was essential to enforcement of such restrictive measures. Few legal challenges were raised against these measures, given the widespread legitimacy that they enjoyed and the very obvious nature of the emergency. The New Zealand experience of the COVID-19 lockdown confirms that law is as much about legitimacy as it is legality and crucial to the former is the element of trust.

Recovery Plans

Although the COVID-19 crisis is often styled as a health disaster, in practice, this is not the case in New Zealand. Although the hazard is health-related, New Zealand's successful elimination strategy has meant that the disaster itself is economic and social. This reality was recognized early by the government, and compensation for stringent lockdown measures adopted has formed a crucial part of the overall response. A wide-ranging economic package was therefore adopted to support citizens who endured economic and social disadvantages during lockdown. This came in diverse forms, crucial to retain community support for the lockdown and emphasizing the community-focused nature of the government's elimination strategy. For example, the Winter Energy Payment was doubled during lockdown, a COVID-19 Income Relief Payment was introduced, and rent increases and evictions were prohibited for six months. In addition, partnerships were established with local organizations to support and finance the housing of homeless people during the period of lockdown (Corlett 2020). However, the largest economic support came in the form of a wage subsidy scheme allocated to finance the wages of employees of business that lost revenues due to the pandemic. To be eligible, businesses had to have lost over 30% of their revenue in comparison to the previous year; to keep their staff employed; to pay their staff at least 80% of their usual salary but not under the minimum wage; and the business had to pass on the full amount of the subsidy to their employees. The initial package of NZD5 billion grew to NZD13 billion, and the original period of 12 weeks was extended to another 12 weeks as well, as re-used in the following local lockdowns in September 2020 and February/March 2021.

In addition, two financial supports have been adopted to respectively bolster and enhance employment rate on a longer-term basis and to combat violence against women. First, in response to the economic fallout following COVID-19, the Aotearoa | New Zealand government announced a NZD 50 billion fund to rescue the economy and bring the unemployment rate back up down to 4.2% within two years. In particular, the government has invested NZD 3.3 billion into infrastructure projects, which are to be fast-tracked under emergency legislation (Logan 2020). This initiative, termed the "Shovel-Ready Projects," aims to create jobs by stimulating the workforce, in particular, the construction industry, and by supporting the broader community. However, this particular recovery initiative has been criticized for inadequately providing gendered responses in situations of crisis and urgency (Hayes and Masselot 2020).

Second, the COVID-19 government response has included legal and budgetary provisions toward tackling increased violence against women resulting from lockdown. Unlike the economic response, this initiative builds on existing strategies that place gender at the center of the policy design. Building on the Domestic Violence Victims' Protection Act, adopted in 2018, to help victims of violence remain in employment and find a way out of violence (NZ Law Society 2018; Masselot 2020), the government has allocated substantive funding toward the support of services for victims or survivors of family violence (Ministry of Social Development 2020). The package includes services for perpetrators and provides a long-term approach to ensure safer and healthier homes (Beehive 2020). These legal and budgetary initiatives aim to not only provide women with the essential support needed but also contribute to a reduction of family and sexual violence. The allocation of funds toward the issue of domestic violence is especially significant in this period of economic crisis as it aims to aid women's recovery from the mental and physical effects of violence, enabling them to gain independence and get back on their feet. In a time of economic uncertainty, it is important that victims of family violence are supported in the employment field to ensure that they are not faced with compounded disadvantages such as loss of hours or redundancy.

These financial support mechanisms have not been without their problems, with the auditor general in particular expressing a degree of concern around potential abuse of the government's largess. There have also been a number of controversies around large companies accepting financial compensation from the government while posting significant profits. This has led to reputational damage to the companies concerned, and a number have been quick to return money that the public perceives as unfairly received. However, both the coalition government and the Labour government that succeeded it have clearly been of the view that economic risk outweighed any risk that some companies would abuse the system for their own gain. This approach looks to have been justified, as the "team of 5 million" appears still to be holding firm, as the arrival of vaccines in New Zealand herald, if not the beginning of the end, then at least the end of the beginning.

Conclusion

Overall, it can be asserted that New Zealand's higher level of trust in public officials (including both the government and health practitioners) provided a basis for the delivery of a pandemic response that it was ill-prepared for. This level of trust allowed the central government, led by the Prime Minister, to bridge the gaps in the legal, administrative, and health systems which left Aotearoa | New Zealand vulnerable to novel coronavirus pandemics (and other disasters).

This trust was not misplaced, and despite the odd misstep, the New Zealand governments' response has led to widespread acceptance of the unprecedented restrictions placed upon its citizens. Excellent communication from Prime Minister Ardern to the community fostered the idea of a team effort that allowed for the mitigation of structural weaknesses, in particular, the vulnerability of the health system. Although decision-making was centralized, it had strong inclusive flavors which itself fed back into an enhanced legitimacy of, and trust in, the decision-making power of the leadership. The proof of this was evidenced in Labour's astonishing electoral victory in November 2020. New Zealand thus fits into the hypothesis where there is low administrative policy capacity, high inclusiveness, and high trust can compensate for structural deficiencies through centripetal response plans. The government's decision to work as a "team" in-stilled a level of widespread national and community pride in the response which has sustained it during the pandemic thus far and allowed New Zealand to over-come systemic vulnerability. Although this approach has a concerning reliance upon individuals to deliver and act upon the "team" rhetoric, it has nevertheless served New Zealand well during the current epidemic. This model may not be transferrable to future disasters and pandemics, given the inherent systemic weaknesses that exist beneath it, but in the present situation, few kiwis would have it any other way.

Acknowledgment

The authors wish to acknowledge the financial support of QuakeCoRE (the New Zealand Centre for Earthquake Resilience) and the academic support of colleagues in LEAD (The Institute of Law Emergencies and Disasters) at the University of Canterbury in preparing this chapter.

Notes

1 New Zealand has adopted a Four-Level COVID-19 Alert System (https://covid19. govt.nz/). Each Alert Level tells people what measure they need to take. At Alert Level 1, individuals should stay home if they are unwell, wear face covering on public transport, maintain good hygiene, and keep track of their movement through the COVID tracer App or manually. In contrast, at Alert Level 4, personal freedom can be restricted: people are instructed to stay home in their bubble; travel is severely limited across the country; all gatherings are cancelled, and all public venues are closed; businesses are closed except for essential services (e.g., supermarkets, pharmacies, clinics, petrol stations, and lifeline utilities); educational facilities are closed; rationing of supplies and requisitioning of facilities are possible; healthcare services are reprioritized. At all Alert Levels, there are stringent border restrictions including health screening and testing for almost all arrivals and managed isolation or quarantine for anyone who is not travelling quarantine-free.
2 As of February 2021, the total number of persons who have died of COVID-19 in New Zealand is 26.
3 On March 24, 2021, the New Zealand government announced quarantine-free travel from Niue, which was followed by agreements with Australia (April 18, 2021) and the Cook Islands (May 17, 2021). The Australian arrangement has been suspended several times due to COVID-19 outbreaks in various Australian states.
4 The population density in New Zealand is 18 per km^2.
5 Geoffrey Palmer famously described New Zealand's Parliament as the "fastest legislature in the west" (Palmer 1979).
6 https://covid19.govt.nz/alert-system/about-the-alert-system/.
7 The government consulted a range of experts in the civil service, the administration, and the Universities.
8 https://www.miq.govt.nz/.

References

Ardern, Jacinda 2020. April 21st. Press Conference.
Baker, Michael G., Amanda Kvalsvig, Ayesha J. Verrall, Lucy Telfar-Barnard, and Nick Wilson. 2020a. "New Zealand's elimination strategy for the COVID-19 pandemic and what is required to make it work." *The New Zealand Medical Journal (Online)* 133 (1512): 10–14.
Baker, Michael G., Nick Wilson, and Andrew Anglemyer. 2020b. "Successful elimination of Covid-19 transmission in New Zealand." *New England Journal of Medicine* 383 (8): e56.

Baker, Michael G., Nick Wilson, and Tony Blakely. 2020. "Elimination could be the optimal response strategy for covid-19 and other emerging pandemic diseases." *British Medical Journal* 371–375.

Beehive. 2020. *Next steps to end family and sexual violence: Budget 2020.* At https://www.beehive.govt.nz/release/next-steps-end-family-and-sexual-violence-budget-2020

Blainey, Geoffrey. 1966. *The tyranny of distance: How distance shaped Australia's history.* London: MacMillan.

Blair Cameron. 2020. "Captaining a Team of 5 Million: New Zealand Beats Back Covid-19, March –June 2020." Innovations for Successful Societies, Princeton University. At https://successfulsocieties.princeton.edu/sites/successfulsocieties/files/NewZealand_COVID_FInal.pdf

Caracciolo di Torella Euegenia., and Annick. Masselot. 2020. *Caring responsibility in EU law and policy: Who cares?* Oxon: Routledge.

Chapple, Simon., and Kate. Prickett. 2019. *Who do we Trust in New Zealand? 2016 to 2019*, Institute for Governance and Policy Studies, Victoria University of Wellington. At https://www.wgtn.ac.nz/__data/assets/pdf_file/0011/1762562/trust-publication-2019.pdf

Chaudhry, Rabail, George Dranitsaris, Talha Mubashir, Justyna Bartoszko, and Sheila Riazi. 2020. "A country level analysis measuring the impact of government actions, country preparedness and socioeconomic factors on COVID-19 mortality and related health outcomes." *EClinicalMedicine* 25: 100464.

Collinson, Anna. 2020. "Covid: Lockdown had 'major impact' on mental health." BBC News 21 October. At https://www.bbc.com/news/health-54616688

Cooke, Robin. 1990–91. "Introduction." *New Zealand Universities Law Review* 14 (1): 1–8.

Corlett, Eva. 2020. "Covid-19 lockdown: Nearly 1000 motel units available for homeless." *New Zealand Herald*, April 12. At https://www.nzherald.co.nz/nz/news/article.cfm?c_id=1&objectid=12324268

Dunstan, Kim. 2020. "About 250,000 visitors in New Zealand." Statistic New Zealand, 25 March. At https://www.stats.govt.nz/news/about-250000-visitors-in-new-zealand

Franks, Josephine. 2020. "IMDb users review New Zealand's coronavirus daily briefing: 'Favourite show of 2020'." 13 August. At https://www.stuff.co.nz/entertainment/122432961/imdb-users-review-new-zealands-coronavirus-daily-briefing-favourite-show-of-2020?rm=a

Gilby, Lynda. 2021. "New Zealand beat Covid-19 without a vaccine: this is how they did it." *The Loop ECRP's Political Science Blog.* At https://theloop.ecpr.eu/the-covid-19-pandemic-how-new-zealand-got-the-response-right/?fbclid=IwAR1AKzTJTnuyWBSWEyeQCtBS-gnJt-PvoiHcC0l8WE7hbQ3nP8KLDBvVszI

Global Health Security Index. 2019. At https://www.ghsindex.org/wp-content/uploads/2019/10/2019-Global-Health-Security-Index.pdf

Health and Disability System Review. 2020, May. *Health and Disability System Review – Final Report – Pūrongo Whakamutunga.* Wellington: HDSR. At www.systemreview.health.govt.nz/final-report.

Hopkins, W. John 2020. "Smoke, Mirrors and Legal Uncertainty: The Rights and Wrongs of New Zealand's CoVID-19 Response" in *Governing the Crisis: Law, Human Rights and COVID-19* 2021, ed. Kirchner, Stefan 232–248. Lit verlag: Münster.

Hopkins, W. John 2016. "The First Victim—Administrative Law and Natural Disasters." *New Zealand Law Review* 23 (1): 189–211.

Ince Yenilmez, Meltem. 2020. "The Covid-19 pandemic and the struggle to tackle gender-based violence." *The Journal of Adult Protection* 22 (6): 391–99.

Jamieson, Thomas. 2020. "Go hard, go early: Preliminary lessons Rom New Zealand's response to COVID-19." *The American Review of Public Administration* 50 (6–7): 598–605.

Kipp, Robert. 2016. "From cold war to Canterbury: The New Zealand experience in emergency management." PhD Thesis, University of Canterbury.

Lancet, The. 2020. "Facing up to long COVID." *Lancet (London, England)* 396 (10266): 1861.

Logan, Tom. 2020. "'Shovel-ready' projects ignore important aspects of community resilience." The Conversation. At https://www.canterbury.ac.nz/news/2020/shovel-ready-projects-ignore-important-aspects-of-community-resilience.html

Masselot, Annick. 2019. "Visions for gender equality post-2020: How to improve the interaction between legal instruments (EU acquis) and policy-making (communication, funding programme, European semester)?" in *New Visions for Gender Equality 2019*, eds. Niall Crowley & Silvia Sansonetti, 9–13. SAAGE –Scientific Analysis and Advice on Gender Equality in EU. Luxembourg: Publications Office of the European Union.

Masselot, Annick 2020. "Employment law." *New Zealand Law Review* 2 (21): 257–77.

Masselot, Annick, and Maria Hayes. 2020. "Exposing gender inequalities: Impacts of Covid-19 on Aotearoa | New Zealand employment." *New Zealand Journal of Employment Relations* 45 (2): 57–69.

Ministry of Social Development. 2020. *Funding for family violence services through Budget 2020*. At https://www.msd.govt.nz/about-msd-and-our-work/newsroom/2020/funding-for-family-violence-services-through-budget-20.html

New Zealand Law Society. 2018. *Domestic violence victim protection bill passes*. At https://www.lawsociety.org.nz/news/legal-news/domestic-violence-victim-protection-bill-passes/

O'Connor, Helen, W. John Hopkins, and David Johnston. 2021. "For the greater good? Data and disasters in a post-COVID world." *Journal of the Royal Society of New Zealand* DOI: 10.1080/03036758.2021.1900297.

Palmer, Geoffrey 1979. *Unbridled power? An interpretation of New Zealand's constitution and government*. Wellington: Oxford University Press.

Peters, B. Guy. (2015). "Policy capacity in public administration." *Policy and Society* 34 (3–4): 219–28.

Smyth, Jamie 2020. "New Zealand's 'go hard and early' Covid policy reaps economic rewards." *The Financial Times* 17 December. At https://www.ft.com/content/b8c4ab58-99db-4af2-9449-5fd70a9235ce

Statistics New Zealand. 2018. "Census ethnic group summaries." At https://www.stats.govt.nz/tools/2018-census-ethnic-group-summaries

Statistics New Zealand. 2020. "Māori population estimates: At 30 June 2020." 17 November. At https://www.stats.govt.nz/information-releases/maori-population-estimates-at-30-june-2020

Transparency International. 2020. "Corruption perceptions index." At https://www.transparency.org/en/cpi/2020/index/nzl

United Nations. 2018 "Revision of World Urbanization Prospects" *United Nations: New York, NY, USA* (2018) at https://www.un.org/development/desa/publications/2018-revision-of-world-urbanization-prospects.html.

Weekes, John 2021. "Covid 19 coronavirus: Anger at breach, fears about 'conspiracy theories' during lockdown." *New Zealand Herald*, 28th February 2021. At https://www.nzherald.co.nz/nz/covid-19-coronavirus-anger-at-breach-fears-about-conspiracy-theories-during-lockdown/FD37KPUOA7AN3FVCCFMJMSJFHI/

Wilson, Suze. 2020. "Three reasons why Jacinda Ardern's coronavirus response has been a masterclass in crisis leadership, The Conversation." At https://theconversation.com/three-reasons-why-jacinda-arderns-coronavirus-response-has-been-a-masterclass-in-crisis-leadership-135541

World justice project. 2020. At https://worldjusticeproject.org/our-work/research-and-data/wjp-rule-law-index-2020

Cases

R v Pora [2001] 2 NZLR 37 (CA).

Taylor v New Zealand Poultry Board [1984] 1 NZLR 394.

4
Centrifugal Responses

9

OF "HERD IMMUNITY" AND INOCULATION INVESTMENT

The British Response to COVID-19

Theofanis Exadaktylos

Two news stories dominated headlines in the United Kingdom (UK) on January 31, 2020. The first was the final day of Britain as a European Union (EU) member state and the end of the transition period following the formal withdrawal of the country from the EU. The second was the return of a half-empty flight from Wuhan evacuating British citizens and their families from the new coronavirus-hit Chinese province. The plane landed in the Midlands, and six buses with 83 evacuees were paraded on their way to a quarantine facility at the Wirral near Milton Keynes.[1] These people were about to spend the next two weeks isolated to avoid spreading the new coronavirus in Britain. This chapter explores the British government response as the new coronavirus started spreading in Europe and in Britain and as the pandemic evolved since February 2020 and into spring of 2021.

The chapter builds on the arguments around the interaction of policy styles with trust to propose that the overall response of the UK was in line with its adversarial policy style. In conjunction with lower levels of trust in government, the style led to a centrifugal approach that first sought to react to the information influx and then calculate the political costs. The aim was to avoid taking full responsibility of the management of the crisis by diffusing decision-making to different executive authorities around the country, depoliticize experts, and underscore people's 'patriotic duty' and personal responsibility.

The chapter is organized as follows: The first section discusses the dominance of the Westminster model of policymaking and its relevance to policy styles. It continues with the analysis of the UK response to the pandemic in four periods: (a) the outbreak of the pandemic that led to the first national lockdown; (b) the easing of measures in light of the summer season; (c) the second national lockdown and the hope for an open Christmas season; and (d) the third national lockdown which took the country the longest as vaccination started to roll out

DOI: 10.4324/9781003137399-13

leading to the announced roadmap for a return to 'normalcy.' The concluding section reflects on the variation observed in these periods which cover just about the first year of the pandemic in Britain. Centrifugalism can explain this variation including the many conflicting messages, the U-turns, and the final realization of how the measures should have worked. It should be noted that the chapter does not evaluate success or failure.

The Westminster Model of Policymaking Eroded?

The UK was once considered a prototype country for the application of the concept of 'policy style.' In some early conceptualizations, Richardson (1982) argued that policy decisions would converge toward that national style; that is, a policymaking paradigm, whereas styles would diverge across countries depending on national institutional settings. The UK was one of the first countries where this idea was academically applied to explain policymaking under standard operating procedures. Richardson and Jordan (1979) argued that, in the case of the UK, shared norms and understanding of both policy problems and solutions created established ways of doing things, and hence policy progress would be incremental rather than radical stepping carefully on previously established knowledge. Following the comparative benchmark across two dimensions (anticipatory vs. reactive and exclusive vs. inclusive) that Richardson had developed, the UK was classified as reactive and more top-down-driven and branded as the "Westminster" model. In other words, given the institutional arrangements in the UK, solutions were sought only when a problem emerged. Decisions were driven by a small centralized policymaking community based in Westminster with pre-existing consensus in the way of doing things between social partners and stakeholders. Nonetheless, during Thatcher's premiership in the 1980s, there was an intentional shift to increase exclusion of interest groups and concentrate power at the center of government. This effectively turned consensus-seeking from pluralism into plurality of voices.

Policy styles are not perennial, and new paradigms of policymaking can emerge given the presence of political entrepreneurship and ideological approaches to problem-solving. As New Labour came to power in 1997, it brought along changes in the administration of a seemingly unified nation. Responding to calls for greater autonomy of the home countries of the UK as well as long-term concerns over the decision-making dominance of Whitehall (and by extension, England), Tony Blair pushed a devolution strategy (Flinders 2010). Devolution started with Scotland in 1999 and progressively moved to Wales and Northern Ireland in variable degrees of self-government and different levels of executive capacities. This move inevitably created new centers of power and a need to revise the Westminster model back to a policy-community-oriented and consensus-seeking form for policies pertaining to the whole of the UK. Home countries would be able to set their own rules as they saw fit within specified limits. This way of doing things, of course, came with some additional resources and the desire of the home countries to acquire even more authority within their jurisdiction. Yet, even in this seemingly new policy style, the shadow of previous practices meant that high-level policy problems were still solved in a top-down manner, centrally at Whitehall (Jordan and Cairney 2013). Effectively, the backsliding toward the 'impositional end of the policy style spectrum' aligned with the traditional Westminster model (Richardson 2018a), combining the high administrative capacity of the British civil service and the low inclusion of different actors in decision-making. The shift was influenced largely by the return of the Conservative Party in power since 2010 and austerity-driven policy design (Richardson 2018b). The latter has been cited as the reason for the demise of the National Health Service (NHS); an issue which the chapter will discuss in a later section.

For the purposes of this book, policy capacity incorporates: (a) technical skills and competences; (b) adequate resources; and (c) political support to legitimate capacity. Higher autonomy, more expert staffing, and more cooperative aspirations indicate higher policy capacity. Inclusion covers the way interests are mediated. Inclusiveness (or absence of) affects adherence by the public, extent of political conflict, and effectiveness of policy especially in times of crisis. High inclusiveness can make measures more effective, whereas low inclusiveness may take away ownership of policies from social actors, that is, they have not been consulted or agreed with the policy. Considering policymaking practices since 2010, the UK can be firmly classified as having a policy style of higher administrative policy capacity with low inclusiveness of social actors and hence be branded as 'adversarial.' This is aided by the country's majoritarian/winner-takes-all tradition which has been effectuated further by the success of the Conservative Party over the last decade in securing working majorities in Parliament. The 'adversarial' nature of British policymaking creates clear winners and losers, and fingers can be pointed at easily when failure arises, and success can be easily credited too.

The nature of the relationships between policy actors and citizens builds on trust and hence, it is an important intervening dimension within policymaking. In times of crisis, trust is the factor that allows a leap of faith by citizens to experts but also to those in the leadership side of policymaking. In times of crisis, citizens' trust is skewed toward political leaders with a simple request: the government should be seen as doing something (Chatzopoulou and Exadaktylos 2021). Considering that the pandemic as a crisis is not a result of management failure by the government, being seen as responding to the crisis may be sufficient to elicit additional trust in political actors and increase the rally-round-the-flag effect.

Urgency and uncertainty of policymaking during a pandemic crisis shortens the time period citizens have to make sense of the world, to absorb information and make rational decisions. Trust, therefore, becomes an important factor in the way governments are able to handle such crises but also in the way that citizens perceive the effectiveness of government policy in that time frame. In the UK, for example, the longstanding reputation of the NHS and the appreciation shown to it by the British public create a strong mode of confidence in the abilities of the NHS, despite problems in delivering day-to-day services. On the other hand, in the past decade, trust in government has been declining in the UK, particularly in the aftermath of the 2016 decision to withdraw from the EU. Finally, there is relatively high social trust in Britain, that is, in the way people trust others. Hence, in the context of the pandemic, political trust will be diffused across the government (in protecting citizens), the health system (in saving lives), and the citizens (in terms of private responsibility). The expectation is one suggesting that while all eyes will fall on the government to provide 'trusted' direction, confronting the pandemic will truly fall on the competence of doctors and nurses, but also on the ability of the public to challenge the government and support each other.

Perhaps, this is the combination that helps understand better the rationale behind the UK government's response to the pandemic but also some of the framing of the decisions or the expectation on people's behavior and toleration for constraints. In addition, lack of clear guidance allows the government to diffuse responsibility and blame at a later stage. Therefore, the government will have centrifugal tendencies, rely on the personnel on the ground and on citizens' self-responsibility, and put up the experts as a smokescreen.

Evidence for this chapter mainly includes government documents related to the policy plans outlined in the context of the pandemic. The analysis of press releases, policy documents, government papers, and other communication memos at the national and local level allows a thorough examination of the policy style over time. The period under examination commences in February 2020, when cases started burgeoning in the UK and finishes in February 2021 when the plan to normalcy was announced. It incorporates three critical junctures to assess variation in the response: (a) relaxation of first lockdown (Summer 2020); (b) imposition of second lockdown (November 2020); and (c) third lockdown before Christmas coinciding with the inoculation program starting in Britain. There are two interesting charts that help in understanding further the UK response. Figure 9.1 juxtaposes the recording of daily cases and the decision to increase or decrease restrictions. Figure 9.2 gives the same story but from the point of view of the daily recorded deaths. This seems to be an even more accurate picture linking deaths with decision-making (Figures 9.1 and 9.2).

From 'Herd Immunity' to a Lockdown: British Centrifugalism

The UK found itself entangled in the global outbreak of the pandemic just few weeks following its departure from the EU (January 31, 2020). Following a turbulent period as a result of the UK's EU Referendum, the new Conservative government under the leadership of Boris Johnson had promised stability with a firm hand on Brexit and a so-called "end to austerity" (Atkinson 2019). Nonetheless, the main criticism after almost ten years of Conservative governments and a stark financial austerity program was that health inequalities had widened in the UK, and the health of the nation had deteriorated, with life expectancy

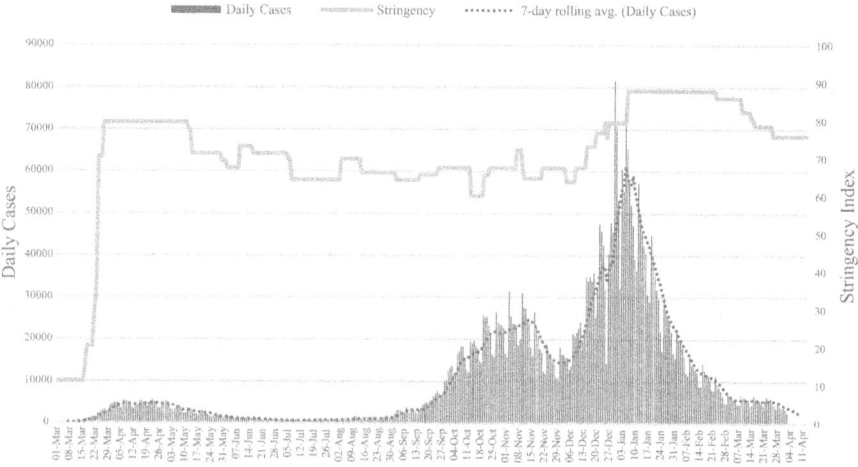

FIGURE 9.1   Daily Cases Versus Stringency of Measures.

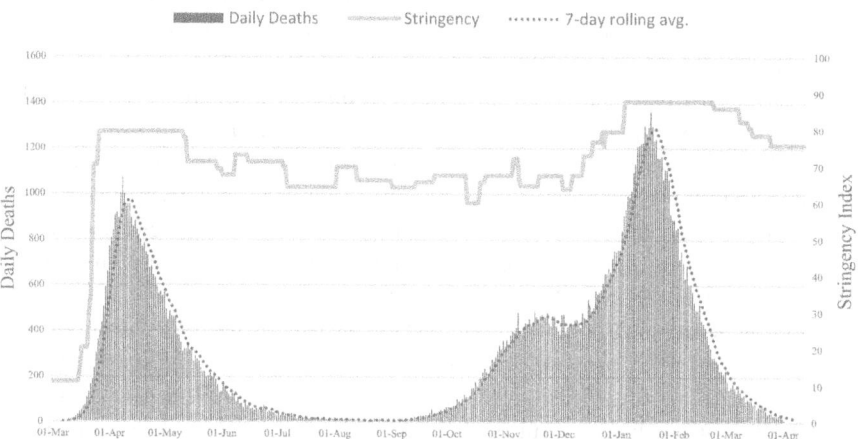

FIGURE 9.2   Daily Recorded Deaths Versus Stringency of Measures.

having stalled for the first time since 1900 (Iacobucci 2020). In a press conference on February 25, 2020, Professor Sir Michael Marmot discussing the review of his 2010 Marmot Report commented that austerity had taken a 'significant toll' on equality and health, arguing that England had lost a decade and had 'made a series of wrong decisions in 2010 that have contributed to this' (Bodkin 2020).

By the end of February, the coronavirus pandemic was already knocking on the UK's door albeit with just nine confirmed cases (Public Health England (PHE) 2020), and while this report suggested that levels of preparation in Britain had to be ramped up, the government was projecting a message of protection measures based on personal hygiene and traveling restrictions to and from the worst-affected countries in the world. The extent and evolution of the pandemic in the rest of Europe was raising alert. The NHS was based on strong medical expertise of staff and technological capabilities, but it was identified early on that it would be unable to cope with a crisis similar to Italy (Buckingham 2020). The effects of the adversarial policy style were hitting home: the pro-activity of the UK was based on a flu pandemic plan revised in 2014 (Public Health England 2014), and despite the evolution of the coronavirus pandemic, the UK was holding off in preparing the system with additional intensive care unit (ICU) beds.[2] It was only on March 13 that the government announced the building of seven temporary Nightingale Hospitals in England to treat coronavirus patients; the first one completed in London two weeks later. These rapidly constructed critical care facilities increased ICU capacity by more than 3,600 (Flynn et al. 2020).

At the start of the pandemic, there was a combination of high institutional capacity and low trust in the government's capacity to handle the emerging crisis. The government had hit rock bottom in terms of trust in 2019 (34%)[3] mainly as a result of the uncertainty over the Brexit negotiations, yet the public still trusted the commitment of NHS staff (doctors, 95% and nurses, 93%), the truthfulness of civil servants[4] (65%), and the public (65%).[5] The government on its part relied on PHE to create the awareness campaign and guidance notes producing an Action Plan on March 3, 2020 (Department of Health & Social Care 2020) pursuing a centrifugal strategy in its policy response. It maintained the centralization of decision-making, but relied on the work of multiple health agencies and the devolved administrations. Going forward, this would prove beneficial to avoid taking the blame for any wrong action, especially following hard criticism on the Prime Minister's absence from the Civil Contingencies Committee (COBRA)[6] meetings and public view and the initial ideas of creating 'herd immunity' (Calvert et al. 2020).

Following its adversarial policy style and lower trust, Britain was prompted to more centrifugal plans as expected. Despite centralization of decision-making, since the introduction of devolved administrations in 1999, which Flinders (2010) highlights as 'bi-constitutionality,' there is a 'concurrent development of consensual devolved regimes and a majoritarian UK central government' (Jordan and Cairney 2013: 234). But that does not happen in high-profile, high-conflict policy issues, where the central government still pursues a top-down policy style and especially in times of crisis that involve tough choices with more winners and losers (Jordan and Cairney 2013: 254). Decisions in the context of the pandemic crisis involved choices of who would be tested and treated, identification of priority groups and key workers, and minimization of the impact of the virus on the UK population.

The UK followed a steep hierarchy in terms of who defines the problem and makes decisions but allowing scope for manoeuver by the devolved administrations in Scotland, Wales, and Northern Ireland. Despite the UK's response having evolved since the outbreak and into the lockdown phase, the message remained fairly consistent with high profile public campaigns and slogans for instructions that the public should follow. This was largely orchestrated through daily press conferences since March 16, 2020, frequently led by the Prime Minister (until he tested positive for coronavirus on March 27)[7] and alternating key ministers accompanied by the Chief Medical Officers (CMOs) (Tomkins 2020). Measures were portrayed as being driven by science to avoid blame, hence the change of heart from initial ideas of 'herd immunity' to 'lockdown'—a polyphonous approach that allowed the government to suggest that decisions were based on evidence, but ultimately, their hands were tied to bad or good science. Finally, the intensity or stringency of the measures to protect the public against coronavirus followed a slow and very gradual increase before the government proceeded to a full lockdown. Fines for breaking the measures were introduced, largely monitored by the police force, and on many occasions imposed, but the responsibility fell heavily on the British public to exercise their common sense. This was made even more important following criticisms on many occasions where high profile ministers, scientists, and government advisors admitted to breaking the lockdown measures with a number of excuses (Cartwright and Rose 2020). On two occasions, this criticism was targeted at Dominic Cummings, Downing Street's top advisor, who was found in breach of travel restrictions and was recorded commenting on herd immunity about the insignificance of pensioners losing their lives.[8]

Nonetheless, following the publication of the Coronavirus Action Plan (Department of Health & Social Care 2020) on March 3, the government's response was to be guided by international developments, advice of the World Health Organization (WHO), and the expertise of Scientific Advisory Group for Emergencies (SAGE) who would provide data modeling. The government would continue to be advised by the four CMOs (in England, Wales, Scotland, and Northern Ireland) who would also give the direction travel of the policy response to the health and social care systems and government agencies across the UK. According to the same paper, the structure of command would come centrally from the Department of Health and Social Care (DHSC). Decisions would be based on advice by the CMOs and SAGE as a 'single source of co-ordinated scientific advice [...] to decision makers' (Department of Health & Social Care 2020, 22). The NHS would deliver health care in England and Wales and PHE technical expertise for planning and delivery. A tripartite partnership between DHSC, PHE, and NHS England was established responsible for the strategic oversight and direction of the response but with centrifugal tendencies with similar arrangements for the devolved administrations in the other nations of the UK. PHE and its counterparts in the other devolved administrations would lead on expert advice.

The Action Plan also outlined the chain of command when looking at local and regional responsibilities, where local organizations would work jointly with Local Resilience Forums, Local Health Resilience Partnerships (England and Scotland), the NHS (Wales), and Emergency Preparedness Groups (Northern Ireland) (Department of Health & Social Care 2020: Annex A). But this multi-agency working structure left some decision-making to the local level for the best distribution of resources to serve the best outcomes for the local areas, including support through quick guides provided by NHS England on the increased demand for their services locally. This is important, as discretion was offered in local decision-making despite the highly centralized decision-making mechanisms led by DHSC and the government. Social care would also be decentralized to an extent on the back of local authorities, private, and third-sector bodies but reporting to the local health authorities.

Despite all this planning, there was a considerable delay, with the first set of substantial measures announced on March 16, 2020, focusing on the protection of vulnerable groups, on the restriction of non-essential travel and non-essential contact and mass gatherings in sporting events, claiming that the timing was such because of the difficulty and disruption this measure would bring to people's lives. The rationale offered was one of slowing the spread, reducing the peak, and giving the NHS the chance to cope with the increasing cases (Prime Minister 2020a). Developments were rapid since then, with the second set of measures coming few days later on March 22 for shielding the vulnerable and closing schools (Prime Minister 2020b) and on March 23 for closing non-essential shops, playgrounds, and places of worship and introducing hard social distancing measures with limited time spent outdoors only for exercise purposes once a day (Prime Minister 2020c). Since then, and according to the Stringency Index by Oxford University (Hale et al. 2020), the UK remained under strict lockdown for approximately ten weeks (index of 75.93).

Returning to the adversarial policy style, given the low inclusion in policy-making in the UK in times of crisis a highly centralized response would be the primary focus. On the flip side, given the high institutional capacity of the UK in terms of expertise, advisory bodies, and institutional structures, the UK could also be expected to have a more decentralized strategy leaving considerable room to the local authorities. Hence, why were there such variant patterns of policy response in the UK? The determining factor is trust: trust in government interacts to refract the impact of policy styles. In the case of the UK, while trust in government remained relatively low and the capacity of the NHS has decreased in the past decade as a result of austerity and underfunding, the public rests their trust on the doctors and nurses of the NHS. Hence, the government initially showcased a centralized policy response on the one hand, but with a degree of decentralization back to doctors and experts to gain the public's support, while at the same time ensuring some blame avoidance as actions were seen to be driven by science.

The 'Easy Times': Too Early, Too Fast?

The first lockdown in the UK lasted for approximately ten weeks. During this time, the pressure to reopen economic activity was high, and returning to normalcy became the primary focus of the Conservative government. The economic support measures were due to lapse in June 2020, and the government appeared not to want to foot the financial impact bill for too long, sticking to its original plan. The policies to contain or mitigate the effects of the pandemic from June 10 onward, since the UK adopted a more decentralist approach to adjusting policies, followed the demand by the devolved administrations to have a higher say for their local jurisdictions. For example, the hospitality sector opened up at different times for England (July 4), Scotland (July 15), Wales (August 3), and Northern Ireland (July 3) (Flynn et al. 2020). This was a result of the variable speed at which the pandemic was evolving but also a means to keep better control of resources in smaller communities. This was also evidenced in England, where certain areas were forced back into local lockdowns, especially in the North.

In the meantime, the exceptionally good weather did not help containment efforts as people largely ignored social distancing, alongside the seemingly positive messages around the drop of daily cases and deaths (Figure 9.1 and 9.2) and international travel resuming to allow holidays abroad. The so-called 'travel corridors' were opened early in July to the delight of holidaymakers. According to the statement submitted to the House of Commons by the Transport Secretary, Grant Shapps (2020), this was a decision 'guided by science' where the Department for Transport 'worked closely with health and policy experts from across government' to ensure minimal risks and helping the re-opening of travel and tourism. The travel corridors were to operate under scrutiny by PHE and the CMO in assessing levels of infections, trends in cases, and deaths as well as testing capacity of foreign countries. The rules would apply to England, but the devolved administrations were allowed to set out their own approaches (Shapps 2020). Unfortunately, the mechanisms to monitor the self-isolation period for those returning were not sufficient and that led to the importing of additional cases and variants from abroad. However, the policy became quite reactionary and unclear once the second wave started to hit Europe from August 2020 onward.

Finally, the government decided to extend the job retention schemes and the business support schemes that it set out during the first lockdown period, further adding pressure to maintain the economy open as much as possible (UK Government 2020a, b, c). The Chancellor of the Exchequer, Rishi Sunak, announced the 'Eat Out to Help Out' scheme on July 15 to run in August, advertised as discounts (covered by the Government) on meals at coffee shops, pubs, and restaurants to boost sales and revenues in the much-battered hospitality sector. According to the report by Her Majesty's Revenue and Customs (HMRC) Department, there were almost 50,000 businesses making claims through the scheme, and the pay-outs reached almost £850 million, increasing every week throughout August (UK Government 2020d). This translated into more than 160 million meals.

Combining the reinvigoration of the hospitality sector figures for August with the ability of foreign travel meant an inevitable spike in recorded cases. The UK was not out of the woods in the summer, and the government was reacting once again to, rather than proactively preventing, the second wave. By September, it was clear that restrictions would return. Back to linking policy style to trust, trust in the government's ability to handle the pandemic had been declining steadily since the beginning of the crisis. While in April 2020, 69% trusted the UK government to control the spread of the virus; by July 2020, this figure had dropped to 50% (Duffy 2020). This was further pronounced by evidence that during the first lockdown, trust in others was double the trust in government figures (Parsons and Wiggins 2020).[9]

Post-Halloween Terror: A Second Lockdown

When autumn began, the rising cases and subsequent deaths already signaled the start of the second wave (Figure 9.2). The UK government, however, appeared once again quite reluctant to impose a lockdown. It was not until late September that the government pre-empted the possibility of new restrictions as workers were called back home, and the government's job retention scheme was extended. Already, SAGE, as an expert body, was warning the government to act quickly to avoid a second lockdown (Wise 2020). In its 10-point plan, SAGE called for immediate measures to be reviewed when a functional testing system could be in place (SAGE 2020a), attributing the spike to the indoor service in pubs and restaurants, and the fact that workplaces had not been COVID-19-proof. Professor Stephen Reicher, leading the SAGE plan, suggested that the government was wrong in blaming people for breaking the rules, but rather that the public was encouraged to do things that exposed people more (such as eating out or going to work). The report also highlighted that 46% of workplaces had not taken social distancing measures. Schools should operate with more digital resources, and colleges and universities should have only online teaching. This latter point became more evident as universities commenced semesters with face-to-face teaching resulting in high mobility of younger persons around the country. By the end of September, more than 40 universities reported COVID-19 outbreaks within just one week of teaching.[10]

Unfortunately, this call was largely ignored following the adversarial policy style in UK policymaking, with the government instead announcing a three-tier system for restrictions in England. SAGE had already outlined the worst-case scenario in July, arguing that more than 85,000 deaths could be predicted until March 2021, pointing out that hospitalization could rise to 356,000.[11] Nonetheless, the Centre for Global Health at the University of Edinburgh, which collaborates with WHO, suggested that there was reliable scientific evidence showing a very large second wave was under way (Mahase 2020). In its latest report, SAGE recommended a two-week circuit breaker during the October break for schools to reduce transmissions (SAGE 2020b), but again, the advice was largely ignored. A member of the Scientific Pandemic Influenza Group on Modelling suggested that regional 'firefighting techniques' that the government was implementing were pointless, and there was the urge to move to something more national. The chair of the British Medical Association's (BMA) London branch was also pointing to the stress factor of new cases on the NHS, urging the government to 'get its act together and deliver a fit-for-purpose test, trace and isolate system' and to improve public health messaging (Mahase 2020).

On Halloween evening, Prime Minister Johnson announced the inevitable: a four-week national lockdown to 'prevent a medical and moral disaster for the NHS' (Prime Minister 2020d). The Prime Minister defended the government's decision for a local and a regional approach passionately as 'the right thing to do,' further accentuating the centrifugal element of the policy response in the UK. He pointed out the cost of the restrictions on jobs and livelihood and that the government hoped that 'strong local action [and] strong local leadership […] could get the rates of infection down' (Prime Minister 2020d). This presented yet one more U-turn by the government which failed to acknowledge the expert advice, bring the economy to the forefront over public health, and diffuse decision-making to a degree down to the local level.

Such developments had detrimental effects on public trust as demonstrated by a study by King's College London and Ipsos MORI at the end of November 2020 (Duffy 2020). The study reported only 38% trusting the government's ability to manage the pandemic, with a further 57% saying that they do not trust the government to control the spread of the virus. In addition, 68% agreed that the government's response had been confused and inconsistent. A further 40% thought that the government's plan was not adapting to new scientific evidence with only 27% saying it did. That was a considerable shift from the start of the pandemic when these numbers were 15% and 58%, respectively. Finally, more than two-thirds believed that the government had not sufficiently prepared for the second wave. These results suggest that centrifugalism was the only way the government could use to diffuse blame and shift more responsibility locally and to the general public.

The Virus that Stole Christmas: Lockdown 3.0

When the second lockdown was lifted on December 2, the UK had indeed managed to bring the cases down and flatten the curve once more (Figures 9.1 & 9.2). In his Winter Plan statement, Prime Minister Johnson reflecting on the effects of the second lockdown appeared once again optimistic, giving out a new message to the public that the bad days were not gone just yet. Johnson praised the breakthroughs in treatment, testing, and vaccines predicting that such advances would reduce the need for restrictions in early 2021. He announced that the Oxford-AstraZeneca vaccine was going to become available and that the government had already ordered a total of 350 million doses, preparing the NHS to roll out the inoculation program (Prime Minister 2020e). Amongst others, the PM also announced additional powers to the local authorities to enforce the new stricter three-tier system of restrictions and additional training to officers on how to respond to breaches of the restrictions. This again emphasized the centrifugal approach of the UK, which alongside references to the coordination with the devolved administrations showcase the persistence of a particular policy style.

The hope of the government in the beginning of December was to ensure that people would have some flexibility to see their loved ones and enjoy Christmas with some constraints. PM Johnson was firm that a new lockdown would be out of the cards (Prime Minister 2020e). This firmness soon turned into a third lockdown just few weeks later, as analyzed in this section. However, seeing how trust in the government's ability to deal with the pandemic had collapsed in the months leading to November, the PM was quick to underscore the need for the public to keep 'sensible precautions' and that the new tougher tier-system was driven by 'scientific advice.' This latter comment was interesting given the government's persistent disregard for scientific recommendations earlier.

On December 8, Britain commenced its vaccination program, albeit not with the homegrown Oxford-AstraZeneca, but the German Pfizer/BioNTech vaccine.[12] In his December 16 statement, PM Johnson praised the NHS for delivering almost 140,000 doses already, but flagged the failure of certain regions in England to control the rates of infection. Soon, London went in the red, and a new Tier 4 category was introduced, tightening further the rules for Christmas. A new variant, branded as "Kent variant," was booming with infections, and the curve had started to increase once more (Chowdhury et al. 2021). The PM highlighted how vital it was that 'everyone exercise[d] the greatest possible personal responsibility' in light of Christmas adding that, alongside the devolved administrations, they 'decided that the overall situation [was] worse and more challenging than we had hoped when we first set the rules' (Prime Minister 2020f). Scientists were already warning about the advent of a third wave in the New Year as a result of having relaxed the measures earlier despite what data suggested (Wilson 2020). The message was clear: Christmas had just been stolen by the virus. But in terms of the response, the message was still largely unclear, leaving a number of parameters to the judgment of ordinary citizens. Keeping laws the same, a vague 'smaller and shorter Christmas' was requested, 'minimising the number of people to meet,' avoid traveling from a 'high prevalence to a low prevalence area' and to 'think carefully about avoiding crowds in the Boxing Day sales' (Prime Minister 2020f).

Unfortunately, the calculated centrifugalism instead of a change in policy style had dire effects in its ability to avoid further measures. On January 4, 2021, the PM announced that the country was yet again entering a third lockdown without an advertised end in sight, but a vague promise of a review in the middle of February. The rapid rise in infections, deaths, hospitalizations, and rates of spread due to the new 'Kent variant' was making the management of the crisis extremely difficult under the previous measures. Almost 82,000 new cases had been registered on December 29, which was double the daily rate reported in the previous 14 days. The four UK CMOs had advised raising the alert from Level 4 to Level 5, indicating that if no action had been taken, the capacity of the NHS would be more than full within 21 days (Prime Minister 2021a). In light of this advice, the new restrictions were tougher than before with limitations on practically all activities. They were announced on the same day as the Oxford-AstraZeneca vaccine arrived and just a day after schools were meant to start.

The third lockdown in the UK was marked by the roll-out of the vaccination program and hopes that the end of spring would find the country in a much better position. Starting with the inoculation program, the government perceived the vaccine as the biggest weapon against the pandemic but also a benchmark for reviewing the lockdown measures and other restrictions. The DHSC, however, had been planning the program since the start of the pandemic, demonstrating possibly one of the few, if not the only, occasions where proactive planning was at play. On the same mindset, the government had already signed contracts with AstraZeneca and Pfizer already in June 2020, securing valuable doses early on, months before the EU managed to secure its contracts (Baraniuk 2021). A task force was set up in May 2020, comprising scientists and logistics experts to organize the vaccination program, and the Medicines and Healthcare Products Regulatory Agency (MHRA) was asked to follow swift procedures in approving and authorizing the use of vaccines.

Conclusion: How Has Policy Style and Trust Informed the UK's Response One Year On?

There is no denying that the initial response by the UK was based on an adversarial policy style that, combined with a relatively low trust to government, led to a centrifugal response to diffuse responsibility and avoid direct criticisms of poor crisis management. The impact of the pandemic has been profound in the UK. What began as a strategy for achieving herd immunity turned into a national standstill of economic and social life three times in a year. The many unknown properties of the pandemic alongside ill-prepared or irrelevant mechanisms of crisis management led to the adversarial policy style of the UK casting the wrong kind of shadow in the UK's response. The involvement of the devolved administrations in the response added a further level of complication in ensuring a clear message and a strategy for public consumption.

It is clear that the first national lockdown decision, despite coming in late after abandoning the idea of 'herd immunity,' helped keep cases low. However, the decision to lift measures early and without appropriate monitoring mechanisms and clarity of guidance for the public meant that the spread of the virus was more covert and circulating within the community in a dormant fashion. This was particularly evident from the fact that different areas within the country despite moving at different paces of infection rates operated under the same national rules. The second observation was that the reaction of the government was again delayed despite early signals in September 2020 that the second wave had arrived, revealing limited lesson-drawing. Once more, the government's response was relying too much on reaction rather than prevention and on the public's perception of responsibility. But the public was profoundly confused as the government kept sending vague signals. In light of collapsing trust in government by November 2020, this combination gave the public a free hand in deciding what was best for themselves and without decisions being guided by expert opinion.

On reflection, despite the delayed response in March 2020, Britain managed to bring deaths considerably down (Figure 9.2) spreading waves of optimism within government that the situation was under control. This blissful ignorance, however, and further encouragement to the public to enjoy the outdoors and go on holiday abroad meant that, when cases spiked again in September, the government was unprepared to tackle the second wave. Reacting to pressures from the economy and local authorities, diffusing responsibility to the public and ignoring calls from experts, the government was again delayed in tightening measures making the waves of deaths in the winter of 2020/2021 inevitable. Confirming the expectation, the adversarial style cast a long shadow in the British response overall with trust becoming a catalyst in determining the direction of travel. The UK maintained centralized elements but diffused responsibility and tasks to the devolved administrations and local authorities to save face. Low trust in its ability to perform meant that the government sought other support from doctors and nurses and local authorities who had a better overview of the situation on the ground. It was only in February 2021, when the vaccine roll-out and lesson-drawing from past mistakes unlocked a clearer and more transparent centrifugal response in terms of guidance, messages, and decision-making.

Notes

1 Coronavirus: Britons evacuated from Wuhan arrive at quarantine facility, BBC website January 31, 2020, https://www.bbc.co.uk/news/uk-51318691.
2 https://www.weforum.org/agenda/2020/03/look-inside-london-nightingale-temporary-hospitals-coronavirus/.
3 https://data.oecd.org/gga/trust-in-government.htm.
4 For the purpose of this chapter, Public Health England (PHE) can be considered as one of the bureaucratic elements of the government.
5 https://www.ipsos.com/ipsos-mori/en-uk/trust-politicians-falls-sending-them-spiralling-back-bottom-ipsos-mori-veracity-index.
6 The Civil Contingencies Committee is also known as COBR or COBRA (an acronym on their situation center meeting room Cabinet Office Briefing Room A).
7 https://www.theguardian.com/world/2020/apr/05/timeline-boris-johnson-and-coronavirus.
8 Dominic Cummings was found to have breached coronavirus rules, having traveled from London to Durham, claiming that he wanted to get an eye test and was recorded outlining the government's strategy as "herd immunity, protect the economy and if that means some pensioners die, too bad" (Shipman and Wheeler 2020).
9 Parsons and Wiggins (2020) used an 11-point scale to measure trust, showing that trust in government declined following the easing of lockdown, particularly, in England. The government scored between 5 and 6 on average ratings, whereas 'others' scored between 7 and 7.5.
10 Covid: About 40 universities report coronavirus cases. https://www.bbc.co.uk/news/uk-54322935.
11 SAGE. Covid in winter 2020, a worst-case scenario. Spectator 2020 October 29. https://www.spectator.co.uk/article/classified-covid-in-winter-2020-a-worst-case-scenario.
12 Covid-19 vaccine: First person receives Pfizer jab in UK. https://www.bbc.co.uk/news/uk-55227325.

References

Atkinson, Andrew. 2019. "Johnson victory Heralds gradual end to U.K.'s era of austerity", *Bloomberg*, 14 December 2019, https://www.bloomberg.com/news/articles/2019-12-14/johnson-victory-heralds-gradual-end-to-u-k-s-era-of-austerity.

Baraniuk, Chris. 2021. "Covid-19: How the UK vaccine rollout delivered success, so far", *The BMJ*, 18 February 2021, 372 (n421), https://www.bmj.com/content/372/bmj.n421.

Bodkin, Henry. 2020. "'Lost decade' condemned as life expectancy stalls", *The Daily Telegraph*, 25 February 2020, https://www.telegraph.co.uk/news/2020/02/25/lost-decade-condemned-life-expectancy-stalls/.

Buckingham, Helen. 2020. "Coronavirus: How will the NHS cope?", Nuffield Trust comment. 21 February 2020, https://www.nuffieldtrust.org.uk/news-item/coronavirus-how-will-the-nhs-cope.

Calvert, Jonathan, George Arbuthnott and John Leake. 2020. "Revealed 38 days; when Britain sleepwalked into disaster. Boris Johnson skipped five Cobra meetings on the virus, calls to order protective gear were ignored and scientists' warnings fell on deaf ears. Failings in February may have cost thousands of lives", *The Sunday Times*, 19 April 2020, pp. 6–7.

Cartwright, Edward and Jonathan Rose. 2020. "We asked people if they were breaking lockdown rules before and after the Dominic Cummings scandal – here's what they told us", *The Conversation*, 3 June 2020, https://theconversation.com/we-asked-people-if-they-were-breaking-lockdown-rules-before-and-after-the-dominic-cummings-scandal-heres-what-they-told-us-139994.

Chowdhury, Jitesh, Simon Scarr, Andrew MacAskill and Andrew R.C. Marshall. 2021. "Variant of concern: How a deadly and more contagious variant of the coronavirus tore through the UK and across the world", 26 March 2021, https://graphics.reuters.com/HEALTH-CORONAVIRUS/UK-VARIANT/ygdpzgblxvw/.

Department of Health & Social Care. 2020. "Coronavirus action plan: A guide to what you can expect across the UK", Policy Paper, 3 March 2020, https://assets.publishing.service.gov.uk/government/uploads/system/uploads/attachment_data/file/869827/Coronavirus_action_plan_-_a_guide_to_what_you_can_expect_across_the_UK.pdf.

Duffy, Bobby. 2020. "The UK government's handling of the coronavirus crisis: Public perceptions", The Policy Institute, King's College London, 6 December 2020, https://www.kcl.ac.uk/policy-institute/assets/the-handling-of-the-coronavirus-crisis.pdf.

Flinders, Matthew. 2010. *Democratic Drift*. Oxford: Oxford University Press.

Flynn, Darren, Eoin Moloney, Nawaraj Bhattarai, Jason Scott, Matthew Breckons, Leah Avery and Naomi Moy. 2020. "COVID-19 pandemic in the United Kingdom", *Health Policy and Technology*, 9(4): 673–691, https://doi.org/10.1016/j.hlpt.2020.08.003.

Hale, Thomas, Samuel Webster, Anna Petherick, Toby Phillips and Beatriz Kira. 2020. *Variation in government responses to COVID-19 version 6.0*, Blavatnik School of Government Working Paper (May 25, 2020), www.bsg.ox.ac.uk/covidtracker.

Iacobucci, Gareth. 2020. "Marmot 10 years on: Austerity has damaged nation's health, say experts", *British Medical Journal*, 368: m747, 25 February 2020.

Jordan, Grant and Paul Cairney. 2013. "What is the 'dominant model' of British policy-making? Comparing majoritarian and policy community ideas", *British Politics* 8(3): 233–259.

Mahase, Elisabeth. 2020. "Covid-19: UK government must 'get its act together' as modelling suggests 85,000 deaths in second wave, experts say", 30 October 2020, *The BMJ*, 371 (m4242), https://www.bmj.com/content/371/bmj.m4242.

Parsons, Sam and Richard D. Wiggins. 2020. *Trust in government and others during the COVID-19 pandemic - Initial findings from the COVID-19 Survey in Five National Longitudinal Studies*. London: UCL Centre for Longitudinal Studies.

Prime Minister. 2020a. PM statement on coronavirus: 16 March 2020, https://www.gov.uk/government/speeches/pm-statement-on-coronavirus-16-march-2020.

Prime Minister. 2020b. PM statement on coronavirus: 22 March 2020, https://www.gov.uk/government/speeches/pm-statement-on-coronavirus-22-march-2020.

Prime Minister. 2020c. PM statement on coronavirus: 23 March 2020, https://www.gov.uk/government/speeches/pm-address-to-the-nation-on-coronavirus-23-march-2020.

Prime Minister. 2020d. Prime Minister's statement on coronavirus (COVID-19): 31 October 2020, https://www.gov.uk/government/speeches/prime-ministers-statement-on-coronavirus-covid-19-31-october-2020

Prime Minister. 2020e. PM statement on COVID-19 Winter Plan: 23 November 2020, https://www.gov.uk/government/speeches/pm-statement-on-covid-19-winter-plan-23-november-2020.

Prime Minister. 2020f. Prime Minister's statement on coronavirus (COVID-19): 16 December 2020, https://www.gov.uk/government/speeches/prime-ministers-statement-on-coronavirus-covid-19-16-december-2020.

Prime Minister. 2021a. Prime Minister announces national lockdown: 4 January 2021, https://www.gov.uk/government/news/prime-minister-announces-national-lockdown.

Public Health England. 2014. Pandemic Influenza Response Plan 2014. 13 August 2014, https://assets.publishing.service.gov.uk/government/uploads/system/uploads/attachment_data/file/344695/PI_Response_Plan_13_Aug.pdf.

Public Health England. 2020. Health Protection Report. Vol. 14: issue 4. 26 February 2020, https://www.gov.uk/government/publications/health-protection-report-volume-14-2020/hpr-volume-14-issue-4-news-25-and-26-february.

Richardson, Jeremy J. (ed.) 1982. *Policy Styles in Western Europe*. London: Allen & Unwin.

SAGE. 2020a. "Measures to avoid a national lockdown: An emergency ten point plan", 20 September 2020, www.independentsage.org/wp-content/uploads/2020/09/Emergency-Plan-PUBLISHED.pdf.

SAGE. 2020b. "Emergency Plan", 16 October 2020, https://www.independentsage.org/wp-content/uploads/2020/10/Emergency-plan-Oct-2020-FINAL.pdf.

Shapps, Grant. 2020. Statement on Travel Corridors. https://www.gov.uk/government/speeches/travel-corridors.

Shipman, Tim and Caroline Wheeler. 2020. "Coronavirus: Ten days that shook Britain – and changed the nation forever", 22 March 2020, *The Sunday Times*, https://www.thetimes.co.uk/article/coronavirus-ten-days-that-shook-britain-and-changed-the-nation-for-ever-spz6sc9vb.

Tomkins, Leah. 2020. "Where is Boris Johnson? When and why it matters that leaders show up in a crisis", *Leadership*, 1–12, early view https://doi.org/10.1177/1742715020919657.

UK Cabinet Office. 1999. "White paper: Modernising government. London: 30 March 1999", https://webarchive.nationalarchives.gov.uk/20131205101137/http://www.archive.official-documents.co.uk/document/cm43/4310/4310.htm.

UK Government. 2020a. "Financial support for businesses during coronavirus (COVID-19)", https://www.gov.uk/government/collections/financial-support-for-businesses-during-coronavirus-covid-19#support-for-small-and-medium-sized-businesses.

UK Government. 2020b. "Coronavirus grant funding: Local authority payments to small and medium businesses", https://www.gov.uk/government/publications/coronavirus-grant-funding-local-authority-payments-to-small-and-medium-businesses.

UK Government. 2020c. "Guidance: Get a discount with the Eat Out to Help Out Scheme", https://www.gov.uk/guidance/get-a-discount-with-the-eat-out-to-help-out-scheme.

UK Government. 2020d. "Eat Out to Help out Statistics", https://www.gov.uk/government/statistics/eat-out-to-help-out-statistics/eat-out-to-help-out-statistics-commentary.

Wilson, Clare. 2020. "Highlight: Countries across Europe are taking very different approaches to the festive period", *New Scientist* 248 (3312): 12–13.

Wise, Jacqui. (2020). "Covid-19: Act now to avoid second lockdown, says Independent SAGE", 21 September, *The BMJ*, 370 (m3695), https://www.bmj.com/content/bmj/370/bmj.m3695.full.pdf.

10

THE BREAKDOWN OF COOPERATIVE FEDERALISM

Brazil's Response to the COVID-19 Pandemic

Valesca Lima and José de Arimatéia da Cruz

Introduction

Since the outset of the COVID-19 pandemic, countries have implemented health strategies to prevent the further spread of the virus, requiring each one of them to respond with multiple efforts to prevent illness and death. While some national governments actively followed the World Health Organization (WHO) recommendations, most jurisdictions adopted some level of control on the outcomes of the pandemic, even if it took a while for countries to find their foot and somewhat control the situation. But, tragically, for the 194,976[1] people who died in Brazil as a consequence of the virus by the end of 2020, the country's response to the pandemic has been one of horror and neglect. This makes Brazil the second country with the second highest number of cases of COVID-19 after the United States, as the country became a global epicenter for the COVID-19 pandemic rate of infection and deaths. This chapter examines the Brazilian government responses to the health crisis, covering the first year of the pandemic.

The spread of the coronavirus pandemic raises questions about States capacity in crisis management. Despite its continental proportions and large population, Brazil's policy capacity is high, even if facing several policy implementation challenges. The country has one of the most substantial public infrastructures in the world, including free universal healthcare, universal primary education, a comprehensive cash transfer program, mass social housing, and decentralization of several public services (Paim et al., 2011; Loureiro et al., 2020; Tikkanen, 2020). The health structure, in particular, has performed relatively well in previous epidemics, such as Zika, Chikungunya, and flu (Teixeira et al., 2018), but it has not been able to respond to the COVID-19 public health emergency. Conversely, to its high capacity, inclusion and political trust are low. First, because Brazil has a strong concentration of power in the hands of the executive (presidential system)

DOI: 10.4324/9781003137399-14

and weak inclusion of social actors in policymaking, which leads to poor mediation. Second, Brazil has historically low levels of institutional trust (Rennó et al., 2011). The high levels of perceived corruption undermine the credibility of Brazilian institutions and may have significantly increased mistrust in government over the years (Avritzer and Rennó, 2021).

The failed response to COVID-19 pandemic is not only due to the lack of adoption of the health protocols established by the WHO. Brazil's disastrous approach incentivized the spread of COVID-19 among its own population with an anti-science-based approach to combat COVID-19, poor management, confusing public statements, and a very adversarial approach to the media. Despite the country's well-respected publicly funded health care system, the *Sistema Único de Saúde* (SUS, Unified Health System), the Federal administration led by the President Bolsonaro failed to take the proper actions necessary to address the pandemic. In his anti-science and hubris approach, Bolsonaro downplayed the disease when it first arrived in Brazil, calling it a "gripezinha" ("light flu"). He openly discouraged social distancing, downplayed the threat posed by the virus, ridiculed public health officials' concerns, railed against lockdowns, presented falsehoods, therefore undermining subnational public health policy and delegitimizing health specialists in his own administration.

But how was one person alone able to cause this level of undemocratic response to the pandemic paired with political and social disruption? Bolsonaro was certainly the face of the coronavirus-denial movement worldwide, and as populist leader in a power-concentrating regime, Bolsonaro was able to exert the strategies and deeds of populism. With a strong cult of personality (his supporters call him "mito" or "legend") and an anti-establishment and patriotic discourse, he has stretched the rule of law to its limits and opened a pathway to an institutional reform without mediation or institutional checks and balances. His political influence in the pandemic comes from the manipulation of the cooperative model of federalism adopted in the country, which Bolsonaro has systematically undermined and tried to turn it into hierarchical mode with less funding, less policy articulation, and even less political negotiation. His push for a Dual Federalism model led to a centrifugal COVID-19 policy approach and great levels of conflict and incoordination with subnational administrations. In this chapter, we argue that (a) the Federal administration systematically promoted the spread of the virus and (b) even if Bolsonaro has deliberately harmed the responses to the pandemic by dismembering the federative pact, cooperative federalism has been upheld by the Supreme Federal Court (STF), and as a consequence, new subnational actors have emerged from this process to reinforce previous policy styles that work. We use a historical–institutional analysis to examine how Bolsonaro's government influenced policy responses to the pandemic via the "Dual Federalism" or in the Brazilian case, "Bolsonaro's federalism" (Abrucio et al., 2020; Censon and Barcelos, 2020), a concept that entail the disengagement of the Federal Government with states and municipalities, devolution of power, and more responsibilities for subnational administration. We make use of official documents published by the Brazilian

Federal Government, states, and municipalities; public statements by Bolsonaro and health officials; scientific reports and documents produced by national health and research organizations, such as the University of São Paulo (USP) and the WHO, to sustain my analysis. Together, these documents provide the evidence needed for an examination of change in policy style in the past decades and also to analyze the overall government's response to the pandemic.

This chapter is organized as follows: the next section addresses the way Dual Federalism has been slowly unfolding, and it is now a fully fledged model under implementation clashing with the federal cooperative model. We then move to analyze how the "Bolsonaro's federalism" was implemented, the conflicts it caused, and the consequences of its implementation. We continue to examine the conditions that allowed this to happen in a context of low political trust. Finally, in the conclusion, we reflect on the changes of policy styles over time and on the new subnational leadership actors that emerged from the health crisis and future research.

Federalism and Policymaking—Dualism in the Brazil's COVID Response Leading to Low Trust

The re-emergence of debates on state capacity for public policy amid a global health crisis is justified by its practical importance in implementing social and health protection policies, saving lives, sustain development, and lasting consequences of the pandemic. Once again, States established themselves as the main actors in charge of dealing with the pandemic, mobilizing national sentiments on a large scale. The intervening state was claimed even by the neoliberals (Bringel and Pleyers, 2020, p. 17). While it is well-know by now that the political response to the pandemic varied according to institutional capacity, the autonomy of the political actors implicated—and even according to the effective belief in the deadliness of the virus (Schaefer et al., 2020), Brazil's misguided and uncoordinated response to the COVID-19 pandemic went against the expected policy style of early intervention and national coordination observed in previous health crises (Teixeira et al., 2018). The problem now, as emerging research has started to highlight, is largely due to intragovernmental conflicts, originating from a clash between two models of cooperative federalism or dual federalism (Censon and Barcelos, 2020; Schaefer et al., 2020).

According to Pierson (1995), there are two primary forms of federalism that impact public policies, the dual and cooperative models. Dual federalism is based on hierarchy, modeled from top-bottom, where each federation member has strong autonomy over different areas to prevent the centralization of power. Federative coordination would be only contingent, circumstantial and detrimental to efficient decision-making and resource allocation (Abrucio et al., 2020). Among the countries organized under a federative model, the US epitomized the case of dual federalism. In turn, the cooperative federal model shares authority and combines it with subnational autonomy and national coordination, blending both centralized (e.g. economic decisions) and decentralized actions (e.g. policy implementation). Cooperation often involves citizen inclusion via participation in policymaking. This may take the form of intergovernmental forums, such as local policy councils, participatory budget, and mini-publics, that can lessen or even thwart unilateral decisions (Gaventa, 2006, Lima, 2019; Schnabel, 2015), including the possibilities of states and municipalities to strive for their own economic and social development (Ribeiro, 2018).

Historically, Brazil has experienced those two models. Cooperative federalism was adopted after the 1930 Revolution that seized power from the First republic, but the Getúlio Vargas Administration deformed it into a centralism that snatched the autonomy of member states. With the 1937 Constitution, centralization was back, and member states were required to reproduce the rules defined by the Union (Ribeiro, 2018). This pattern of centralization persisted during the military regime (1964–1985). In the re-democratization process, intergovernmental relations changed, starting from the decline of authoritarian rule and culminating in the new 1988 Constitution, when Brazil returned to a cooperative federalism after years of institutional darkness under the military dictatorship.

As a cooperative federation, Brazil's institutional design centered on intergovernmental coordination, in which the authority of the Union is combined with subnational autonomy for countrywide coordination in various areas, including the elaboration and implementation of public and social policy. In this approach, coordination became imperative, and that is the "spirit" of the 1988 Brazilian Federal Constitution, where despite the autonomy of subnational governments, they still need federal policy coordination (Censon and Barcelos, 2020).

Institutional design and policy styles are not a fixed feature, but are contingent on the correlation of political forces at a given historical–conjunctural moment and on the political and economic context in which public policies are introduced (Loureiro et al., 2020). Since re-democratization, all Federal administrations have respected the constitutional perspective of cooperation. While right-wing presidents Collor de Mello and Fernando's overall policy agenda focused on increasing state capacity via international investments, open economy, and established a few national policy councils, the left-leaning Workers Party focused on a mix of social policies to fight poverty to improve the life conditions of the poor, with the creation of several structural of citizen participation, welfare programs, and neo-developmentalism political economy based on commodities cycle. Decentralization was very much increased during Workers' party administration (2003–2016), which included the progressive construction of state and municipality capacities in several policy areas.

But, since 2014, Brazil has undergone dramatic waves of turbulence and instability, with election results questioned, the impeachment process of Dilma Rousseff, and continuous and recurrent episodes of political crisis coupled with the most serious economic recession in Brazilian history (Avritez and Rennó, 2021, p. 12). It is in this context of intense political, economic, and social deterioration that a right-wing extremist, Jair Bolsonaro, was elected. With an antidemocratic, militarist, and openly conservative agenda, the current president has strived for democratic destabilization, as he has consistently attacked democratic institutions, championed authoritarianism, threatened political opponents with violence, and encouraged right-wing radicalism among his supporter base. Thus, the pandemic coincides with a crisis of democracy, further exacerbating the process of authoritarianism and blame game put forward as the Federal administration concretely attempts to change federalism and consequently the style of policymaking in the country.

Bolsonaro's federalism (Abrucio et al., 2020) is guided by a heavily centralized and hierarchical vision on issues with a national and dualistic impact on intergovernmental relations, which decreases the federal government's stake in mitigating territorial inequalities and assisting subnational governments. In practice, it is characterized by a trickle-down approach in which there is less federal involvement in public policy, clearly highlighted in his slogan "Mais Brasil, Menos Brasília" (direct translation, "More Brazil, Less Brasilia," Brasilia is where the seat of the government is located).

According to Abrucio et al. (2020, p. 669), Bolsonaro's federalism is based on three pillars. First, Bolsonaro's federalism advocates for a devolution of responsibilities from the Federal Government to local governments without funding or assistance, including drastic funding reduction. Second, Bolsonaro's federalism reinforces dualism through an autocratic concentration of decisions that affect subnational entities, leaving hardly any room for dialogue, negotiation, or participation of states in federal programs. Third, Bolsonaro's federalism is a carbon copy of former president Trump's policy during his administration in which intergovernmental confrontation and the struggle against real or imagined adversaries are continuous. Furthermore, the persistent attack against perceived enemies feeds the rhetoric of war that stir up his supporters and stamp out an anti-system position against "tudo que está aí" ("everything out there"), as Bolsonaro frequently says. The greatest among these perceived enemies are the institutions themselves and their respective leadership since the Bolsonarist approach to presidentialism repudiates institutional negotiation and the checks and balances of the Brazilian state, including federalism (Abrucio et al., 2020, p. 699).

The two forms of federalism exist in parallel to each other and often in conflict over who has power and who does not. That is, the Federal administration is trying to change the rules of the game and therefore purposely feeding low trust in government responses. Translated into practice, the administration made clear that it would not act decisively on the pandemic, as it claimed it was the responsibility of subnational governments to act.

The devolution of social policy is a key strategy in Bolsonaro's government, as the president has consistently challenged the cooperative approach. This shifting of responsibilities has helped the president to avoid blame for the disastrous pandemic response, as he places the blame for its erratic response to the COVID-19 on governors and mayors, without taking any responsibility for the several mistakes that occurred. This misguided reorientation of policies, priorities, and funding has directly impacted the pandemic response, as Bolsonaro's discourse has been largely accepted by a relatively big part of the population that distrust the political class. Furthermore, the economic downturn caused by the COVID-19 pandemic has also contributed to the undermining of the population's confidence in some Brazil's political and civil institutions.

Brazil's COVID-19 Response—Breaking Away with Previous Policy Style and Misalign of Critical Policy Steps

Three types of evidence support the argument that Bolsonaro's administration purposefully broke away with the previous policy styles of federal cooperation by undermining public health advice. Here, we explore a set of acts and omission related to the Federal's administration strategy of obstructing preventive behavior. This involves government acts and statements to obstruct subnational government endeavors to manage the pandemic, federal normative acts, including inadequate, delayed legislation, and presidential vetoes, and propaganda against public health (Ventura et al., 2021). The confluence of those acts led to the rapid spread of the virus.

Government Acts

On February 25, 2020, Brazil's public health officials announced that Latin America had its first COVID-19 case, when a male resident of São Paulo arriving from Italy tested positive for the virus. A month later, all 26 states plus the Federal District reported COVID-19 cases. Lacking a national contingency plan to curb the spread of the virus, the pandemic triggered a variety of responses. State and municipal officials pushed forward with their own plans as a persistent political divide took form. Between March 12 and March 21, nearly, all state governors mobilized to install health policies according to WHO's international guidelines. Through a declaration of a state of emergency on their own, local officials imposed varying levels of closures and restrictions on schools, intercity public transportation, shops, bars, large social events, parks, and beaches. On March 20, Brazil's federal government declared a countrywide state of emergency which lifted expenditure ceilings with newfound funding routed into a special pandemic war budget (IMF, 2020; Paraguassu and Eisenhammer, 2020). By March 19, 2020, land borders were partially closed, while incoming foreigners traveling by air were banned on March 30 (Salcedo et al., 2020). But this only lasted for a short while as the administration started to challenge the constitutionality of lockdowns and travel bans in the Courts.

Since the outset of the pandemic, Bolsonaro's administration defended the theory of "herd immunity," in line with its policy of non-intervention and little responsibility. The theory of herd (or collective) immunity spreading is the belief that the "natural immunity" can be the result of from the virus infection and would protect individuals and lead to the control of the pandemic. This theory has not been confirmed scientifically, but this did not prevent the world leaders to try to implement, such as Boris Johnson in the UK (see Chapter 9). The WHO does not endorse this approach. Herd immunity is a concept only achievable through vaccination, not by exposing people to the pathogen that causes the disease (WHO, 2020). Nevertheless, the government was both openly pursuing a strategy of promoting the spread of COVID-19 under the misguided theory despite the clear guidelines from WHO. In the state of Amazon, in the North of the country, the health system collapsed due to the extreme high number of cases by a new highly contagious variant borne out in that location. The result was a massive death toll of gigantic proportions occasioned by the lack of social distancing, lockdowns, and other public health measures. The governor of Manaus (the capital of Amazon) was a hardcore bolsonarist and ignored the seriousness of the pandemic. This lack of action, in combination with other factors, including the belief in of herd immunity and use of unproven pharmaceuticals—such as chloroquine, ivermectin, and azithromycin, the infamous "Covid Kit"—is likely to have contributed to the severity of the outbreak and related deaths (Buss et al., 2020; Lalwani et al., 2020; Malta et al., 2021). As a pandemic policy, "herd immunity is another word for mass murder," as explained by the president of the ACCESS Health International[2] with serious political and policy implications.

In contrast to all types of public health policy implemented in the country before, the policy was to transmit instructions on how to be brave and face the virus instead of enforcing behaviors that helped contain and mitigate the effects of the pandemic. The only measures suggested was the so called "vertical isolation" where only the most vulnerable were put in isolation, which had little to no acceptance. A second measure was a purported "early treatment" with provenly ineffective drugs (COVID kit). In addition, the government exhibited lack of sensitivity by trivializing the deaths and damage caused by the disease. In addition to remaining silent about the COVID victims and survivors, the federal government promoted the idea that only elderly people or people with comorbidities and those without access to "early treatment" would die (Ventura et al., 2021, p. 16).[3]

Devaluing Brazil's federal system of government and in response to Rio's governor declaring the closing of Rio's airports due to the pandemic, Bolsonaro issued an executive order that concentrated the power of the federal government to adopt measures that could restrict the transport of goods, the movement of people, and the maintenance of services during the COVID-19 pandemic. Four days later, a federal court prohibited the federal government from adopting measures contrary to social isolation as a way of preventing COVID-19. Bolsonaro also issued a decree declaring exempting churches and lottery houses from state and municipal health regulations by classifying them as essential services. Again, a federal court suspended the decree ruling that it violated federal law (Mello, 2020).

In the absence of a pandemic response plan,[4] it was up to governors and mayors to define and execute preventive health measures. Those varied from state to state, with a varied of stringency level among states and municipalities. As of May 2020, only 11 of the 26 federation members had sanctioned some form of lockdown.[5] But where implemented, these measures were systematically obstructed by the Federal administration justified by the supposed opposition between health protection and the safeguard of the economy, which included spreading the idea that quarantine measures cause more damage than the virus, and that they—and not the pandemic—would cause hunger and unemployment (Ventura et al., 2021). Placing all the blame for the health and economic crisis in the governor and mayors, Bolsonaro said: "(…) The population wants to go back to work, unfortunately a few governors, a few mayors insist on issuing decrees forcing these people to stay at home."[6] The Federal administration was alerted several times about the nonexistence of national plan and strategic guidelines to manage the pandemic, as well as the lack of a coordinated and comprehensive communication plan, which could compromise the costs and results of efforts against the pandemic (Ventura et al., 2021). A national communication was only presented after judicial deliberation, when Federal Public Prosecutor Office determined that the Federal Government present, within ten days, a National Communication Plan for facing the pandemic, including a timeline of action and a specific date for the initial implementation of the plan.[7] In a similar fashion, transparency of information suffered an attempted obstructions, when the cumulative number case and death counts stopped being published in the official heath minister website—a clear attempt to distort the actual pandemic numbers. A court order forced the Federal government to continue publishing the information.[8]

Federal Normative Acts

The normative pandemic acts were collected and analyzed by the project "Rights in the pandemic: Mapping the impact of Covid-19 on human rights in Brazil," coordinated by professors from the University of São Paulo (USP). The project found that in the federal level alone, 3,049 normative acts were published (laws, provisional measures, decrees, ordinances, resolutions, etc.) related to the pandemic in 2020 (Ventura et al., 2021). While this number seems an impressive legislative repertoire, the report calls attention to the series of decrees that expanded the list of activities considered essential during the pandemic and a series of vetoes to proposed bills introducing minimal obligations to states and municipalities to fight the virus. Draft bills mandating the use of masks faced several second rounds of vetoes within the constitutional deadlines for passing a bill. These actions show the escalation of political confrontation between the Federal administration and the Legislative and Judiciary powers and also the state and municipal powers that wanted to adopt preventive health measures to contain the spread of the virus, eliminating any possibility of good communication and cooperation with subnational actors.

Other normative acts included the declaration of emergency ('state of public calamity'), leading to the initiation of extensive economic measures in an attempt to preserve workers' positions and incomes (IMF, 2020). Beginning in March, Brazil's government increased lines of credit and established monetary transfers for formal, informal, and low-income workers (the "auxílio emergencial" or "emergencial social benefit"). The government eased taxes across the board and lowered import levies on essential medical supplies. Despite these gradual measures, tensions rose between state governors and the president as political influence regularly interfered with public health measures. This likely contributed the decling of public approval of President Bolsonaro's work between April and August (see Figure 10.1).

The low and inadequate funds allocated for financing health actions were included in these normative actions, but several governors and mayors reported that resources—both funding and PPE materials—were not reaching them. Regionally, Brazil has significant resource-centered bureaucratic agencies which could have helped Brazil tackle the pandemic. Fund-to-fund transfer, for example, is part of the healthcare institutional arrangement enshrined in the 1988 Constitution. This transfer delays were unusual for the SUS, considering its long trajectory of operational fund-to-fund transfers (Bertoni, 2020). The amount of money transferred was often challenged, as the federal government often reported high fund transfers that were later not confirmed by governors and mayors. Sixteen of the 25 state governors signed a collective statement challenging the data released on social media by the President regarding the amount of funding made available to states.[9] The 2020 budget for COVID-related actions

unrealistically and irresponsibly disregarded the needs for the acquisition of vaccines, diagnostic kits and supplies; sustainability and maintenance

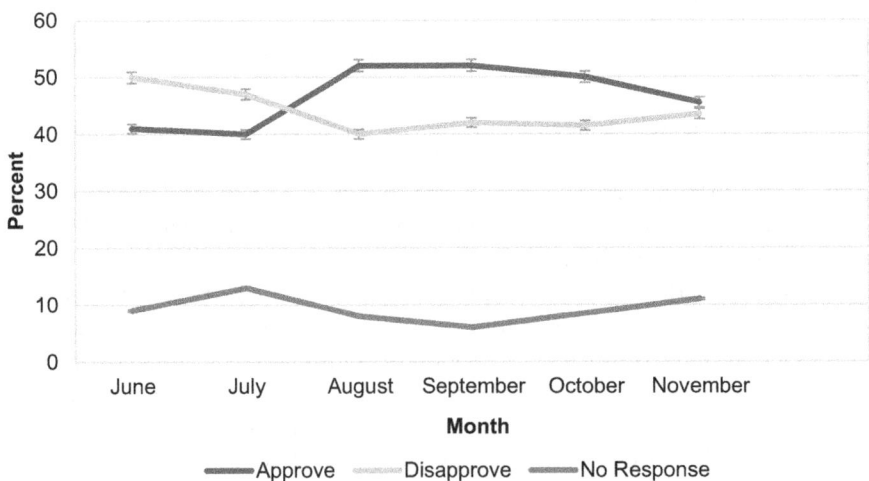

FIGURE 10.1 Approval Ratings for President Bolsonaro (June–November 2020).

of services provided by the SUS, such as clinical and ICU beds, medical equipment, care for COVID-19 sequelae, supressed demand for outpatient and hospital procedures.

(Ventura et al. 2021, p. 154)

Discourse against Public Health

Previous pandemic response frameworks in Brazil had a relatively strong information-based policy style, in which the government invested resources in treatment and research but also in public awareness campaigns to make its policies known and understood. In contrast, Bolsonaro's administration not only had no clear communication plan[10] but also actively shared propaganda against sound public health advice, including an anti-vaccine, anti-social distancing, anti-quarantine, and anti-mask discourse. Table 10.1 shows the percentage of mask adherence in South American and African countries. From these data, it is possible to observe that where the use of facemask was mandatory, mask adherence was often much higher. In Brazil, only 45.5% reported wearing a mask at the time of the survey, which is much lower than in Asian countries and Latin neighbors, such as Peru 99.8% and Ecuador (91.7%). This survey data suggest that the Federal Government anti-mask approach was largely accepted and followed by parts of the population (Gramacho et al., 2021; Kalil, 2021). This negligent behavior is likely to be connected to the low adherence to facemask use specially in the initial periods of the pandemic (Fodjo et al., 2020).

The president personally urged people to not comply with social distancing and other measures to slow down the spread of the virus. Not only did Bolsonaro challenge the other two branches of government in a federal system in which power sharing and checks and balances are one of its main pillars, but he also ignored the advice from some of health officers and went to the

TABLE 10.1 Survey characteristics and overall adherence to mask-use for COVID-19 prevention in selected countries

Country	Participants who reported using face mask: N (%)	Face mask-use mandatory at the time of survey
Brazil	(45.7%)	No
Democratic Republic of Congo	(43.2%)	Yes
Ecuador	(91.7%)	No
Mozambique	(93.9%)	Yes
Peru	(99.7%)	Yes
Somalia	(51.2%)	No
Thailand	(94.0%)	Yes
Uganda	(32.7%)	No
Vietnam	(99.4%)	Yes

Source: Adapted from Fodjo et al. (2020). Period of survey vary from April 3, 2020 to June 8, 2020.

public with his own erroneous messages regarding vaccination and COVID-19 pandemic. For example, on March 24, 2020, on a televised pronouncement, Bolsonaro stated that under his government, the main objective had been to minimize the "panic and hysteria" regarding the COVID-19 pandemic. He also directly criticized the Brazilian media for spreading "lies and fantasy" about the pandemic in Brazil and its consequences. In a very confrontational and adversarial manner, Bolsonaro criticized those that criticized him. In a speech in Porto Seguro, Bahia, Bolsonaro stated:

> Some say that I am setting a bad example. Either you are an imbecile or the idiot who is saying that I set a bad example. I already had the virus. I already have antibodies. Why do I have to be vaccinated?
>
> *(CM, 2020)*

Despite Brazil's universal healthcare apparatus containing an epidemiological surveillance system, professionals expressed early concerns following healthcare budget cuts prior to the pandemic's onset. Brazil's hospitals held an impressive ICU bed count of 21 per 100,000 residents (roughly twice that of Italy, France, or Spain), but only one-tenth of beds were installed in public hospitals (Sandy and Milhorance, 2020). Most Brazilians rely exclusively on the SUS. The SUS is guaranteed by the Federal Constitution of 1988, in its Article 196, by means of Law 8,080/1990. The SUS is the only public health system in the world serving more than 190 million people, 80% of them depend exclusively on it to any health care.

But Bolsonaro is not the only one on his administration attacking science and public health expertise. Other health authorities aligned with his agenda created confusion and distrust among the Brazilian population regarding the efficacy of public health advice. The country had four health ministers since beginning of the pandemic,[11] showing the tumultuous state of the Federal administration in a moment when the health minister should be working at full capacity. Two of the ministers, Henrique Mandetta and Nelson Teich, were sacked by Bolsonaro due to clashes related to the management of the pandemic especially when it came to coordinating actions between Union, states, and municipalities, funding for the SUS as a necessary institutional arrangement to federative coordination and implementation of health restrictions. The other two ministers shared the Federal administration's anti-science approach, defending Bolsonaro's pro-COVID speeches, while upholding pseudo-scientific discourses and promoting the use of miraculous drugs. Even the health experts composing the national team of COVID actions were politicized medical professionals[12] showing that the current institutional structure of the Federal administration was instrumental to erode the political trust in health experts and likely to have collaborated to the low level of compliance among the population.

Another example was the online campaign encouraging people to return to work amid the pandemic, which sometimes included the hiring of social media influencers. On March 28, a federal judge ordered the federal government not to carry out a publicity campaign "O Brasil Não Pode Parar" (Brazil Cannot Stop) urging the population to defy social distancing recommendations and go about their lives with confidence. The president's Communication Office had already published two social media postings with that slogan. The president's son, Senator Flavio Bolsonaro, had distributed a video with the federal government logo that was supposedly part of the campaign (Human Rights Watch, 2020). The Federal Public Prosecutor's Office asked for the suspension of the campaign, arguing "that the campaign conveys misleading advertising, violating the merely informational nature imposed by the Federal Constitution, by disseminating, without solid scientific evidence and in non-compliance with the technical consensus and international recommendations on the matter (…)" (as translated by Ventura et al., 2021).

Trust in the Political Institutions During a Health Crisis

Even before the pandemic, decline of trust in political institutions was observed Brazil. Citizens' lack of trust opened the space for the election of a populist incumbent who thrives on divisive discourses. The failed response framework of the Federal administration added to an ongoing crisis in democracy, which, combined with authoritarian attitudes and irresponsible public health policy decisions at the national level, resulted in general decrease in trust in the healthcare system. In turn, this combination resulted in a sharp disassociation between responsible administration of a health crisis and an effective pandemic response.

Low trust in government played a significant role in determining how different countries performed in containing and responding to the COVID-19 pandemic, especially in those countries that had not recently experienced deadly outbreaks in the past. Better appreciating the role of government trust can help countries prepare for, and respond to not only the current pandemic but also those still to come (Bollyky et al., 2020). While Brazil had a consistently positive trajectory of health crisis strategies—including prevention, treatment, and vaccination—the Federal Administration's inability and unwillingness to spearhead a national pandemic strategy weakened the Brazilian population confidence on the federal government's ability to exercise its most fundamental function: protect the people against this disease. By touting chloroquine as a cure for COVID-19 despite several studies questioning the credibility of such claims (Samuels and Kelly, 2020) and side-stepping public health officials' recommendations to address the pandemic head on, Bolsonaro's actions proved to be inefficient, confusing, and utterly irresponsible, opening the door for several accusation of "genocide" and other crimes.[13]

Emerging Actors—STF, Governors, and Organizations

As noted elsewhere in this volume, policy styles cast long shadows in many directions. Even with attempts from different sides of the Federal administration to erode health policy and construct a new one based on an extreme form of dual federalism with a central authorit, part of previous policy styles remained. In the Brazilian case, the analysis shows that policy styles change over time but also that relatively stable, persistent modes of policy deliberation endure. While the pro-COVID policy of the Federal administration caused an incalculable damage to the population with its anti-scientific approach, the actions of some particular actors help to mitigate an even-worse pandemic scenario. Three of them have been central to uphold the democratic and cooperative values of the federal pact.

The first one is the STF. The Court has been one of the main political target of Bolsonaro for supporting health measures, upholding decisions that forced the Federal government to fulfill its coordination role, and decisions for the maintenance of a joint approach among federation members. Some Court verdicts were critical for the adoption of health measures, including verdicts on the sharing of responsibilities among the Federal and subnational entities, to protect indigenous health, delivery of ventilators to state governments, and determination for the government to elaborate a national vaccination plan on time (see Ventura et al., 2021 for a complete timeline of those decisions). Some have argued that Brazilian federalism is in fact undergoing a process of reinforcement because STF decisions unequivocally granted more power to governors and mayors on health-related public policies issues (Bustamante et al., 2021).

The second group of actors is the state and local authorities that began to take initiatives to address the pandemic and fill the gaps left by the Federal government. Some states and municipalities, for example, developed their own vaccination plans and started to negotiate the import and production of vaccines, as it was the case of the states of São Paulo and Maranhão. Of note are the Fórum de Govern adores (Governors' Forum), and the Consórcio Nordeste (Consortium of the Northeast States) which strengthened horizontal cooperation and filled gaps left by the Federal Government with regionally coordinated actions of quarantine and social isolation that counterweight discourses and presidential decisions.

The third group of actors consists of are health, professional, research, and civil society organizations that resisted, criticized, debated, campaigned, evaluated, and demanded a proper plan of action to face the pandemic. Some of those organizations are the Brazilian Bar Association (OAB) which brought several petitions to the STF related to the poor management of the pandemic. In addition, the National Federation of Municipalities (CNM), the National Council of State Secretaries of Health (Conass), and the National Council of Municipal Secretaries of Health (Conasems) developed scientific reports and technical documents among its members to facilitate subnational cooperation (Censon and Barcelos, 2020).

Together, those actors collaborated to counterbalance the damage the Bolsonaro's federalism caused to cooperative federalism and its associated policy styles. This response to the COVID-19 pandemic shows that the Federal administration policy style and lower trust prompted the construction of more decentralized response plans because the Union refused to act, giving way to a new types of regional leadership and some level of trust in political institutions. For now, it is unclear whether the cooperative federal model will be further shaped by the current Federal government approach of top-down centralized response policies in some area but not in others.

Conclusion

This chapter analyzed how Brazil's Federal administration fomented low political trust via poor decisions that led to an uncontrolled pandemic. The low level of trust in public officials, including both the government and health officials, provided a basis for pandemic response that was inefficient and demanded new types of coordinated action without the participation of the national government. This centrifugal approach gave way to news types of regional leadership that helped to somewhat address the impact that the political neglect of public health amidst a health crisis.

Whereas it is hard to predict how far cooperative federalism can resist in an exceptionally hostile environment for national cooperation, the impacts of Bolsonaro's federalism on policy are likely to be long-lasting. Nevertheless, regional leaders used this critical moment to create opportunities for overcoming limits to existing policymaking and respond to the fragmentation of policy styles. In a way, some policy norms and structures remained in place, thanks to the democratic institutions that despite being under constant political attack, were able to guarantee that core constitutional values are defended.

While those findings have the potential to worry those that observe the slow deterioration of the democracy in the Brazil, including its uneasy position on the international stage on several issues, (e.g. Amazon devastation, attacks on indigenous people, misogynist, and racist remarks), they also show that federative dynamics are far from static, that policy styles can be forcibly changed quickly under authoritarian governments but that strong, high capacity states can stand up to attack on democratic institutions. Besides keeping an eye opened to what kind federalist pact will be dominant in Brazil in the years to come, an interesting area of further research is the systematic study of changes in federal dynamics at the regional and local levels in the post-pandemic context, both in Brazil and other federal states.

Notes

1   Number from the University of Oxford "Our World in Data" project. As of February 2021, one year after the beginning of the pandemic, the number of deaths increased to 321,515 deaths. At the time of the writing, September 2021, the number of cumulative deaths is reaching the devastating mark of 600,000 deaths.
2   CNN Brasil: https://edition.cnn.com/world/live-news/coronavirus-pandemic-10-14-20-intl/h_571c71aa21a9a2a0d0aadd95af67a022.
3   Of note, we mention the disturbing footage of Bolsonaro making an impression of someone infected by COVID-19 gasping for air (https://www.youtube.com/

watch?v=g4K_WlfUhuI) and his comments on people who "would not stop whining" at the Covid death toll ("Until when will you keep crying?" https://www.theguardian. com/world/2021/mar/05/bolsonaro-brazil-covid-coronavirus-death-toll).
4 The Comitê de Combate ao Covid (Covid combat committee) was only created in March 2021, one year after the outset of the health crisis.
5 https://noticias.uol.com.br/saude/ultimas-noticias/redacao/2020/05/09/saiba-onde-ja-foi-decretado-o-lockdown-no-brasil.htm.
6 "'Thursday Live' with the president on transmitted on Facebook, February 2nd, 2021." Available at: https://www.youtube.com/watch?v=sA1AJ1NuDP4.
7 https://stf.jusbrasil.com.br/jurisprudencia/1222866415/arguicao-de-descumprimento-de-preceito-fundamental-adpf-829-rs-0052170-2520211000000.
8 CNN - Brazil resumes publishing Covid-19 data after court ruling: https://www. bbc.com/news/world-latin-america-52980642.
9 Reuters: https://www.reuters.com/article/saude-covid-bolsonaro-estados-idLTAK-CN2AT2TJ.
10 An actual plan was only published when the vaccination program started in late December 2020.
11 They were Henrique Mandetta (January 2019 to April 2020), Nelson Teich (April to May 2020), Eduardo Pazzuelo (May 2020 to March 2021), and Marcelo Queiroga to date.
12 https://www.cnnbrasil.com.br/politica/apelidada-de-capita-cloroquina-secretaria-da-saude-depoe-a-cpi-na-quinta-20/.
13 Indigenous Brazilians accuse Jair Bolsonaro of genocide at ICC: https://www.dw.com/en/indigenous-brazilians-accuse-jair-bolsonaro-of-genocide-at-icc/a-58810568.

References

Abrucio, Fernando Luiz, Eduardo José Grin, Cibele Franzese, Catarina Ianni Segatto, and Cláudio Gonçalves Couto. 2020. 'Combating COVID-19 under Bolsonaro's Federalism: A Case of Intergovernmental Incoordination'. *Revista de Administração Pública* 54 (4): 663–77.

Avritzer, Leonardo, and Lucio Rennó. 2021. 'The Pandemic and the Crisis of Democracy in Brazil'. *Journal of Politics in Latin America*. Online First. https://doi.org/10.1177/1866802X211022362.

Barbosa, Rafael. 2020. 'Governo Bolsonaro é aprovado por 52% e desaprovado por 41%, diz PoderData'. *Poder360*, 14 October 2020. https://www.poder360.com.br/poderdata/governo-bolsonaro-e-aprovado-por-52-e-desaprovado-por-41-mostra-poderdata/.

Bringel, Breno, and Geoffrey Pleyers. 2020. 'Introducción: La Pandemia y Sus Ecos Globales'. In *Alerta Global*, edited by Breno Bringel and Geoffrey Pleyers, 9–32. Políticas, Movimientos Sociales y Futuros En Disputa En Tiempos de Pandemia. Buenos Aires: CLACSO.

Buss, Lewis F., Carlos A. Prete, Claudia MM Abrahim, Alfredo Mendrone, Tassila Salomon, Cesar de Almeida-Neto, Rafael FO França, et al. 2020. Three-quarters attack rate of SARS-CoV-2 in the Brazilian Amazon during a largely unmitigated epidemic. *Science* 371 (6526): 288–292. doi: 10.1126/science.abe9728

Bustamante, T., P. N. M. Meyer, and F. Tirado. 2020. 'Opposing an Idle Federal Government'. *Verfassungsblog* (blog). https://verfassungsblog.de/opposing-an-idle-federal-government/.

Censon, D., and M. Barcelos. 2020. 'The Role of State in the COVID-19 Pandemic Crisis Management: Different Views about Federalism and the Relations between Federal Government and Municipalities'. *Revista Brasileira de Gestao e Desenvolvimento Regional* 16 (4): 35–48.

Faria de Moura Villela, Edlaine, Rossana Verónica Mendoza López, Ana Paula Sayuri Sato, Fábio Morato de Oliveira, Eliseu Alves Waldman, Rafael Van den Bergh, Joseph Nelson Siewe Fodjo, and Robert Colebunders. 2021. 'COVID-19 Outbreak in Brazil: Adherence to National Preventive Measures and Impact on People's Lives, an Online Survey'. *BMC Public Health* 21 (1): 152.

Fodjo, Joseph Nelson Siewe, Supa Pengpid, Edlaine Faria de Moura Villela, Vo Van Thang, Mohammed Ahmed, John Ditekemena, Bernardo Vega Crespo, et al. 2020. 'Mass Masking as a Way to Contain COVID-19 and Exit Lockdown in Low- and Middle-Income Countries'. *Journal of Infection* 81 (3): e1–5. https://doi.org/10.1016/j.jinf.2020.07.015.

Gaventa, J. T. 2006. 'Triumph, Deficit or Contestation? Deepening the "Deepening Democracy" Debate'. IDS Working Paper (264), Brighton.

Gramacho, Wladimir G., and Mathieu Turgeon. 2021. 'When Politics Collides with Public Health: COVID-19 Vaccine Country of Origin and Vaccination Acceptance in Brazil'. *Vaccine* 39 (19): 2608–12.

Human Rights Watch. 2020. 'Brazil: Bolsonaro Sabotages Anti-Covid-19 Efforts'. *Human Rights Watch* (blog). 10 April 2020. https://www.hrw.org/news/2020/04/10/brazil-bolsonaro-sabotages-anti-covid-19-efforts.

Kalil, Isabela, Sofia Cherto Silveira, Weslei Pinheiro, Álex Kalil, João Vicente Pereira, Wiverson Azarias, and Ana Beatriz Amparo. 2021. 'Politics of Fear in Brazil: Far-Right Conspiracy Theories on COVID-19'. *Global Discourse* 11 (3): 409–25.

Lalwani, Pritesh, Bárbara Batista Salgado, Ivanildo Vieira Pereira Filho, Danielle Severino Sena da Silva, Thiago Barros do Nascimento de Morais, Maele Ferreira Jordão, Aguyda Rayany Cavalcante Barbosa, et al. 2021. 'SARS-CoV-2 Seroprevalence and Associated Factors in Manaus, Brazil: Baseline Results from the DETECTCoV-19 Cohort Study'. Paper ID 3795816. Rochester: SSRN.

Lima, Valesca. 2019. *Participatory Citizenship and Crisis in Contemporary Brazil*. 1st ed. 2020 edition. US: Palgrave.

Loureiro, M. R., F. L. Silva, A. V. Aranha, and F. Calabraz. 2020. 'Building Policy Capacity within Contextual and Political Boundaries: An Analysis of Policies in Fiscal and Social Areas in Brazil (1988/2016) | Revista Do Serviço Público'. *Revista Do Serviço Público* 71 (SE): 7–37.

Malta, Monica, Steffanie A. Strathdee, and Patricia J. Garcia. 2021. 'The Brazilian Tragedy: Where Patients Living at the "Earth's Lungs" Die of Asphyxia, and the Fallacy of Herd Immunity Is Killing People'. *EClinicalMedicine* 32: 100757. doi:10.1016/j.eclinm.2021.100757

Mello, Igor. 2020. 'Coronavírus: Justiça Proíbe Bolsonaro de Adotar Medidas Contra Isolamento Em Igrejas e Lotéricas'. https://noticias.uol.com.br/cotidiano/ultimas-noticias/2020/03/27/justica-suspende-decretos-de-bolsonaro-que-liberavamigrejas-e-lotericas.htm?cmpid=copiaecola.

Paim, Jairnilson, Claudia Travassos, Celia Almeida, Ligia Bahia, and James Macinko. 2011. 'The Brazilian Health System: History, Advances, and Challenges'. *The Lancet* 377 (9779): 1778–97.

Paraguassu, L., and S. Eisenhammer. 'Brazil Cuts Growth, Sees Coronavirus Quickly Ravaging Health System'. Reuters. https://www.reuters.com/article/uk-health-coronavirus-brazil-idUKKBN2172PO.

Pierson, Paul. 1995. 'Fragmented Welfare States: Federal Institutions and the Development of Social Policy'. *Governance* 8 (4): 449–78.

Rennó, L., A. E. Smith, M. Layton, and F. B. Pereira. 2011. *Legitimidade E Qualidade Da Democracia No Brasil – Uma Visao Da Cidada*. 1ª edição. São Paulo, SP, Brasil: INTERMEIOS.

Ribeiro, Ricardo Lodi. 2018. 'Do federalismo dualista ao federalismo de cooperação – a evolução dos modelos de estado e a repartição do poder de tributar'. *Revista Interdisciplinar do Direito – Faculdade de Direito de Valença* 16 (1): 335–62.

Samuels, E., and K. Meg. n.d. 'Analysis | How False Hope Spread about Hydroxychloroquine to Treat Covid-19 — and the Consequences That Followed'. *Washington Post*. 17 September 2021. https://www.washingtonpost.com/politics/2020/04/13/how-false-hope-spread-about-hydroxychloroquine-its-consequences/.

Schaefer, Bruno Marques, Roberta Carnelos Resende, Sara de Sousa Fernandes Epitácio, and Mariah Torres Aleixo. 2020. 'Government Actions against the New Coronavirus: Evidence from the Brazilian States'. *Revista de Administração Pública* 54 (5): 1429–45.

Teixeira, Maria Glória, Maria da Conceição Nascimento Costa, Enny Santos da Paixão, Eduardo Hage Carmo, Florisneide Rodrigues Barreto, and Gerson Oliveira Penna. 2018. 'The Achievements of the SUS in Tackling the Communicable Diseases'. *Ciência & Saúde Coletiva* 23: 1819–28.

Tikkanen, Roosa. 2020. 'International Health Care System Profiles Brazil'. 5 June 2020. https://www.commonwealthfund.org/international-health-policy-center/countries/brazil.

Ventura, Deisy de Freitas Lima, Fernando Mussa Abujamra Aith, Rossana Rocha Reis, André Bastos Ferreira, Alexia Viana da Rosa, Alexsander Silva Farias, Giovanna Dutra Silva Valentim, and Lucas Bertola Herzog. 2021. 'LexAtlas C19- Brazil - The Timeline of the Federal Government's Strategy to Spread Covid-19'. University of São Paulo.

WHO, World Health Organisation. 2020. 'Coronavirus Disease (COVID-19): Herd Immunity, Lockdowns and COVID-19'. https://www.who.int/news-room/q-a-detail/herd-immunity-lockdowns-and-covid-19.

11

THE U.S. RESPONSE TO THE COVID-19 PANDEMIC

Incoherent Leadership, Fractured Federalism, and Squandered Capacity

Kristin Taylor, Rob A. DeLeo, Deserai A. Crow and Thomas A. Birkland

Overview of U.S. Policy Style

Categorizing a single, distinctive American policy style is extraordinarily difficult, a testament to the highly decentralized system of government codified by the United States Constitution. On the one hand, the US Constitution divides power between the national government and the states, thus creating a complex and often overlapping governance process encompassing 50 subnational units plus an ever-expanding national government. States themselves encompass diverse institutional norms, rules, and cultures that not only promote divergent policy outcomes but often radically different styles and approaches to making public policy (Peters 2019).

On the other hand, the Constitution divides government power between executive, legislative, and judicial branches of government. In doing so, it allows each branch of government to serve as a check on the other branches while, somewhat inadvertently, establishing various distinct policy venues (Calef and Gobble 2007). Because this structure exists at both the national and state levels, the U.S. system amounts to a dizzying array of different institutional locations, each of which has its own unique policymaking style. Commenting on the peculiarities of the U.S. system, Peters (2019) writes:

> It is almost impossible to identify a single style that can characterize the federal government, the 50 states (plus the District of Columbia), and the roughly 89,000 local governments. And even individual institutions within those numerous governments may have their own cultures and policymaking styles.
>
> *(p. 180)*

DOI: 10.4324/9781003137399-15

In spite of these challenges, we rely on the decentralized policy style to examine the U.S. response to the COVID-19 pandemic to understand how well the theory holds up in the context of a crisis. One of the major challenges this case wrestles with when applying the lens of a decentralized policy style for the U.S. response to COVID-19 is the absence of political partisanship in the framework. As indicated throughout the following discussion, partisan differences were a key determinant of how state governments as well as the national government responded to the pandemic.

This chapter begins with an assessment of the distinctive features of the American policy styles, drawing largely from Peters' (2019) investigation of policy capacity and inclusivity in the American state. Our analysis of policy styles pays particularly close attention to the administrative capacity of the American state as well as its inclusiveness or the extent to which policymakers regularly consult with interest groups, activists, the public, and other members of the community. We then explore the intersection of the U.S. policy style and trust both for the policymakers and the medical community.

The balance of the paper is devoted to a detailed case study of COVID-19 policymaking in the U.S., including federal and state actions during the crisis. Our case study consists of four distinct but interrelated parts: (1) a detailed analysis of the coordination structure used to organize state and national operations during the pandemic; (2) an investigation of policymaker communications during the pandemic; (3) an assessment of the stringency of various COVID-19 interventions; and (4) an examination of the degree of decentralization in the U.S. government's response to the COVID-19 pandemic. We conclude by considering the larger theoretical implications of our case for the policy styles literature.

Defining the American Policy Style: Capacity and Inclusivity

Broadly speaking, U.S. government can be characterized as being reactive, meaning that the state does not readily seek out problems. This characteristic is partially attributed to the American electoral system, in which legislators are perpetually focused on re-election (Mayhew 2005), and voters are said to be myopic (Healey and Malhotra 2009), meaning that they only reward elected officials for reacting to problems that have an immediate impact on their daily lives as opposed to addressing emerging issues that may—or may not—affect constituents months or years in the future.

These same features tend to result in reactive policymaking at the subnational level, although there have been notable exceptions. Calef and Goble (2007) suggest caution when applying the policy styles concept in subnational settings, noting that "there is considerable policy variance across industrial sectors within each country (Kitschelt 1991), and in the United States different policy outcomes occur at the national and state levels" (p. 27). For example, the authors show that the state of California was anticipatory in its promotion of electric and hybrid vehicles, adopting policies and regulations that made the state an international forerunner in the movement to curb air pollution.

Building on this framework, the following section further analyzes the U.S. policy style. We pay particularly close attention to the difference in administrative policy capacity and degree of inclusivity. Given the degree of decentralization within the U.S. system described here, it is virtually impossible to account for policy styles of every unit of government. As such, our analysis focuses primarily on the national government and tries to draw some fairly broad generalizations about state activity. But it is important to bear in mind that, when we refer to "the state" in the United States, we are describing a very complex system in which there is no one single actor to which we can point as *the* state.

Administrative Policy Capacity

Despite its tendency toward reactive policymaking, the American policy system enjoys fairly high administrative capacity relative to other countries. Unlike in other countries, much of that policy capacity resides in the legislature, which seeks to act as a balance to the executive branch. While Peters (2015) suggests that the U.S. Congress has willingly shed some of its own policy capacity through internal budget cuts, thereby shifting to a reliance on lobbyists and technical experts to provide information, as opposed to internal information gathering entities, the legislature remains an important driver of policy change at the national level. This dynamic has, at least historically, been particularly pronounced in the health care and public health domains, which tends to provide a myriad of opportunities for experts to exert influence on the composition and design of important policies (Jacobs and Skocpol 2015).

This expert influence over health care and public health communities has been shown to persist in some, but certainly not all, subnational settings. States differ tremendously in terms of their level of professionalization. Whereas some states have robust healthcare infrastructures in which bureaucrats readily engage experts (DeLeo and Donnelly 2017), others have shirked the growth of the administrative state, failing to respond to federal incentives and even balking at important federal mandates. Meanwhile, the federal government has done little, if anything, to bolster the administrative capacity of laggard states and has made significant cuts to important state public health preparedness funding programs since roughly 2010, including the Hospital Preparedness Program (HPP) and the Public Health Emergency Preparedness (PHEP) programs.

No organization better exemplifies the high administrative capacity of the U.S. healthcare system than the Centers for Disease Control and Prevention (CDC). The so-called "sentinel" of American public health (Etheridge 1992), the CDC is responsible for guiding the country's global disease surveillance efforts, identifying threats, and initiating response planning. So powerful is the influence of the CDC and its supporters that it has even stimulated moments of anticipatory policymaking by the federal government, which are typically quite rare. In anticipation of a potential H5N1 avian influenza pandemic, the George W. Bush administration requested several billion dollars to fund pandemic preparedness programs. Agency officials, including the Secretary of Health and Human Services Michael Leavitt, lobbied for a host of statutory changes aimed at strengthening the nation's public health infrastructure, including the Pandemic and All-Hazards Preparedness Act (PAHPA) (PL 109–417), which centralized public health emergency response activities within HHS, and the Public Readiness and Emergency Preparedness Act (PREPA) (PL 109–148), which shielded vaccine manufacturers from liabilities arising from drugs created to combat a novel disease. This flurry of policy activity occurred despite the fact that the novel influenza outbreak was largely isolated to parts of Asia (DeLeo 2018).

Although the much-feared avian influenza pandemic never happened, the various plans and policies created during the Bush Administration proved instrumental in helping the U.S. navigate the 2009 swine influenza pandemic under the Obama Administration, which resulted in an estimated 12,000 deaths— far fewer than the more 90,000 deaths projected by the President's Council of Advisors on Science and Technology (McNeil 2010).

Good public policy capacity can be undermined by uneven political leadership, and even the public health domain is not immune to the reactive tendencies of the American state. History is littered with examples of American politicians either ignoring or outright denying pressing emerging public health issues until they have reached a full-blown crisis. For example, former President Ronald Reagan knowingly ignored the AIDS epidemic for more than four years despite pleas from the public health community to invest resources in combating the devastating disease. The Reagan "administration, unlike earlier ones, has been reluctant to request funds from Congress for research and services during an epidemic; President Reagan did not even mention AIDS in public until January 1986" (Fox 2005). Fox notes that the HIV/AIDS epidemic struck as the health policy establishment was shifting attention away from infectious disease and more toward chronic conditions, including conditions that were claimed to stem from "lifestyle choices" such as smoking, poor nutrition, and even HIV/AIDS.

Complicating matters further, anticipatory policy making has, at times, backfired for U.S. policymakers. Fearing the outbreak of a novel strain of swine influenza at an Army base in New Jersey foreshadowed a global pandemic, former President Gerald Ford launched an ambitious nationwide vaccination campaign. The pandemic never came to fruition; however, the hastily made vaccine resulted in nearly 450 cases of Guillain-Barré syndrome, a paralyzing nervous system disorder, and more than 30 deaths.

Overall, administrative policy capacity in the United States was relatively robust for public health in the time leading up to the COVID-19 pandemic, although with certain caveats. The first is that the U.S. system creates varying degrees of subnational capacity in spite of significant policy capacity at the national level. The second is that the public health policy domain is subject to political costs, namely the reluctance of policymakers to divert scarce resources to preparation for an event that may not occur at all or that will occur at some undetermined point in the future.

Inclusiveness

The American system enjoys modest inclusivity, particularly at the subnational level where myriad policy venues provide avenues for citizens and organized interests to advocate for their preferred policy alternatives. Kingdon (2011) drew on Cohen, March, and Olsen's "garbage can model of organizational choice," and its assumption of "fluid participation" in the policy process to describe a process within which participants come and go in the policy process, although the fluidity of that participation does vary by policy domain. Peters (2019) suggests that the courts are the primary participatory mechanism at the federal level, adding that partisan gridlock has effectively stunted the ability to usher major reforms through the U.S. Congress. Furthermore, Peters documents the rise of what he calls adversarial legalism or the growing reliance on the courts to block substantive policy change, suggesting that the courts play a central role in shaping and resolving important policy issues, also making it extraordinarily difficult to pass major reforms.

This characterization is consistent with trends in federalism in the United States, where there is increasing party polarization within states, resulting in legislative gridlock, and increased adversarial litigation of policies within state and federal courts (Goelzhauser and Konisky 2019). Under adversarial systems, attorneys and legal professionals seek to influence the trajectory of policy change. Their influence is exerted throughout the policy process including during the agenda setting, policy adoption, and program implementation stages. This dynamic, in turn, further reinforces incremental and reactive policy reform due to the difficulty of passing major reforms in the face of near certain adversarial litigation.

Concurrently, the U.S. enjoys a fairly robust NGO/civil society sector, which has been shown to play an important role transmitting public concerns to policy elites. Of course, these actors readily engage the court system; however, they also provide testimony and lobby on behalf of their constituencies. Civil society organizations and advocacy NGOs in the U.S. have grown significantly since the 1980s and with that growth came rapid professionalization of the sector (Dunlap and Mertig 1992; Kraft 2015). Although there is significant variation in the technical, personnel, and fiscal capacity of these organizations, many have come to engage in the policymaking process with equivalent levels of expertise and experience as industry, science organizations, and other traditional 'insider' groups that tend to have more influence over policy decisions (Maloney, Jordan, and McLaughlin 1994). The actors considered insiders to governmental decision-making processes typically use strategies (e.g., lobbying) that draw upon their relationships with decision-makers and their subject-matter expertise (Maloney, Jordan, and McLaughlin 1994; Dur and Mateo 2013; Binderkrantz,

Christiansen, and Helboe 2015), while 'outsiders' often have lower capacity and less prior experience and often must rely on harnessing external attention (e.g., protests or media campaigns) to pressure decision-makers since they do not enjoy the same level of access or expertise as insiders (Binderkrantz 2005; Nownes and Freeman 1998). While there is overlap in the strategies used and considerable variation in civil society capacity in the U.S., the sector is far more professionalized than in many national contexts and has significant access to decision-makers in the policy process.

Trust in U.S. Government and Health Care Systems

Political trust in government is generally low in the United States. Historically, Americans have had a less negative view of their local and state governments compared with their attitudes toward the national government (Peters 2019). This trend began in the 1980s and has been attributed to public perceptions of the economy, scandals in government, and crime (Chanley, Rudolph, and Rahn 2000). Although trust in government may be low in the United States, it is different from active distrust of the U.S. government (Cook and Gronkey 2005). The effect is that Americans are skeptical of government but are not hostile toward it. According to a survey conducted by the Pew Research Center (2019), 35% of Americans were confident that elected officials acted in the public's best interests, and this was far less than businesses or the media. The low levels of trust in government manifest in some policy domains particularly, after major disasters and crises, like Hurricane Katrina, public trust in government at all levels is low (Nicholls and Picou 2013).

The COVID-19 pandemic has only exacerbated American's distrust of government. Only 42% of Americans believe that the government has done a good job handling public health threats according to Pew. In fact, as of September 2020, only 20% of Americans indicated that they trust the federal government (Pew Research Center 2020). By contrast, a separate Pew study fielded on the cusp of the COVID-19 pandemic indicated that most have high levels of trust in medicine and medical science. Public perception of doctors was highly positive: 74% of Americans thought that doctors almost always have the best interest of their patients in mind, and 57% of Americans believed that doctors do a good job at diagnosis and treatment (Pew Research Center 2020). Moreover, most Americans (68%) had a positive perception about medical research scientists and their ability to research and investigate disease and treatments. These favorability ratings appear not to be political or at least partisan; Democrats and Republicans both have roughly the same positive perceptions of doctors. But while Americans trust physicians and medical researchers, most Americans (83%) also report knowing little to nothing about the work of medical researchers. This lack of knowledge is consistent with what is known about epistemic communities (Haas 2007; Dunlop 2010), the workings of which are generally unseen to and unknown by the public.

When taken in sum, Americans have low levels of trust and confidence in government but high levels of trust in the medical field. Given that low levels of political trust can diminish administrative capacity and make problems more intractable (Rothstein 2012; Exadaktylos and Zahariadis 2014), such public tendencies are problematic for the policy style of the United States and its response to the COVID-19 pandemic. It implies that American distrust of government would diminish the state's administrative capacity to be effective in the face of the pandemic. However, we expect that low levels of trust may not necessarily be the same for all levels of government. Although public confidence in subnational governments follows the pattern of trust in national government, Americans generally have higher confidence levels in state and local governments (Wolak and Palus 2010).

Furthermore, lack of knowledge about the medical research community could contribute to low understanding of and compliance with the recommendations made by medical professionals related to curbing the virus, including the methods and conditions under which the virus is transmitted, the efficacy of mask-wearing, and safety and efficacy of vaccines. While public opinion polling reflects increasing acceptance of the COVID-19 vaccine, in February 2021, 39% of Americans still stated that they would not get the COVID-19 vaccine (Pew Research Center 2021). Low levels of trust in government coupled with a lack of public knowledge about the medical research community creates a potentially confounding policy problem around the federal and state governments' efforts to achieve widespread vaccination.

The COVID-19 Pandemic Response in the United States

The U.S. response to the coronavirus pandemic has, by all accounts, been very poor. The U.S., as of February 15, 2021, had the eighth highest per-capita case rate for COVID-19 and the highest rate of all large nations. The U.S.'s cumulative case rate at 83,667 per million persons is substantially greater than that of the European Union (47,000).[1] This high case rate means that the U.S. has recorded more COVID-19 deaths than any other country in the world. At the time of this writing, more than 425,000 have succumbed to the virus, accounting for nearly one-fifth of all global COVID-19 fatalities. For context, Brazil is the only other country to eclipse 200,000 deaths; its per-capita case rate is similar to that of the EU. The total number of U.S. fatalities will exceed 500,000 deaths in February or March 2021, a number sufficient to reduce life expectancy by an entire year, the largest single-year decline since World War II (Marchione 2021).

There are four important elements to the pandemic response that shed light on the decentralized policy style of the U.S.: the coordination of the response within government, the communication of risk, the degree of policy stringency that the national and subnational governments undertook, and the degree of centralization in the government's response to the pandemic. Until January 20, 2021, the national government's response to the pandemic was characterized by an initial lack of urgency at the national level that evolved into a flood of misinformation and lies, leaving many state and local governments to fend for themselves throughout the crisis. The transition from the Trump Administration to the Biden Administration has indicated that the national government has shifted its position to be more proactive and science-based in its handling of the response to the pandemic. What remains unclear at this writing is the extent to which these failures are the result of the structure and composition of the U.S. system of government or are primarily idiosyncratic features of the managerial incompetence that characterized the Trump Administration. Furthermore, political divisions about the COVID-19 pandemic that existed prior to the election of President Joe Biden remain, as evidenced by high levels of vaccine hesitancy among Republicans (Kaiser Family Foundation 2021).

Coordination Structure

In the case of COVID-19 in the U.S., it is important to make the distinction between the existing coordination structures that were in place and the failure to effectively use these structures. In the time leading up to the COVID-19 pandemic, the U.S. federal government had the capacity to initiate an effective, coordinated response to a widespread public health crisis. However, this capacity to provide a coordinated response was squandered.

As previously noted, the George W. Bush Administration devoted billions of dollars to pandemic preparedness programs within the U.S. Department of Health and Human Services. The 2003 H5N1 pandemic led to the passage of the Pandemic and All-Hazards Preparedness Act (PL 109–417), which effectively centralized public health emergency response responsibilities within the U.S. Department of Health and Human Services (HHS). Under this legislation, HHS is the lead coordinating authority, and under this law, the Director of HHS has wide-ranging authority to declare a public health emergency, thereby preempting state policies addressing pandemic emergency response. Subsequently, the Obama Administration relied on the previous federal policies for pandemic planning to respond to the 2009 H1N1 swine flu pandemic. The response was considered to be fairly successful, with the exception of vaccine acquisition and distribution.

When taken in sum, the George W. Bush and Obama administrations demonstrated that the United States had the administrative capacity, at least in the terms of the legal and governing authority, to provide a coordinated response in which the national government would lead in a public health emergency. In the 2009 swine flu pandemic, the U.S. federal government demonstrated its ability to address capacity issues, like governing authority, and avoid creating a political climate in which the prospect of a pandemic became politically intractable. The transition of pandemic preparedness planning from the Bush to Obama Administrations demonstrates that coordination of pandemic response need not be an intractable issue.

This capacity went unused in the COVID-19 pandemic response. While there was a *de jure* capacity for greater coordination, the *de facto* response was one that was decentralized and, most specifically, disorganized. This was not for want of being informed about the possibility of such a pandemic. The Obama Administration briefed some incoming senior Trump Administration officials and worked through a pandemic scenario (Collman 2020; Toosi, Lippman, and Diamond 2020), but, to the extent that anything was learned by the participants in that briefing, its fundamentals were not applied to the emerging crisis. From the beginning of the pandemic in March 2020, the federal government failed to provide a coherent strategy to respond to the pandemic, effectively ignoring existing planning and preparedness and politically undermining steps that states could take blunt the effects of the virus as it spread (Mervosh et al. 2021). Moreover, the federal guidelines around testing in the early stages of the pandemic proved to reveal a failure in coordination among the Centers for Disease Control testing guidelines, the approval of tests by the Food and Drug Administration, and inaction within HHS (Shear et al. 2020).

While the federal government was unable to use existing administrative capacity to coordinate a response to the pandemic, states were left to go it alone. The result was a haphazard response that is frustrating but not entirely unusual in the fragmented system of the U.S. federal government. Effectively, fragmented federalism means that states adopt a patchwork of policy standards and implementation across the country (Bowling and Pickerill 2013). Inasmuch as the federal coordinating capacity is centralized, the nature of governance and politics in the U.S. is one of fragmentation and political polarization (Goelzhauser and Konisky 2019).

In April 2020, the Trump Administration effectively ceded authority to respond to the pandemic to state governors (Shear et al. 2020). The resulting coordination can only be characterized as highly decentralized and politically fragmented. For example, in some states like New York, California, Massachusetts, and Michigan, governors were proactive in implementing measures to curb the spread of the virus, often with negative political consequences from the federal government (Shear, et al. 2020). Meanwhile, in numerous other states, the coordinated response was almost non-existent, with economic concerns about specific sectors of the economy holding primacy over public health (Mervosh et al. 2021).

Finally, the pandemic has also revealed widespread structural deficiencies within the country's institutions of public health. In the early stages of the pandemic, the country struggled to acquire basic personal protective equipment (PPE), forcing doctors in some hospitals to request donations or, worse yet, reuse certain items like N95 respirator masks. Testing remained woefully inadequate for the first year of the pandemic. In late 2020, an analysis by researchers at Brown and Harvard Universities found that the U.S. should be doing roughly three times as many daily tests conducting to adequately control the outbreak (Stein 2020). And while the vaccination campaign remains ongoing as of this writing, the Trump Administration's early roll-out was marred by blunders, including an exhaustion of reserves in January 2021, despite assurances from the Trump Administration that the public would be readily able to obtain vaccinations. In February and March 2021, the Biden Administration worked to bolster those vaccine supplies (Department of Health and Human Services 2021).

In the COVID-19 response, the U.S. had the administrative capacity to provide a centralized, coordinated response, and yet, it failed to do so. There are many competing and intervening explanations why: a failure of leadership in the Trump Administration, a lack of governing experience, and a denial and ignorance of facts and scientific evidence. However, through the lens of policy styles, public trust in government remains a promising explanation. Because of a lack of public trust, fostered by political polarization and a patchwork of responses to varying degrees of effectiveness, coordination was highly decentralized. Moreover, the efficacy of this decentralized response is one that is undermined by the political blame directed at state governors who were trying to address pandemic disease (Mervoskh et al. 2021). We would expect that public trust in government would be low when basic public health protective measures, such as promoting social distancing and mask-wearing, and limitations on particularly risky business operations were viewed by federal leaders as a threat to their political position.

Since taking office in January 2021, President Joseph Biden has introduced a pandemic response plan that centralizes coordination of the pandemic response at the national level by mandating mask-wearing in federal buildings and on interstate travel, setting national guidelines for school re-openings, invoking the Defense Production Act to increase vaccine production, and promising reimbursements to states that choose to use the National Guard to distribute vaccines (Biden 2021). However, given the extreme amount of discontent in the American electorate, public trust in government will likely remain low in the months ahead. Moreover, given the attempts of the Biden Administration to use existing governing authority as a potential source of capacity to centralize coordination, the future efficacy of the pandemic response policies remains to be seen.

Communication

Communication is a critical component of response to any crisis or disaster. This is especially true when the information is complex, and the message receiver (the public) has the ability to mitigate their risks through certain actions that must be communicated by experts and elected officials. The crisis communication in public health literature suggests that there are a number of critical components to effective communication of risk-related information during a crisis. Organizations (the government in the case of COVID-19) "should attempt to provide sufficient information in a timely manner to the public … should attempt to provide information that is accurate and non-contradictory to the public … [and] can spawn controversies by engaging in speculations" (Weible et al. 2020).

Evidence from research also supports these practices, indicating that using deliberately constructed messages based on tested models of crisis risk communication can lead to greater individual intentions to engage in risk mitigating behaviors. One such communication model—the IDEA approach to crisis risk communication—includes four elements that communicators should consider: (1) helping message recipients internalize the potential impact of the risk or crisis event, (2) identifying modes of communication about risks that are appropriate for the audience and crisis situation, (3) developing clear, succinct, and accurate messages about the risk faced, and (4) clearly stating actions that individuals can take to reduce their risks (Sellnow, Lane, Sellnow, and Littlefield 2017). These attributes of effective crisis risk communication can be summed as: "Be truthful, honest, frank, and open … Coordinate, collaborate, and partner with other credible sources … Communicate clearly and with compassion" (Covello 2003). When messages about risk during a crisis are consistent, clear, and simple, they are more likely to be understood by the public. When they are communicated by trusted experts or other messengers, they are more likely to be considered valid.

None of these best practices were followed by the Trump Administration throughout the first year of the pandemic. Communication about COVID-19 cases, causes, transmissibility, and testing was inconsistent from the early stages of the pandemic. The Trump Administration did not provide information about the virus when it first began to spread in the U.S., and President Trump and his aides gave conflicting information to the expert scientists (Lopez 2020). Early press briefings attempted to play down the virus, often attempting to divert attention from the virus and toward economic indicators which, at the time, looked favorable for the president (see, e.g., Irwin 2020). In February 2020, Trump falsely promised that the virus would disappear in the spring (Schafenberg 2020) and, less than a month later, questioned the accuracy of World Health Organization (WHO) data (Chalfant 2020).

False claims and inconsistent communication about the pandemic fostered political conflict. As the pandemic rolled on, President Trump turned his ire toward recommended practices. Trump instead infamously touted the drug chloroquine's potential for fighting the virus. Demonstrating the danger of fractured and inaccurate communications approaches, CNN reported, "Health officials in Nigeria have issued a warning over chloroquine after they said three people in the country overdosed on the drug, in the wake of President Trump's comments about using it to treat coronavirus" (Busari and Adebayo 2020). Despite planning for a coordinated response that was grounded in prior pandemic experience and scientific expertise, when COVID-19 arrived in the U.S., resources were not used planned.

Given the policy style of the U.S. where diffuse decision-making is commonplace and given that the national government—and the executive branch in particular—is expected to serve as an exemplar of good communication practices during crises, the uncoordinated communication and falsehoods from federal officials sowed confusion among state policymakers and the public. The effects on the U.S. government's capacity to respond to the pandemic were manifold. First, the lack of urgency communicated by the executive branch appears to have permeated the legislative branch as well, at least during the early stages of the pandemic. Aside from a handful of statements in favor or opposition to President Trump's initial travel ban (Allasan 2020), the legislative branch effectively failed to articulate how it planned to support pandemic preparedness efforts until at least late February or early March 2020.

Second, state-level officials (Faussett and Bosman 2020) as well as the general public (Evanega et al. 2020) were similarly confused and had to act independently of the federal government since they had no consistent information from the federal government to assist in their risk mitigation, COVID-19 response, or future scenario planning. In many instances, state interventions fractured along party lines as governors ideologically aligned with the President Trump adopted far less stringent interventions compared to their counterparts in Democratic-governed states.

Third, communication from the Trump Administration in 2020 left the public confused and uncertain about how best to protect themselves. A 2020 study by researchers at Cornell University found that nearly 37% of coronavirus misrepresentations could be tied to President Trump, and that only about 16% of the media articles reporting on the coronavirus included a fact checking component, suggesting much of this misinformation made it to the public (Evanega et al 2020). Experts chided President Trump's mixed messaging, noting that it undermined the adoption of critical public health interventions.

Stringency of Measures

COVID-19 policy stringency in the United States has varied over time. We rely on the policy stringency index for COVID-19 compiled by Hale and colleagues (2020), which measures the general strictness of policies that are intended to restrict individual behavior, like stay at home orders and so-called lockdowns. The index reflects U.S. national policy stringency and the variation of state policies, containing measures for closures of schools and workplaces, prohibitions of public events, limits to the size of gatherings, and issuances of stay at home requirements and travel restrictions. At the outset of the pandemic, policy stringency was rather low until mid-March 2020 when closures and policies intended to limit individual behavior quickly picked up and were adopted. By this time, the COVID-19 Government Stringency Index rated the United States 72.96 out 100. This stringency remained consistent until states and local governments relaxed restrictions, reducing the stringency index 62.5 by September. As case counts began to rise, in the late fall, policy stringency increased again to 75.46. As of February 16, 2021, according to the Oxford COVID-19 Government Response Tracker (https://covidtracker.bsg.ox.ac.uk/), the overall stringency of COVID-19 policies in the United States was 68.08, compared to 86.11 in the UK, 83.33 in Germany, 75.46 in Canada, 71.76 in Mexico, and 63.89 in France.

As mentioned elsewhere, there are notable differences between national COVID-19 response policies and subnational policies in the U.S. Policy stringency varied from one state to another as governors were left to their own devices to respond to the crisis. At the beginning of 2021, 41 states had a stay at home order eased or lifted, 4 put a new stay at home order in place, and 6 states had taken no action (Kaiser Family Foundation 2021). Furthermore, the stringency of limits on social gatherings varied among states with three states prohibiting all gatherings, 10 states limiting gatherings to ten or fewer people, 20 states limiting gatherings to 20 or fewer, two states limiting to 25 or fewer, 7 states limiting gatherings to 50 or fewer, and 19 states that placed no limits on gatherings.

Finally, face-covering requirements are one policy with remarkably variable degrees of stringency among the states (Table 11.1). Although the majority of states (39) had some form of mask-wearing requirement in place, some states loosened the stringency of mask-wearing to only certain types of employees or devolved authority to require mass to local governments. The implication for policy stringency is that while most states undertook a centralized approach to determining what the standards should be for mask-wearing in public places, some states did not. There are two potential explanations. First, as mask-wearing is viewed as politically unpopular in some states, those state governors were reluctant to impose a requirement at all. Or, second, state governors were reluctant to make a potentially unpopular mask requirement and left it up to local governments to use their political and administrative discretion regarding mask mandates.

TABLE 11.1 Face-covering requirements by state as of February 17, 2021

Face-covering requirement	States
No Requirement	South Dakota, Florida, Missouri, Montana, Oklahoma
Allows Local Officials to Require for General Public	South Carolina, Tennessee
Required for Certain Employees	Nebraska, Idaho, Alaska
Required for Certain Employees; Allows Local Officials to Require for General Public	Georgia, Arizona
Required for General Public	Arkansas, Wyoming, Utah, Iowa, North Dakota, Ohio, Indiana, Mississippi, Kansas, Wisconsin, Virginia, Colorado, Louisiana, Maine, Maryland, Alabama, Delaware, Washington, California, North Carolina, Connecticut, District of Columbia, Illinois, Kentucky, Michigan, Minnesota, Nevada, New Mexico, Oregon, Pennsylvania, Rhode Island, Texas, Massachusetts, Hawaii, New Jersey Vermont, West Virginia, New Hampshire, New York

Source: Adapted from the Kaiser Family Foundation 2021.

Degree of Centralization

In the case of the COVID-19 pandemic in the United States, policy capacity to respond to the problem is highly centralized, but political trust is very low. There were established response plans, and the federal government's public health agencies had experience in responding to infectious disease outbreaks in the past. The Department of Health and Human Services had prepared to respond and lead the effort during a pandemic. Moreover, the federal government has authority to centralize and marshal resources under the Defense Production Act (PL 81–774, 50 U.S.C. 4501 et seq.) emergency procurement procedures with the Federal Emergency management Agency, and distribute resources from the U.S. federal stockpiles. However, almost none of this occurred during the Trump Administration save the efforts under Operation Warp Speed to support the development of a vaccine.

However, given the low public trust in government and misinformation noted above, the policy style of the United States during the COVID-19 pandemic has been one of a *centrifugal response*. In what could be characterized as a blame avoidance tactic, the Trump Administration through its own inaction delegated, in effect, the handling of the crisis to states and governors, which served as an attempt to avoid political consequences for the botched U.S. response. Furthermore, it allowed President Trump and his administration to assign blame to state governors for more stringent policy responses that were politically unpopular: closure of bars and restaurants and stay at home orders in particular. Compounding the challenge from the state level, these unpopular measures were more appropriately within the states' power (known as the police power) under the American constitutional system than they were within the federal government's remit. As a result of low levels of public trust in government, Americans have been left to rely on their trust in medical doctors and hospitals to diagnose, treat, and care for the sick during the pandemic.

The policy style, given the capacity and previous experience of the U.S., should have been one of centralization, inclusion of states, and high levels of trust in the government's ability to perform. However, given that national capacity to centralize a response went unused, conflicting and misleading information was communicated to states and the public, and President Trump's management focused on avoiding blame, centralization is not what occurred. What remains to be seen is how the Biden Administration will rely on the centripetal policy style that exists on paper rather than the centrifugal policy style that has characterized the U.S. response to the COVID-19 pandemic in its first year.

Conclusion

We consider the decentralized policy style of the United States in the COVID-19 pandemic response in this chapter. Existing research suggests that the U.S. lacks a cohesive policymaking style (Peters 2019). As such, it is no surprise that we did not find the policy styles framework to be a tidy fit for the U.S., especially in the context of public health policymaking during regular conditions. We expected that given the decentralized policy style, the response in the U.S. should have been characterized by high inclusiveness of decision-making where the "key political actors" are the politicians and the public (Howlett and Josun 2018). This means that politicians and the public should enjoy a more central role in policy-making than bureaucrats while possessing a high degree of governing capacity to respond to the crisis. We found that there was a high degree of inclusiveness due to devolution of responsibility to the states while fostering political partisan polarization.

The challenge of using the policy styles framework is only magnified in the context COVID-19. There are two important ways in which the decentralized policy style did not work well in this case. First, the framework does not speak to leadership in a way that was useful for analyzing national policy choices, particularly choices that devolved most power and authority for the pandemic response to states. What remains unclear is whether this is a weakness in the framework, a weakness in the application of the framework during a crisis, or an artifact of an unconventional President of the United States. President Trump not only undermined the existing strengths with the coordination and response infrastructure of the U.S. by effectively abdicating any responsibilities of the federal government but also systematically spreading misinformation about the disease itself and public health best practices. Put differently, President Trump operated outside of the bounds of core democratic norms, let alone institutional structures designed to enhance the federal government's capacity to manage large-scale crises within a highly decentralized federal system. In this respect, COVID-19 potentially represents a poor test case of the enduring nature of the U.S. policy style.

Second, the policy styles framework does not help unpack the implications of political partisanship and polarization in the pandemic response either from the federal to state levels of government or from one state to another. The partisan differences, particularly for the stringency of mask-wearing, were considerable in this case study. Future development of the policy styles framework should be cognizant of the need to address partisan politics. We have argued that public trust in government, or lack thereof, has been at the intersection of partisan politics and policy style. Future work using the policy styles approach must account for the relationship between political party and public trust in government.

Finally, the U.S. response to the COVID-19 pandemic has evolved over time. The Biden Administration has attempted to reverse nearly all policies and approaches used by the Trump Administration, so it is possible that the pandemic response may shift dramatically in 2021. President Biden has emphasized his commitment to rebuilding trust and relying on the science in his decision-making, while taking steps to reassert the federal government's role in guiding state action, particularly with regard to the vaccine roll-out. Time will tell whether these efforts are enough to undo some of the damage caused by the Trump Administration.

Note

1 Data from Johns Hopkins University, via the Our World in Data Website, https://ourworldindata.org/coronavirus-data-explorer, accessed February 16, 2021.

References

Allassan, Fadel. 2020. "How Congress Is Responding to the Coronavirus Outbreak." *Axios.* https://www.axios.com/congress-coronavirus-response-china-12a33f56-f2c4-4f2b-beec-0f8329a3d813.html.

Apuzzo, Matt, and Selam Gebrekidan. 2020. "Can't Get Tested? Maybe You're in the Wrong Country." *The New York Times.* https://www.nytimes.com/2020/03/20/world/europe/coronavirus-testing-world-countries-cities-states.html.

Biden, Joe. *National Strategy for the COVID-19 Response and Pandemic Preparedness.* https://www.whitehouse.gov/wp-content/uploads/2021/01/National-Strategy-for-the-COVID-19-Response-and-Pandemic-Preparedness.pdf.

Binderkrantz, Anne. 2005. "Interest Group Strategies: Navigating between Privileged Access and Strategies of Pressure." *Political Studies* 53(4): 694–715.

Binderkrantz, Anne Skorkjaer, Peter Munk Christiansen, and Helene Helboe Pedersen. 2015. "Interest Group Access to the Bureaucracy, Parliament, and the Media: Interest Group Access." *Governance (Oxford, England)* 28(1): 95–112.

Busari, Stephanie, and Bukola Adebayo. 2020. "Nigeria Prepares for Coronavirus Outbreak." *Convolutional Neural Networks.* https://www.cnn.com/videos/world/2020/03/23/exp-nigeria-coronavirus-isolation-center.cnn (March 31, 2020).

Calef, David, and Robert Goble. 2007. "The Allure of Technology: How France and California Promoted Electric and Hybrid Vehicles to Reduce Urban Air Pollution." *Policy Sciences* 40(1): 1–34.

Chalfant, Morgan. 2020. "Trump Disputes WHO's 3.4 Percent Global Death Rate for Coronavirus." *The Hill.* https://thehill.com/homenews/administration/486068-trump-disputes-whos-34-global-death-rate-for-coronavirus (February 24, 2021).

Chanley, Virginia A., Thomas J. Rudolph, and Wendy M. Rahn. 2000. "The Origins and Consequences of Public Trust in Government: A Time Series Analysis." *Public Opinion Quarterly* 64(3): 239–56.

Cohen, Michael D., James G. March, and Johan P. Olsen. 1972. "A Garbage Can Model of Organizational Choice." *Administrative Science Quarterly* 17: 1–25.

Collman, Ashley. 2020. "In 2017, Obama Officials Briefed Trump's Team on Dealing with a Pandemic like the Coronavirus. One Cabinet Member Reportedly Fell Asleep, and Others Didn't Want to Be There." *Business Insider.* https://www.businessinsider.com/trump-appointees-trained-pandemic-response-in-2016-2020-3 (February 24, 2021).

Covello, Vincent T. 2003. "Best Practices in Public Health Risk and Crisis Communication." *Journal of Health Communication* 8: 5–8.

DeLeo, Rob A. 2018. "Indicators, Agendas, and Streams: Analysing the Politics of Preparedness." *Policy & Politics* 46(1): 27–45.

DeLeo, Rob A., and Kevin P. Donnelly. 2017. "Remodeling the Model: Policy Transfer and the Implementation of the Affordable Care Act in Massachusetts." *Polity* 49(1): 5–41.

Department of Health & Human Services. 2021. "Biden Administration Purchases Additional Doses of COVID-19 Vaccines from Pfizer and Moderna." *Hhs.gov.* https://www.hhs.gov/about/news/2021/02/11/biden-administration-purchases-additional-doses-covid-19-vaccines-from-pfizer-and-moderna.html.

Dunlap, Riley E., and Angela G. Mertig. 1992. *American Environmentalism: The U.S. Environmental Movement, 1970–1990.* Philadelphia: Taylor & Francis.

Dunlop, Claire A. 2010. "Epistemic Communities and Two Goals of Delegation: Hormone Growth Promoters in the European Union." *Science & Public Policy* 37(3): 205–17.

Dür, Andreas, and Gemma Mateo. 2013. "Gaining Access or Going Public? Interest Group Strategies in Five European Countries: Gaining Access or Going Public?" *European Journal of Political Research* 52(5): 660–86.

Etheridge, Elizabeth W. 1992. *Sentinel for Health: A History of the Centers for Disease Control.* Berkeley: University of California Press.

Evanega, Sarah, Mark Lynas, Jordan Adams, and Karinne Smolenyak. "Quantifying Sources and Themes in the COVID-19 'Infodemic.'" *Cornell.edu.* https://alliance-forscience.cornell.edu/wp-content/uploads/2020/09/Evanega-et-al-Coronavirus-misinformationFINAL.pdf.

Fausset, Richard, and Julie Bosman. 2020. "What Governor's Say about Trump's Response to Coronavirus." *The New York Times.* March 11. https://www.nytimes.com/2020/03/11/us/coronavirus-governors-trump.html

Fox, Daniel M. 2005. "AIDS and the American Health Polity: The History and Prospects of a Crisis of Authority: AIDS and the American Health Polity." *The Milbank Quarterly* 83(4): Online-only-Online-only.

Goelzhauser, Greg, and David M. Konisky. 2019. "The State of American Federalism 2018–2019: Litigation, Partisan Polarization, and the Administrative Presidency." *Publius* 49(3): 379–406.

Haas, Peter. 2007. "Epistemic Communities." In *The Oxford Handbook of International Environmental Law*, eds. Daniel Bodansky, Jutta Brunnée, and Ellen Hey. Oxford: Oxford University Press.

Hale, Thomas et al. 2020. "Variation in Government Responses to COVID-19." In *Blavatnik School of Government Working Paper*, http://www.bsg.ox.ac.uk/covidtracke.

Healy, Andrew, and Neil Malhotra. 2009. "Myopic Voters and Natural Disaster Policy." *The American Political Science Review* 103(3): 387–406.

Irwin, Neil. 2020. "Coronavirus Shows the Problem with Trump's Stock Market Boasting." *The New York Times.* https://www.nytimes.com/2020/02/26/upshot/coronavirus-trump-stock-market.html.

Jacobs, Lawrence R., and Theda Skocpol. 2015. *Health Care Reform and American Politics: What Everyone Needs to Know, 3rd Ed.* New York, NY: Oxford University Press.

Kaiser Family Foundation. 2021. "State COVID-19 Data and Policy Actions." *Kff.org.* https://www.kff.org/coronavirus-covid-19/issue-brief/state-covid-19-data-and-policy-actions/.

Kingdon, John W. 2011. *Agendas, Alternatives and Public Policies.* 2nd ed. Boston: Longman.

Kraft, Michael E. 2015. *Environmental Policy and Politics.* 7th ed. London, England: Routledge.

Lopez, German. 2020. "Trump's Expert Urged Caution about a Coronavirus Treatment. Trump Hyped It up Anyway." *Vox.* https://www.vox.com/policy-and-politics/2020/3/20/21188397/coronavirus-trump-press-briefing-covid-19-anthony-fauci (March 31, 2020).

Maloney, William A., Grant Jordan, and Andrew M. McLaughlin. 1994. "Interest Groups and Public Policy: The Insider/Outsider Model Revisited." *Journal of Public Policy* 14(1): 17–38.

Marchione, Marilynn. 2021. "US Life Expectancy Drops a Year in Pandemic, Most since WWII." *Apnews.com.* https://apnews.com/article/us-life-expectancy-huge-decline-f4caaf4555563d09e927f1798136a869 (February 20, 2021).

Mayhew, David R. 2004. *Congress: The Electoral Connection, Second Edition*. New Haven, CT: Yale University Press.

Mervosh, Sarah, Mike Baker, Patricia Mazzei, and Mark Walker. 2021. "One Year, 400,000 Coronavirus Deaths: How the U.S. Guaranteed Its Own Failure." *The New York Times*. https://www.nytimes.com/2021/01/17/us/covid-deaths-2020.html.

Mitchell, Travis. 2020. "Americans' Views of Government: Low Trust, but Some Positive Performance Ratings." *Pewresearch.org*. https://www.pewresearch.org/politics/2020/09/14/americans-views-of-government-low-trust-but-some-positive-performance-ratings/.

Nownes, Anthony J., and Patricia Freeman. 1998. "Interest Group Activity in the States." *The Journal of Politics* 60(1): 86–112.

Peters, Guy B. 2015. "Policy Capacity in Public Administration." *Policy and Society* 34 (3–4): 219–28.

Peters, Guy B. 2019. "The American Policy Style(s): Multiple Institutions Creating Opportunities and Gridlock." In *Policy Styles and Policy-Making: Exploring the Linkages*, eds. Michael Howlett and Jale Tosum. London: Routledge, 180–98.

Pew Research Center. 2020. "Intent to Get a COVID-19 Vaccine Rises to 60% as Confidence in Research and Development Process Increases." *Pewresearch.org*. https://www.pewresearch.org/science/2020/12/03/intent-to-get-a-covid-19-vaccine-rises-to-60-as-confidence-in-research-and-development-process-increases/.

Sanders, L. 2020. "Most Americans Don't Trust President Trump for Accurate COVID-19 Information Says CBS/YouGov Poll." *Yougov.com*. https://today.yougov.com/topics/politics/articles-reports/2020/03/24/who-americans-trust-covid (March 30, 2020).

Scharfenberg, David. 2020. "Donald Trump's Coronavirus Advice Just Might Kill Us." *The Boston Globe*. https://www.bostonglobe.com/2020/03/07/opinion/donald-trumps-coronavirus-advice-just-might-kill-us/.

Sellnow, Deanna D., Derek R. Lane, Timothy L. Sellnow, and Robert S. Littlefield. 2017. "The IDEA Model as a Best Practice for Effective Instructional Risk and Crisis Communication." *Communication Studies* 68(5): 552–67.

Shear, Michael D., et al. 2020. "The Lost Month: How a Failure to Test Blinded the U.S. to Covid-19." *The New York Times*. https://www.nytimes.com/2020/03/28/us/testing-coronavirus-pandemic.html.

Shear, Michael D., Noah Weiland, et al. 2020. "Inside Trump's Failure: The Rush to Abandon Leadership Role on the Virus." *The New York Times*. https://www.nytimes.com/2020/07/18/us/politics/trump-coronavirus-response-failure-leadership.html.

Stein, Rob. 2020. "Is Your State Doing Enough Coronavirus Testing? Use Our Tool to Find Out." *National Public Radio*. https://www.npr.org/sections/health-shots/2020/12/22/948085513/vaccines-are-coming-but-the-u-s-still-needs-more-testing-to-stop-the-surge.

Toosi, Nahal, Daniel Lippman, and Dan Diamond. 2020. "POLITICO." *Politico.com*. https://www.politico.com/news/2020/03/16/trump-inauguration-warning-scenario-pandemic-132797.

Weible, Christopher M., et al. 2020. "COVID-19 and the Policy Sciences: Initial Reactions and Perspectives." *Policy Sciences* 53(2): 1–17.

5

Decentralized Responses

12

FOLLOWING THE PUBLIC HEALTH AGENCY'S GUIDELINES

The Swedish Approach to the COVID-19 Pandemic

Evangelia Petridou

Introduction

"We follow the guidelines of the Public Health Agency." Throughout 2020 and into 2021, the preceding sentence had been the standard preamble to any account of individual organizations' narrative of COVID-19-related mitigation measures in Sweden. For the most part, these guidelines have been just that: non-binding, voluntary 'nudges' involving a minimum of interference in the everyday life of the Swedish population (Pierre 2020). Indeed, the Swedish strategy was a departure from that of other European countries, including the Nordic countries. Denmark, Finland, and Norway mandated closures of retail stores and services and lockdown(s) of a varying degree at some point during 2020 (Christensen and Lægreid 2020; Giritli Nygren and Olofsson 2020; Neuvonen 2020). Indeed, the border between Norway and Sweden even in the sparsely populated north of the Scandinavian Peninsula was closed during long periods in 2020 and into 2021.

The decentralized Swedish strategy has not been uncontroversial; it has attracted criticism in the international and domestic media (Savage, Reeves, and Estrin 2020) as well public criticism from experts (see, e.g., Carlsson et al. 2020). It is also true that the number of cases as well as the mortality rate have been higher than those in the neighboring Nordic countries (Johns Hopkins 2021). That said, it is beyond the scope of this chapter—and indeed, this edited volume—to assess the success of the national response. Instead, the purpose of this chapter is to analyze the Swedish pandemic response measures in terms of centralization based on the policy style of Sweden and the concept of trust. In the remainder of this chapter, I first elaborate on the Swedish policy style and discuss the issue of political trust. After a brief note on method and data, I present the Swedish pandemic response contextualized in the preparedness that was in place at its onset. I finish the chapter with a concluding discussion linking the policy style with the response.

DOI: 10.4324/9781003137399-17

Policy Styles and Policymaking in Sweden

The 1982 volume edited by Jeremy Richardson examining policy styles in (Western) Europe included a chapter on Sweden (Richardson 1982/2013). In describing policymaking, almost 40 years ago, Ruin writes:

> In practice, this [that countries have a set of widely accepted ideas regarding governance] has meant that policy-makers, it their day-to-day political decision-making, should seek agreement among participants and avoid conflict; should try to build large majorities for policies rather than force their standpoint on minorities; and compromise rather than cling rigidly to their own policy preferences.
>
> *(1982: 141)*

Ruin (1982/2013) goes on to explain a decision-making process that involves "a multiplicity of participants and as a result, is rather cumbersome" (141). In addition to being open and consensual, Swedish policymaking is oriented toward problem-solving; it is rationalistic in the sense that great efforts are being made to gather as much information as possible about the political issue at hand (Anton 1969; Einhorn and Logue 2003). In other words, it is the opposite of "rash, abrupt, irrational, or indeed, exciting" (Petersson 2016: 651). Even though the degree that Swedish policymaking is open, inclusive, consensual, and deliberative has decreased over past few decades, open conflict is avoided, and inflammatory rhetoric has little place in the process (Petersson 2016).

A deliberative, consensual, problem-solving-oriented, rational policymaking process is a feature of the Nordic corporatist system in general, though differences exist among the Nordic countries explicated by the East–West Nordic model (Ahlbäck Öberg and Wockelberg 2016). The East Nordic administrative tradition is mainly associated with Sweden and to a lesser extent Finland. Sweden is characterized by the absence of formal ministerial rule when it comes to public agencies. In practice, this means that even though public agencies are under a specific ministry, they [public agencies] have considerable leeway when it comes to interpreting laws or exercising public authority (Larsson and Bäck 2008). The responsibility of ministries centers on planning, budgeting, and drafting broad policy guidelines for the public agencies. What is more, the operative autonomy of agencies has increased in the past decades (Einhorn and Logue 2003; Hall 2016; Petridou 2020). This phenomenon is understood as a dual executive or dualism (Hall 2016). In contrast, the West Nordic tradition (Denmark, Norway, and Iceland) implies significant ministerial administration (the 'ministerial model'), which allows for considerable intervention of the ministries in the day-to-day operations of the public agencies (Ahlbäck Öberg and Wockelberg 2016).

The Government Offices [Regeringskansliet] is the central administrative entity with the prime minister as director. The entire office employs some 4600 people (Government Offices of Sweden n.d.), which makes for very small ministries. Conversely, more than 200,000 civil servants are employed in boards and more than 300 government agencies (Larsson and Bäck 2008; Petridou and Sparf 2017; Pierre 2020; Sundström 2016). Public agencies are staffed by experts in an open recruiting process. Their role is to make policy recommendations to the government. The government is not bound by law to follow these recommendations. However, traditionally, this has been the case partly because it is understood that the decisions public agencies make are depoliticized and based on evidence and expertise.

The preparatory work in advance of a government bill takes place within commissions of inquiry, a process accommodated by the small size of ministries. These commissions are appointed by the parliament, always include experts, and generally, their members reflect the parties with seats in the parliament.

The process concludes with the government drafting a bill and submitting it to the parliament (Larsson and Bäck 2008). This consensus-based decision-making model is part of the Swedish duality (Hall 2016). The authors of the commission report have regular meetings and constant negotiations with the politicians who ordered the investigation. In practice, any conflicts regarding the contents of the report are teased out during that time (Petridou and Sparf 2017).

In summary, I posit that the policy style in Sweden is *managerial*. Indeed, policymaking in Sweden is designed to accommodate conflicting interests by seeking compromise so everyone agrees on the output; this is part of the Swedish exceptionality thesis (Pierre 2016). Swedish policymaking is deliberative in the sense that problem-solving is done by technocrats, often in the process of commissions of inquiry and informally from input by agencies (Hall 2016). It is an extensive process during which the proposal is sent out to all relevant organizations for feedback, encouraging a rational debate about the merits of the proposal and finding points of consensus among major parties and interest organizations (Einhorn and Logue 2003). Bureaucracy, in general, has high status in the Swedish administrative system with pronounced extensive accessibility bestowed on the citizens through constitutionally mandated freedom of information, transparency, citizen participation, and user democracy (Kuhlmann and Wollmann 2014). The political system has especially high administrative capacity due to the executive being staffed in an open recruiting process by experts and enjoying unusual autonomy. What is more, it is particularly inclusive, as corporatist systems are, not only because civil society organizations have a seat at the policy making table but also because of institutionalized processes such as the referral process.

Political Trust in Sweden

A high-trust society is almost synonymous with Scandinavia, in general, and the Swedish society, in particular. Some scholars point to the advanced welfare state as the factor that promotes political trust, while others, based on the theory of social capital point to the considerably strong civil society as the explanatory factor for the high levels of political trust in Sweden. Others posit that the advanced welfare state is a result of the high-trust society. This trust is, in turn, a result of a voluntary agreement between the individual and the state, one that strikes a balance between individualism on the one hand and the state as the operationalization of the collective on the other, with long historical roots in Swedish society (see Svedin 2019 for an extensive treatment of trust in Sweden from a historical perspective).

Sweden entered the pandemic with high levels of trust in government at just under 67% in 2018 (Ortiz-Spinoza and Roser 2020). In terms of interpersonal trust, Holmberg and Rothstein (2020) observe a possible recent decrease in trust levels among less socially engaged populations, namely people who are unemployed, supported by welfare benefits, early retirees, and people suffering from poor health.

Two studies conducted in 2020 arrive to slightly divergent conclusions. Esaisson, Sohlberg, Ghersetti, and Johansson (2020) noted a rally-around-the-flag effect, finding that trust in politicians in power, government institutions that handle crisis management, generalized trust in government authorities as well as interpersonal trust (though the latter less so) increased as Sweden moved from the initial to the acute phase of the crisis. Conversely, in a comparative study between Denmark and Sweden, Nielsen and Lindvall (2021) found that Swedes reported trusting the Public Health Agency of Sweden (PHAS) more than the government to guide them safely through the pandemic—at an average of 7.0 and 6.1, respectively, out of a scale from 0 to 10 with three data points during the first phase of the pandemic. The first data point was in late March, the second in late April, while the third one covered the latter part of June. General trust in government averaged 5.3 out of 10 for the period of April and June 2020. Nielsen found that trust declined ever so slightly during that time period, but the effect of the containment policies seems to be marginal. Finally, the authors find that trust seems to be ideologically driven in Sweden, at least to some extent. Left-leaning respondents tended to trust the social democratic government, while the right-wing voters less so, and this cleavage accounts for much of the observed decrease in trust. Unsurprisingly, right-wing respondents trust the public agency more than the government in terms of their ability to deal with the pandemic.

Even though the scale employed by the latter study is not comparable with data available elsewhere, evidence points to declining, but still relatively high levels of political trust in Sweden during the first part of 2020.

Method and Data in Brief

The timeline under examination in this chapter is the entire 2020, covering the first phase of the pandemic, the relative decrease in intensity in the summer, and the second wave in the late fall. The study is based on the analysis of documentary data consisting of governmental documents, including mostly governmental and agency web sites, reports, evaluations, statutes, planning documents, and transcripts of communication to the public.

The Swedish Response to COVID-19

In the following section, I present the Swedish national response to the pandemic including contagion mitigation measures as well as concomitant financial relief measures to businesses and households. I begin with the national framework on preparedness as well as an outline of the health care sector in order to contextualize the measures comprising the response.

Crisis Preparedness

The Swedish crisis management and preparedness system is based on the premise that the whole of society, including the public and private sectors and civil society organizations, must plan for contingencies. When it comes to the public sector, municipalities, county boards, regions, national agencies, and the national government are mandated by law to have competent staff working with contingency management. This includes, *inter alia*, an effective early-warning system, competence in the organization, and appropriate risk and vulnerability assessment mechanisms. The reporting cycle of risk assessments generally follows the mandate period of the government. The municipalities report their assessments to the relevant regional boards, which, in turn, report to the Swedish Civil Contingencies Agency (MSB). The regions also report their assessments to MSB as do some of the national agencies (Swedish Civil Contingencies Agency 2020a).

The 2001 Swedish Commission on Vulnerability and Security (Government Offices of Sweden 2001) proposed three guiding principles, which were legislated shortly afterward: (i) the principle of responsibility, under which entities responsible for an activity during normal times retain this responsibility in crisis or war; (ii) the principle of parity, under which authorities retain their structure and location in crisis or war; and (iii) the principle of proximity, under which crises should be handled at the lowest possible level of government. The fourth principle was added later, that of collaboration. It is not part of the legislation, but, in practice, coordination and collaboration are core administrative organizing principles in Sweden.

The PHAS has an officer on call around the clock. It has the only high-containment laboratory at biosafety level 4 (BSL-4) in the Nordic countries, which is an important part of national preparedness. In order to track and fight communicable diseases, over 60 diseases are monitored via the reporting received in accordance with law and through voluntary notification. This gives PHAS an overview of the epidemiological situation in the country (The Public Health Agency of Sweden 2020a).

PHAS is legally mandated to coordinate preparedness against serious health threats. The pandemic plans are regularly updated and consist of three major documents for preparedness (The Public Health Agency of Sweden 2019a), communication (The Public Health Agency of Sweden 2019b), and access to medication (The Public Health Agency of Sweden 2019c). The agency must evaluate reports from subnational entities and must then determine whether there may be an international threat to human health and, if so, notify the World Health Organization, (WHO) within 24 hours. PHAS is also charged with providing information to relevant agencies, municipalities, and regions of the measures that have been taken.

The National Board of Health and Welfare [Socialstyrelsen] (NBHW) is responsible for supporting the preparedness of the health system. Pandemic scenarios feature in risk- and vulnerability analyses conducted by NBHW, though, indicatively, the threat of a pandemic is treated fairly perfunctorily in the latest analysis dating from 2014 (National Board of Health and Welfare 2014). In the event of an emergency, NBHW must inform the Government Offices and MSB (National Board for Health and Welfare 2020a).

What is more, NBHW is responsible for the development and maintenance of expertise and dissemination of knowledge regarding disaster medicine and emergency preparedness in order to assist the Swedish health system and social services during extraordinary times. The government has commissioned NBHW to coordinate and manage the availability of medicine and medical supplies as needed in a state of heightened alert.

MSB is responsible for helping society prepare for contingencies, including major accidents, crises, and the consequences of war (Swedish Civil Contingencies Agency 2020b). MSB is rarely operative in emergencies but rather supports actors horizontally (other public agencies) or vertically (subnational levels of government).

Collaboration among these agencies at the national level was evidenced in their joint participation in a number of press conferences from the onset of the pandemic and throughout 2020. The elaborate crisis management architecture described above notwithstanding, the first findings of the Corona Commission showed that the regions suffered from an initial lack of personal protective equipment (PPE), reported in early February 2020 by NBHW (Government Offices of Sweden 2020a). Subsequently, the biggest municipalities and regions in Sweden drafted an agreement for the joint procurement of PPE (Swedish Association of Local Authorities and Regions 2020). This speaks to the autonomy of the local level, but also reveals that bigger municipalities with more resources than smaller ones might enjoy more access to more or better crisis preparedness. The Swedish Association of Local Authorities and Regions (SKR) is an organization supporting all regions and municipalities in the country aimed at leveling the playing field among local authorities in terms of competence and resources, even in crisis preparedness.

The Health Care Sector

Sweden has a tax-financed, universal health care system. There has been some degree of privatization when it comes to local health care centers, but hospital and specialty health care is basically public (Blomqvist and Winblad 2014; Rönnestad and Oskarsson 2020). Health care is regulated by the state, while the planning, financing, and provision of health care services are the responsibility of 21 regions. This includes specialist and hospital care, while primary health care is provided in local health care centers. Accessibility of primary care in Sweden continues to be a problem though the quality of specialist and hospital care is very high.

The Swedish health care system is based on the premise that health care must be egalitarian, accessible, evidence-based, effective, and based on people's individual needs. Accessibility is one of the premises of good quality of care according to the Health and Medical Services Act (National Board of Health and Welfare 2020b). However, it is exactly accessibility that has been a longstanding problem in Swedish health care, and attempts to remedy it have spanned decades and include change in legislation, continuous national assessments of waiting times, and steering through contractual agreements between the government and the regions (National Board for Health and Welfare 2020b).

Despite these measures, people in Sweden wait longer for access to primary care and do not have a regular physician assigned to them, though they have a regular local health care center. Compared internationally, fewer people feel that the physician they meet is aware of their medical history. Additionally, people with complex health problems report coordination failures which result in dissatisfaction with the health care they receive (Inspektionen för vård och omsorg 2020; Myndigheten för vård-och omsorgsanalys 2020). Doctors in Sweden report high levels of stress. Compared to ten other western countries, they also see a smaller number of patients during longer visits (about 20–25 minutes in Sweden vs. a 10-to-20-minute average internationally). Finally, Sweden ranked first in the use of digital tools in primary care (Vårdanalys 2020). Availability of intensive care beds was quite low: In 2019, there were 4.89 intensive care beds for adults per 100,000 inhabitants compared to 24.6 in Germany and 20 in the US, while the European average in 2010–2011 was 11.5 (Engerström 2019).

Contagion Mitigation Measures

The measures Sweden adopted to mitigate contagion fall under the following categories: (i) travel advisories (international as well as national, including a ban on incoming international travelers); (ii) COVID-19-related financial support to workers who had either fallen sick or were at risk of contracting the virus; (iii) general regulations regarding hygiene, staying home when having symptoms, and physical distancing; (iv) general regulations about working from home; (v) general recommendations regarding online teaching at high schools and universities; (vi) limits on public gatherings; (vii) limits on restaurant operations; (viii) limits on elder care home visits; (ix) general regulations regarding using mass transportation (National Institute for Economic Research 2020).

Sweden has constitutional safeguards in place against curtailment of civil and political rights—the state does not have the right to declare state of emergency during peace time (Jonung and Nergelius 2020; Petridou 2020). This partly explains the absence of a hard lockdown in the country. Measures in the form of 'national regulations' [allmäna råd] were non-binding and centered on the main message conveyed by public authorities, focusing on personal responsibility for the health of oneself as well as the good of the collective. From March 2020 until December 2020, the PHAS issued COVID-19-related regulations 28 times (Public Health Agency of Sweden 2020a), mostly amending and updating regulations.

Some regulations, such as the prohibition of serving of alcohol after a certain time (enacted in November 2020 following a surge in cases), was a matter of statute (Sveriges Riksdag 2020a). Regulations regarding the number of people allowed to congregate in one place (max eight, also enacted in November 2020) was a regulation not bound by statute (Government Offices of Sweden 2020b). Regardless of the degree to which the regulations were binding, they set to expire at the latest in June 2021 (Folkhälsomyndigheten 2020a) though measures were amended quite frequently.

The nuanced and often-implied expectation of compliance de-coupled from enforcement instruments has created the false impression in international media that Sweden has not enacted any measures at all. Here, I attempt to clarify the different kinds of containment mitigation measures. PHAS issued advice to the public [almänna råd] in a series of official documents called regulations [föreskrifter]. These regulations are expected to be followed by citizens, but they are not accompanied by enforcement mechanisms. Some of these regulations, mainly at the request of the PHAS, became ordinances voted in the Riksdag. Ordinances are laws and include provisions for penalties and enforcements. The table that follows is an overview of contagion mitigation measures (Table 12.1).

Responding to the increase in cases and fatalities in the late fall of 2020, the Swedish government decided on a number of legislative amendments a temporary 'COVID-19 law,' aimed at allowing the national government to legally have the ability to (and enforce) restrictions in gatherings in public places, places where recreational or cultural activities take place, commercial spaces, public transportation, and the hiring of spaces for private gatherings (Sveriges Riksdag 2020b). The law itself (that is, not any measures that may be enforced because of it) was voted to be in effect from January 10 to September 30, 2021, thus limiting the extraordinary (for Swedish standards) powers vested on the national government to eight months.

As mentioned earlier in this chapter, the hands-off approach of the Swedish government has not been without domestic criticism. A number of researchers formed a group called Vetenskapsforum COVID-19 (VFC) [Research Form COVID-19] vociferously opposing PHAS with open letters to one of the most widely read Swedish dailies (Dagen Nyheter) and a web site (www.vetcovid19. se). They advocate a 'zero COVID vision' through a hard —three- to six-week-long lockdown, thorough contact-tracing, and mandatory mask-wearing. In a rebuttal to VFC's 2021 open letter at Dagens Nyheter, an epidemiologist (not working for PHAS) accused the group for being sensationalist, unconstructive,

TABLE 12.1 Overview of Contagion Mitigation Measures

Decision date	Regulations	Laws and ordinances
March		
10	Visits to care facilities are banned	
11		Gatherings over 500 people are banned
13	Wash your hands; avoid close contact with people; stay at home when sick	
16	People over 70 years are urged to limit social contacts	
17	High schools and universities are recommended to switch to online instruction	
19	Avoid non-essential domestic travel	
21		New law giving the government ability to close schools—secondary education is under municipal jurisdiction. The national government gained the legal ability to close down schools during extraordinary times, but it did not do so as a result of the pandemic. The decision remained at the discretion of the municipalities.
21	New rules for restaurants and bars. All guests must sit at a table. Avoid crowding.	
24	Detailed regulations for restaurants and cafés (e.g. buffets are disallowed).	
24	Be careful when exericing or training for sports (e.g., exercise outdoors)	
27		Gatherings over 50 people are banned
30	National strategy for increased testing issued	
31	Internal advisory group installed at PHAS	

(Continued)

Decision date	Regulations	Laws and ordinances
April		
1	National regulations issued by PHAS	
8	PHAS gets access to mobile (anonymized, aggregated) data for the purpose of understanding mobility patterns from the major telephone operator Telia (Note: no tracking phone app was launched in Sweden due to privacy concerns)	
16	Sport events for people born 2002 and later are allowed	
June		
4	Discontinued advice against non-essential travel	
9	Avoid using public transportation. Keep a safe distance between yourself and others inside sports premises. Do not participate in big social gatherings or events.	
11	Avoid using public transportation when you do not have a reserved numbered seat. Choose another means of transportation.	
17		New law on temporary contagion mitigation measures in restaurants and cafés
July		
1		New law on temporary contagion mitigation measures in restaurants and cafés
22	Guidance (information and instructions) regarding contact-tracing	
October		
13	People over 70 years are urged to to avoid social contacts, and to not use public transportation. All people who have (or think they may have) contracted COVID-19 to stay at home and avoid physical contact. PHAS allows regional authorities to enact stricter regulations than the ones applying nationwide (several regions enacted stricter regulations in October and November 2020)	

November

3 Additional and more detailed information campaign aimed at schools

3 New regulations regarding restaurants, cafés, bars, and nightclubs. Max eight people per table. At all events, people must be seated.

18 Temporary change to the alcohol law: Prohibition of the serving of alcohol between 22:00 and 11:00.

December

1 Children to stay at home if someone in the household has COVID-19

3 Recommendation that high schools switch to online instruction

3 Ban on visits in care–homes (qualified)

4 National plan for vaccination issued

8 Advice to limit contacts to a small circle during the holidays

8 More detailed recommendations as part of the general recommendations to the public such as advising against visiting shopping centers.

21 People arriving from the UK are recommended to stay at home for at least seven days and do self-test.

21 Limit on maximum number of people in all public buildings and work places.

22 Changed regulation for restaurants, maximum four people per table.

22 Restaurants and bars must stop serving at 20:00

22 Vaccination started

23 People born prior to 2004 to wear face mask in public transportation during rush hours.

Source: Sparf and Petridou (2021).

and factually selective in their critique (Björkman 2021). In other words, there has been an ongoing public debate in Sweden among public health researchers regarding the appropriateness of the response.

Crisis Communication

The chief epidemiologist Anders Tegnell and, to some extent, the deputy chief epidemiologist Anders Wallensten from PHAS were the main communicators of the Swedish pandemic response when it came to contagion mitigation measures. The first press conference by the Public Health Agency of Sweden together with NBHW took place on February 26 (Folkhälsomyndigheten 2020d) and continued throughout the year. These press conferences were run by agencies—mainly PHAS but included entities, such as the MSB or county governments, if their participation was relevant. In addition to them being broadcast live, they were also available on the agency's YouTube channel (Folkhälsomyndigheten 2020). These agencies published information and updates on their respective websites and social media accounts (Facebook, LinkedIn, Twitter, YouTube). In addition, Sweden has a national online platform, www.krisinformation.se, to communicate official and up-to-date information regarding all hazards, emergencies, and crises. The platform is run jointly by public agencies, and the information is available in Swedish, English, easy-to-read Swedish, and audio. The platform has accounts on Facebook and Twitter. The Swedish Prime Minister held a televised speech to the nation in March and November 2020. Such events are rare in Swedish politics. In both instances, Löfven's message was one of solidarity and individual responsibility, urging citizens to take care of each other (Government of Sweden 2020).

A mass text message campaign was also a means of communication of the national message. On Monday, December 14, a text message was sent to all the registered mobile phone numbers in the country. It read as follows: "Information from the public agencies: Follow the new stricter national regulations and general advice in order to stop the contagion of COVID-19. Read more on the web site krisinformation." The message was minimal and intentionally did not include any links in order to sidestep security concerns. In this instance as well as in all instances when new measures were expected to be announced, PHAS had released information regarding this mass text message ahead of its dispatch in order to prepare the public and minimize confusion. MSB reported 3.5 million visitors to the Krisinformation website on the day the text message was sent out, while the Monday previously that number was 54,000 (Swedish Civil Contingencies Agency 2020c). The text message again evoked the theme of personal responsibility and solidarity that every individual is responsible for the wellbeing of the collective through being careful and following the rules—perhaps, the only chance for compliance in the absence of enforcement instruments. The verb usage had also changed: the modal verb "should" [bör], which had been prevalent in the phraseology of the general regulations had been replaced with the imperative mood, for example "avoid public transportation" or "avoid making new contacts with people during a journey" (Krisinformation.se 2020).

Financial Relief

The Swedish government adopted a series of financial relief measures in anticipation of the economic contraction that was bound to follow the contagion mitigation measures. Twelve budget amendments were approved by Riksdag beyond the two normal occasions (in the fall and spring of the fiscal year) when the annual budget is decided. Measures aimed at supporting households and viable businesses and included transfers for furloughs increased subsidies for sickness periods including doing away with the one-day wait period for sick-leave pay and some subsidies for people in high-risk groups. What is more, measures targeted vulnerable sectors included media and culture, sports, public transportation, railways, airlines and shipping, research and innovation, and higher education (Regeringskansliet 2020c). They included a combined tax reduction of 8.49b SEK, 10.61b SEK, and 16.96b SEK in 2021, 2022, and 2023, respectively (Government Offices of Sweden 2020c). NIER, the National Institute for Economic Research [Konjunkturinstitutet] estimates that the measures taken for 2020 as a result of pandemic outbreak amounted to 194b SEK (National Institute for Economic Research 2020b).

Indeed, the pandemic had a substantial impact on the Swedish labor market in 2020. In March 2020, 42,000 people were furloughed—double as many people as in the worst month during the financial crisis. The unemployment rate of 9.1% in Q3 of 2020 was the highest since the devastating recession Sweden experienced in the 1990s (National Institute for Economic Research 2020b). High unemployment did not affect everyone equally. As we have seen elsewhere, the pandemic exacerbated existing cleavages including generational and educational differentials as well as immigration status. More specifically, the unemployment rate among young people not in school and looking for full-time work was 14%, whereas among older people, unemployment rose at a lower rate. Unemployment among Swedish citizens and residents born outside the country rose to 20.5% in Q3 while dropping to 15.7% in Q4, partly because that group is overrepresented in the transportation, hospitality, and food services industries. Finally, unemployment among people without a high-school diploma rose to 30% during Q3, up from an average of 20% during the 2010s (National Institute for Economic Research 2020b). NIER reports that the Swedish economy recovered at a higher rate than expected in Q3 of 2020 with a GDP increase of about 5% (see also Government Offices of Sweden 2020d). The economic recovery was much slower during Q4 due to the second wave of the pandemic in November 2020.

The Swedish Employment Service estimates that the measures described above softened the effects of the pandemic crisis the labor market. However, the agency predicts that unemployment will rise again in 2021, partly because some people went back to school. This was encouraged by the government through extra funding allocation in the budget both as a short-term and as a long-term solution (Swedish Employment Service 2020).

Evaluation: A Component of the Swedish Policy Style

Evaluations are a standard feature of Swedish public administration. Normally, they are conducted after a process had ended. The drawn-out crisis of the pandemic rendered the evaluation of the national response. First, a commission of inquiry—the Corona Commission was convened to assess the Swedish response to the pandemic (Government Offices of Sweden 2020e). The commission submitted its first findings in the fall of 2020, concluding that the Swedish government failed the people living in elder care. Additionally, Riksrevisionen (The Swedish National Accountability Office) issued a report on the legality of the government's fiscal response to the pandemic in the budget (Swedish National Accountability Office 2020). Finally, a cross-party parliamentary committee was convened in December 2020 with the task of evaluating the work of the Riksdag and the Riksdag Administration during the pandemic (Sveriges Riksdag 2020).

We Follow the Public Health Agency's Guidelines: Discussion and Conclusions

The most prominent features of the Swedish response to the pandemic were the considerable degree of depoliticization of the contagion mitigation measures (as well as the measures aimed at financial support to households and viable businesses) and the decentralized implementation of the national, mostly voluntary guidelines. These features were underpinned by the unspoken agreement between the individual and the state with a long tradition in Sweden: the individual trusts the state to make collective decisions and the state trusts that the individual will, in turn, trust the state and comply with these decisions. In other words, there is a mutual expectation of trust—at least in principle. The high levels of trust amplified the high administrative capacity and high inclusiveness of the policymaking system constituting a managerial policy style to result in a decentralized national pandemic response.

The East Nordic administrative model held even during the protracted crisis of COVID-19. PHAS, operationally autonomous, made decisions regarding the mitigation of contagion, which the government followed, while a considerable increase in public spending throughout 2020 in repeated budget amendments served to counteract the consequences of these measures. The central government (in contrast to Norway [see Sparf, this volume]) refrained from impinging on the autonomy of municipalities, which were free to decide for themselves how to handle the pandemic. This does not mean that the result at the local level was disorderly—rather, municipalities followed the guidelines of PHAS, at times enforcing stricter rules, for example, closing down schools or public swimming pools. The high levels of coordination between the public agencies, the county boards, and the municipalities ensured a fairly uniform approach to the national guidelines (Sparf et al. 2021).

The crisis management rationale in Sweden privileges operations remaining as close as possible to the everyday organizational activities as structures, avoiding extraordinary decision-making structures even during extraordinary conditions such as the pandemic. Notably, this holds even at the local level. In a recent study, Sparf et al. (2021) reported that during 2020, operations and decision-making structures in Swedish municipalities remained as close to business-as-usual as possible, avoiding scaling up to crisis mode. The high levels of administrative capacity underpin decisions based on expert knowledge; high inclusiveness is conducive to incrementalism and perhaps a slow pace of change. At the same time, high administrative capacity and high inclusiveness contribute to the robustness of the policymaking process.

This does not mean that the response to the pandemic remained static. The second wave sweeping the country in the late fall of 2020 saw more stringent (for the Swedish environment) measures, with legally binding regulations including an option to enact a limited 'corona' law, pointing to a level of dynamism in the response to the pandemic. One thing is certain: the findings of the 'corona commission' in addition to those of a host of evaluations of the bureaucratic response at all levels of government will be part of any future policy change when it comes to public health issues, preparedness, and crisis management.

References

Ahlbäck Öberg, Shirin, and Helena Wockelberg. 2016. "Nordic Administrative Heritages and Contemporary Institutional Design." In *Nordic Administrative Reforms: Lessons for Public Management*, eds. Carsten Greve, Per Lægreid and Lise H. Rykkja. London: Palgrave Macmillan. 127–69.

Anton, Thomas J. 1969. "Policy-Making and Political Culture in Sweden." *Scandinavian Political Studies* 4: 88–102.

Björkman, Anders. 2021. "Kritiken mot Sveriges Strategi Blir Inte Bättre av att Upprepas 100 Gånger." *Dagens Nyheter*, April 14. https://www.dn.se/debatt/kritiken-mot-sveriges-strategi-blir-inte-battre-av-att-upprepas-100-ganger/

Blomqvist, Paula, and Ulrika Winblad. 2014. "Sweden: Continued Marketization within a Universalist System." In *Health Care Systems in Europe under Austerity: Institutional Reforms and Performance*, eds. E. Pavolini, and A. M. Guillén. New York: Palgrave Macmillan, 9–30.

Carlsson, Marcus, Lena Einhorn, Fredrik Elgh, Jonas Frisén, Åke Gustavsson, et al. 2020. "The Public Health Agency of Sweden Has Failed —Now The Politicians Must Intervene." *Dagens Nyheter*, April 14. https://www.dn.se/debatt/folkhalsomyndigheten-har-misslyckats-nu-maste-politikerna-gripa-in/

Christensen, Tom, and Per Lægreid. 2020. "Balancing Governance Capacity and Legitimacy: How the Norwegian Government Handled the Covid-19 Crisis as a High Performer." *Public Administration Review* 80: 774–79.

Einhorn, Eric S., and John Logue. 2003. *Modern Welfare States: Scandinavian Politics and Policy in the Global Age*. 2nd ed. Westport, CT: Praeger.

Engerström, Lars. 2019. "Svensk Intensivvårdsmortalitet och Platstillgång i Internationellt Jämförelse." Poster nr: 2886. Svenska Intensivvårdsregister. https://www.icuregswe.org/globalassets/fou/2886-le-poster-sfai-002.pdf

Giritli Nygren, Katarina, and Anna Olofsson. 2020. "Managing the Covid-19 Pandemic through Individual Responsibility: The Consequences of a World Risk Society and Enhanced Ethopolitics." *Journal of Risk Research* 23: 1031–35.

Government of Sweden. 2020. "Prime Minister Stefan Löfvens Speech to the Nation." https://www.regeringen.se/tal/2020/03/statsministerns-tal-till-nationen-den-22-mars-2020/

Government Offices of Sweden. n.d. "The Government of Sweden." https://www.regeringen.se/sveriges-regering/

Government Offices of Sweden. 2001. "Säkerhet i en ny tid." SOU 2001:41.

Government Offices of Sweden. 2020a. "Äldreomsorgen under Pandemin." SOU 2020: 80. https://www.regeringen.se/4af379/contentassets/a8e708fff5e84279bf11adbd0f78fcc1/sou_2020_80_aldreomsorgen-under-pandemin.pdf

Government Offices of Sweden. 2020b. "Regerigens Arbete med Coronopandemin." https://www.regeringen.se/regeringens-politik/regeringens-arbete-med-coronapandemin/

Government Offices of Sweden. 2020c. "From the Budget Bill for 2021: Budget Statement." https://www.government.se/4a73a0/contentassets/ddfaf5ce78494ce991ec231acf9c5b83/summary-budget-statement.pdf

Government Offices of Sweden. 2020d. "Starkare Återhämtning i Svensk Ekonomi än Väntat." https://www.regeringen.se/pressmeddelanden/2020/12/starkare-aterhamtning-i-svensk-ekonomi-an-vantat/

Government Offices of Sweden. 2020e. "Members of the Corona Commission Appointed." https://www.regeringen.se/pressmeddelanden/2020/07/coronakommissionens-ledamoter-utsedda/?TSPD_101_R0=088d4528d9ab2000ecb7d75f1821377a6762afabb87f7bb69fa2e9abba0795654443bb36ec5b7c02089baaee5a1430005acdf69f55118b929e702a87ed1dd3d61062532c87c1f12054ebf1ea57641eb730fc097da43094137ec66791a4748a2c

Hall, Patrik. 2016. "The Swedish Administrative Model." In *The Oxford Handbook of Swedish Politics*, ed. Jon Pierre. Oxford: Oxford University Press. 299–314.

Holmberg, Sören, and Bo Rothstein. 2020. "Social Trust—the Nordic Gold?" Working Paper Series 2020:1. Quality of Government Institute: University of Gothenburg. https://www.gu.se/sites/default/files/2020-05/2020_1_Holmberg_Rothstein.pdf

Inspektionen för Vård och Omsorg. 2020. "Iakttagelser i Korthet." Nr 1/2020. https://www.ivo.se/publicerat-material/iakttagelser-i-korthet/man-tycks-vara-mer-nojda-med-hur-varden-och-omsorgen-samordnas/

Johns Hopkins. 2021. "Corona Virus Resource Center." https://coronavirus.jhu.edu/map.html

Jonung, Lars, and Joakim Nergelius. 2020. "Grundlagen Sätter Ramarna För Sveriges Coronastrategi." *Dagens Nyheter*, Sunday, 2 August. 5. https://www.dn.se/debatt/grundlagen-satter-ramarna-for-sveriges-coronastrategi/

Krisinformation.se. 2020. "Nya Skärpta Nationella Råd." https://www.krisinformation.se/detta-kan-handa/handelser-och-storningar/20192/myndigheterna-om-det-nya-coronaviruset/nationella-rad

Kuhlmann, Sabine, and Hellmut Wollmann. 2014. *Introduction to Comparative Public Administration*. Cheltenham, UK: Edward Elgar.

Larsson, Torbjörn, and Henry Bäck. 2008. *Governing and Governance in Sweden*. Malmö: Studentlitteratur.

Myndigheten för vård- och omsorgsanalys. 2020. "Vården ur Befolkningens Perspectiv: IHP 2020." https://www.vardanalys.se/rapporter/varden-ur-befolkningens-perspektiv-2020/

National Board of Health and Welfare. 2014. "Socialstyrelsens Risk- och Sårbarhetsanalys 2014." https://www.socialstyrelsen.se/globalassets/sharepoint-dokument/artikelkatalog/ovrigt/2014-11-19.pdf

National Board of Health and Welfare. 2020a. "Emergency Preparedness." https://www.socialstyrelsen.se/en/about-us/emergency-preparedness/

National Board of Health and Welfare. 2020b. "Uppföljning och Analys av Överenskommelsen om Ökad Tillgänglighet 2020." Delrapport December 2020. https://www.socialstyrelsen.se/globalassets/sharepoint-dokument/artikelkatalog/ovrigt/2020-12-7066.pdf

National Institute for Economic Research. 2020a. "Makroekonomiska och samhällsekonomiska effekter av de vidtagna åtgärderna för att dämpa Covid-19 i Sverige." Specialstudie, KI 2020:25.

National Institute for Economic Research. 2020b. "Konjunkturläget: December 2020." https://www.konj.se/download/18.3891afad1764bc62ba85729c/1608215087376/KLDec2020.pdf

Neuvonen, Päivi Johanna. 2020. "The Covid-19 Policymaking under the Auspices of Parliamentary Constitutional Review: The Case of Finland and Its Implications." *European Policy Analysis* 6: 226–37.

Nielsen, Julie Hassing, and Johannes Lindvall. 2021. "Trust in Government in Sweden and Denmark During the Covid-19 Epidemic." *West European Politics* 44: 1180–204.

Ortiz-Ospina, Esteban, and Max Roser. 2016. "Trust." Published online at OurWorldInData.org. https://ourworldindata.org/trust [Online Resource]

Petersson, Olof. 2016. "Rational Politics: Commissions of Inquiry and the Referral System in Sweden." In *The Oxford Handbook of Swedish Politics*, ed. Jon Pierre. Oxford: Oxford University Press. 650–62.

Petridou, Evangelia. 2020. "Politics and Administration in Times of Crisis: Explaining the Swedish Response to the COVID-19 Crisis." *European Policy Analysis* 6: 147–58. https://doi.org/10.1002/epa2.1095

Petridou, Evangelia, and Jörgen Sparf. 2017. "For Safety's Sake: The Strategies of Institutional Entrepreneurs and Bureaucratic Reforms in Swedish Crisis Management, 2001–2009." *Policy and Society* 36(4): 556–74.

Pierre, Jon. 2016. "Introduction: The Decline of Swedish Exceptionalism." In *The Oxford Handbook of Swedish Politics*, ed. Jon Pierre. Oxford: Oxford University Press. 1–16.

Pierre, Jon. 2020. "Nudges against Pandemics: Sweden's Covid-19 Containment Strategy in Perspective." *Policy and Society* 39: 478–93.

Richardson, Jeremy (ed). 1982/2013. *Policy Styles in Western Europe.* New York: Routledge.

Rönnerstrand, Björn, and Maria Oskarson. 2020. "Standing in Line When Queues Are on the Decline: Services Satisfaction Following the Swedish Health Care Waiting Time Guarantee." *Policy Studies Journal* 48: 469–93.

Ruin, Olof. 1982/2013. "Sweden in the 1970s: Policy-Making Becomes More Difficult." In *Policy Styles in Western Europe*, ed. Jeremy Richardson. Oxon, UK: Routledge. 141–67.

Savage, Maddy, Philip Reeves, and Daniel Estrin. 2020. "Corona Virus Around the World: Israel, Brazil, and Sweden." *National Public Radio.* July 11. https://www.npr.org/2020/07/11/890078852/covid-19-cases-spike-in-brazil-israel-sweden

Sparf, Jörgen, Evangelia Petridou, Mikael Granberg, and Bearice Onn. 2021. "Pandemi i Det Lokala." Report. Swedish Contingencies Agency. https://rib.msb.se/Dok.aspx?Tab=2&dokid=29763

Sparf, Jörgen, and Evangelia Petridou. 2021. "Sweden: Country Report". Stavanger: University of Stavanger. https://ebooks.uis.no/index.php/USPS/catalog/book/98

Sundström, Göran. 2016. "Administrative Reform." In *The Oxford Handbook of Swedish Politics*, ed. Jon Pierre. Oxford: Oxford University Press. 315–31.

Svedin, Glenn. 2017. "Den Svenska Tillitens Historiska Vagga: Några Kritiska Anmärkningar." *Statsvetenskaplig tidskrift* 119: 781–801.

Sveriges Riksdag. 2020a. "Commission of Inquiry on the Work of the Riksdag During the Corona Pandemic." https://www.riksdagen.se/en/news/2020/dec/21/commission-of-inquiry-on-the-work-of-the-riksdag-during-the-corona-pandemic/

Sveriges Riksdag. 2020b. "Covid Law." https://covidlawlab.org/wp-content/uploads/2021/02/Sweden_2004.04.07_Act_Contagious-Disease-Act_SW.pdf

Swedish Association of Local Authorities and Regions. 2020. "Stärkt samverkan för inköp av bristvaror till kommunerna." https://skr.se/tjanster/press/nyheter/nyhetsarkiv/starktsamverkanforinkopavbristvarortillkommunerna.32758.html

The Public Health Agency of Sweden. 2019a. "Pandemiberedskap. Hur vi förbereder oss – ett kunskapsunderlag." https://www.folkhalsomyndigheten.se/contentassets/b6cce03c4d0e4e7ca3c9841bd96e6b3a/pandemiberedskap-hur-vi-forbereder-oss-19074-1.pdf

The Public Health Agency of Sweden. 2019b. "Pandemiberedskap. Hur vi kommunicerar – ett kunskapsunderlag." https://www.folkhalsomyndigheten.se/contentassets/2f2a536f14e54a83b983594b4b71c3d4/pandemiberedskap-kommunicera-19074-2.pdf

The Public Health Agency of Sweden. 2019c. "Pandemiberedskap. Tillgång till och användning av läkemedel – en vägledning." https://www.folkhalsomyndigheten.se/contentassets/1c7ea06c959541c0bfac32ed4f92f73c/pandemiberedskap-tillgang-anvandning-lakemedel-19074-3.pdf

The Public Health Agency of Sweden. 2020a. "Preparedness." https://www.folkhalsomyndigheten.se/the-public-health-agency-of-sweden/communicable-disease-control/preparedness/

The Public Health Agency of Sweden. 2020b. "Föreskrifter och allmänna råd – covid-19." https://www.folkhalsomyndigheten.se/smittskydd-beredskap/utbrott/aktuella-utbrott/covid-19/foreskrifter-och-allmanna-rad/

The Public Health Agency of Sweden. 2020c. "Folkhälsomyndigheten föreskrifter och allmänna råd om allas ansvar att förhindra smitta av covid-19 m.m." https://www.folkhalsomyndigheten.se/globalassets/publicerat-material/foreskrifter/konsoliderade/hslf-fs_2020_12.pdf

The Public Health Agency of Sweden. 2020d. "Press Release Archive." https://www.folkhalsomyndigheten.se/nyheter-och-press/nyhetsarkiv/2020/

The Swedish Civil Contingencies Agency. 2020a. "Risk- och sårbarhetsanalyser." https://www.msb.se/sv/amnesomraden/krisberedskap–civilt-forsvar/risk–och-sarbarhetsanalyser/

The Swedish Civil Contingencies Agency. 2020b. "About MSB." https://www.msb.se/en/about-msb/

The Swedish Civil Contingencies Agency. 2020c. "Kraftig Ökning av Trafik till Krisinformation.se." https://www.mynewsdesk.com/se/msb/news/kraftig-oekning-av-trafik-till-krisinformation-dot-se-417559?utm_campaign=send_list

The Swedish Employment Service. 2020. "Arbetsmarknadsutsikterna Hösten 2020: Utvecklingen på Arbetsmarknaden 2020–2022." Arbetsförmedlingen analys 2020:12.

The Swedish National Accountability Offices. 2020. "Det Finanspolitiska Ramverket — Regeringens Tillämpning 2020." RIR 2020: 29. https://www.riksrevisionen.se/download/18.78abb6c61764bda823b43426/1608109048035/RiR%202020_29%20Anpassad.pdf

Vårdanalys [Swedish Agency for Health and Care Services Analysis]. 2020. "Vården ur Primärvårdsläkarnas Perspektiv 2019—En Jämförelse mellan Sverige och Tio Andra Länder." Rapport 2020:5 https://www.vardanalys.se/rapporter/ihp-2019/

6
Comparing Responses

13

DIFFERENT GOVERNMENTS, DIFFERENT RESPONSES TO THE COVID-19 PANDEMIC? CONCLUDING REMARKS AND THE WAY FORWARD

Jale Tosun

The term 'crisis' has been used frequently to refer to situations warranting enhanced attention and the adoption of swift and effective responses by policymakers (Boin et al. 2017; Boin and Kuipers 2018; Boin, Lodge, and Luesink 2020). However, despite its prominent use in the literature, in only few cases, the term has been as accurate as with the COVID-19 virus to capture both the characteristics of the problem and the associated problem-solving strategies. This volume edited by Nikolaos Zahariadis, Evangelia Petridou, Theofanis Exadaktylos, and Jörgen Sparf embarked on an intellectual journey to investigate in-depth the responses by national governments to the COVID-19 pandemic through the analytical prism of a crisis. This chapter will summarize and reflect on the insights yielded by the individual country studies and reflect on them in order to further our understanding of policymaking in times of crisis and how national policy styles (Richardson, Gustafsson, and Jordan 1982) and trust in political institutions (Uslaner 2018) shaped the policy responses adopted.

On the one hand, the pandemic *per se* represented a significant challenge to policymakers and policymaking. Especially at the beginning of the crisis, there was considerable uncertainty concerning the characteristics of the virus disease, the threat it entailed to the various groups in society, and which policy measures would be best suited to mitigate its adverse effects (Boin, Lodge, and Luesink 2020). Representing a novel problem, the database on which governments could draw when designing policy responses to COVID-19 was underdeveloped (Capano et al. 2020). Because of the uncertainty, the majority of scientific experts supported the adoption of lockdown-style policies, but they were challenged by a smaller group of scientific experts calling for 'smarter' and less-restrictive policy responses. While diverse views lie at the very heart of scientific debate, the differing opinions created a situation in which policymakers had to justify why they followed the advice by one group of experts and paid less or no attention to the

DOI: 10.4324/9781003137399-19

recommendations by the other (Pamuk 2021). A swift and effective implementation of policies that are accompanied by uncertainty requires elevated levels of trust in political institutions (Capano 2020; Migone 2020).

On the other hand, when analyzing the national policy responses to the COVID-19 pandemic, one also needs to consider that the availability of information, and therefore, the ability to track the governments' (non-)responses was unprecedented. Most importantly, the Center for Systems Science and Engineering at Johns Hopkins University provided real-time data on cases and deaths in all countries around the world, thereby creating a unique context for policymaking and the accountability of policymakers alike. Likewise, the Oxford COVID-19 Government Response Tracker (Hale et al. 2021) documented on a daily basis the policy decisions taken by governments and facilitated a systematic comparison across countries. And the similarly Oxford-based data website Our World in Date published daily information in vaccination progress. The availability of these and similar data sources has arguably affected the politics of COVID mitigation measures (Chakraborty et al. 2021), which, in turn, may have resulted in changes to national policy styles as explained in Chapter 1.

Taken together, not only the pandemic *per se* may have created a challenge to national governments but also the sheer volume and detail of information—and some would add misinformation (e.g., Roozenbeek et al. 2020)—produced and transmitted by the whole range of media. From an analytical viewpoint, national governments did not only have to address the public health challenge related to COVID-19 but also to cope with the fact that their (in)action (McConnell and Hart 2019) was scrutinized very closely by the public in their own countries as well as abroad.

What are the implications of the findings produced by this volume for the usefulness of policy styles and trust in studying the national governments' responses to the COVID-19 pandemic? What are the implications of the findings for theories of policymaking and crisis management? To address these questions, this chapter unfolds as follows. First, it gives an overview of the main insights provided by the individual country chapters. Subsequently, it engages in a comparative discussion of the findings with a view to assess the hypotheses put forward in Chapter 1. Finally, the chapter assesses the value of the contributions of this volume to the study of policy style and presents a research agenda.

Insights from the Comparative Analysis

This section provides background information on the individual countries. Subsequently, it summarizes the findings of the country chapters and then evaluates the hypotheses that guided all empirical contributions to this volume.

Contextualization of the Countries

This volume brought together in-depth investigations of ten diverse governments and how they responded to the COVID-19 crisis in the year 2020. As the crisis extended beyond 2020, this means that in most of the countries studied, the focus was on the first and the second wave of the pandemic. From an analytical viewpoint, it is reasonable to consider the first wave as the critical one since it corresponds to a crisis in the narrow definition of the term. The countries selected for this collection vary along multiple dimensions and therefore offer an appropriate sample for assessing the hypotheses put forward by the editors (see Chapter 1).

The influential volume edited by Richardson (1982), which started the research agenda on national policy styles, already classified the policy styles of Norway, Sweden, and the United Kingdom. Regarding the latter, it should be noted that because of Richardson's leading role in establishing the concept of policy styles and his collaboration with other British scholars such as Grant Jordan (e.g. Jordan and Richardson 1983), from an empirical viewpoint, the British policy style can be considered as the best explored one. Recent studies shed light on how important political events such as devolution (Cairney 2019; Jordan and Cairney 2013) and Brexit (Richardson 2018a; 2018b) changed the British 'negotiation style' (Jordan and Richardson 1982). While for Norway no particular policy style could be identified, Sweden was associated with a reactive and consensus-seeking policy style (Richardson 1982).

Attempting to revive the original concept and to facilitate its applicability beyond Western Europe, Howlett and Tosun (2019; 2021) reformulated the concepted and invited contributions investigating the national policy styles in Brazil (Grin and Abrucio 2019), China (Qian 2019), Turkey (Bolukbasi and Ertugal 2019), the United Kingdom (Cairney 2019), and the United States (Peters 2019). Among many other insights, the country chapters that are part of the collection edited by Howlett and Tosun (2019) indicated that the degree of centralization of political power matters for policymaking, which is also captured by the theoretical framework of the present volume (see Chapter 2). Furthermore, when inspecting the state of research, of the countries included in this collection, the policy style of the New Zealand government received noticeable scholarly attention (see Mazey and Richardson 2020). In stark contrast, the concept of policy styles was never applied to the political systems of Greece and Kenya, making the analysis carried out in this volume very valuable not only for an audience interested in policy responses to the COVID-19 pandemic but also to scholars working on national policy styles.

While a detailed discussion of the policy styles observed for the ten countries goes beyond the scope of this chapter, it should be noted that there is sufficient variation in terms of the degree to which policymakers act on or react to a problem and whether they impose decisions on interest groups or seek consensus with them (Richardson, Gustafsson, and Jordan 1982) or how inclusive policymaking is, and what actors feature prominently in that process (Howlett and Tosun 2019, 2021).

Political trust is another founding block of the conceptual model of this volume. In essence, political trust is about the citizens' belief that the political system or individual political actors such as the government will take decisions and produce outcomes consistent with their expectations (Newton, Stolle, and Zmerli 2018). In contrast to policy styles, which is a qualitative concept, there exist various quantitative indicators for gauging levels of trust in politicians, which allow for empirically demonstrating the cross-country variation. Figure 13.1 is based on data provided by the Global Competitiveness Index of the World Economic Forum and captures the trust in politicians ranging from 1 (low) to 7 (high). The figure reveals that in 2016/2017, the lowest value for trust in politicians was observed for Brazil and the highest for New Zealand. However, the data also shows that trust in politicians was low in Greece and Kenya, whereas it was high in Norway and Sweden.

The editors regard policy capacity to constitute an additional dimension of policy styles. In contrast to the dimensions introduced by Richardson, Gustafsson, and Jordan (1982) and Howlett and Tosun (2019, 2021), there exist various established operationalizations of policy capacity. For the purpose of contextualizing the countries covered in this volume, the Government Effectiveness Indicator by the World Bank appears useful. The composite indicator runs from −2.5 (low capacity) to 2.5 (high capacity) and is available for a large set of countries and for a long period of time (more than two decades). The values presented in Figure 13.2 refer to the year 2019 since it represents the year just before the outbreak of the pandemic. Kenya, Brazil, and Turkey are the three countries with

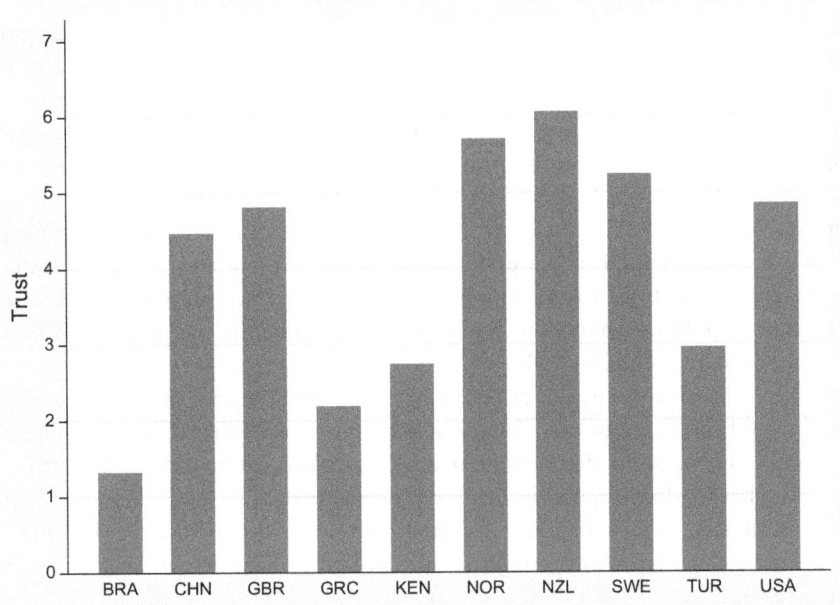

FIGURE 13.1 Trust in Politicians, 2016/2017.

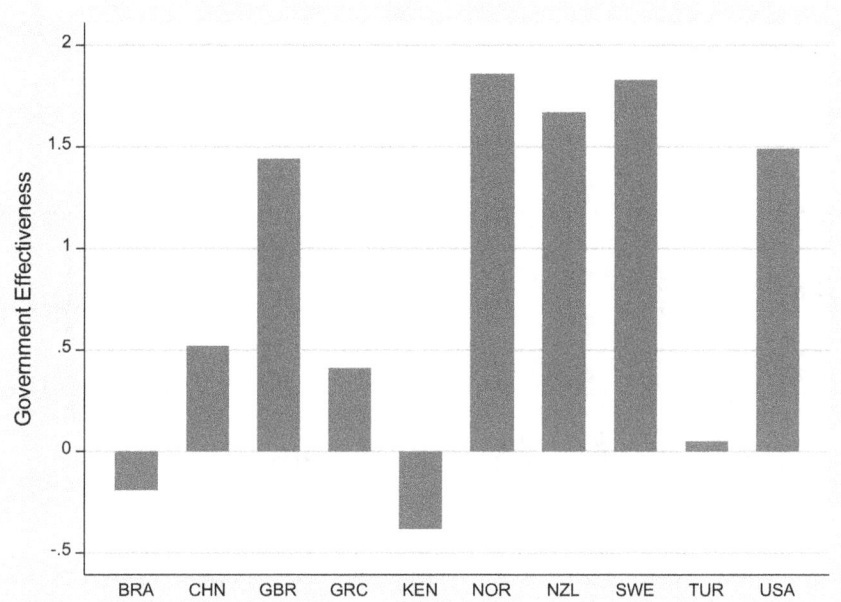

FIGURE 13.2   Government Effectiveness, 2019.

the lowest policy capacity, whereas Norway, Sweden, and New Zealand have the highest level of capacity.

Another indicator that facilitates the systematic comparison of the countries analyzed in this volume refers to the reproduction rates throughout 2020, which is about the number of secondary cases produced by a single infection in a given population (Ahammed et al. 2021). This indicator is useful for understanding how severely the crisis hit the individual countries and also provides an approximation of how consistent the policy response to the crisis was. One could argue that countries with great temporal variation took a less consistent approach than those with little temporal variation. Likewise, we could regard the median reproduction rate as an indicator of how effective the policy responses were in order to stop the spread of the virus.

Figure 13.3 presents box plots with the reproduction rates for the individual countries in 2020. We can infer from the figure that Sweden had the lowest temporal variation and accepted the highest reproduction rate over the observation period. We see greater temporal variation in the reproduction rate of China (judged by the length of the box) and Turkey (judged by the outliers marked by the dots). New Zealand is worth highlighting because it had the lowest median reproduction rate (indicated by the white line inside the box) in 2020, suggesting that the government took a drastic and apparently effective policy response to contain COVID-19.

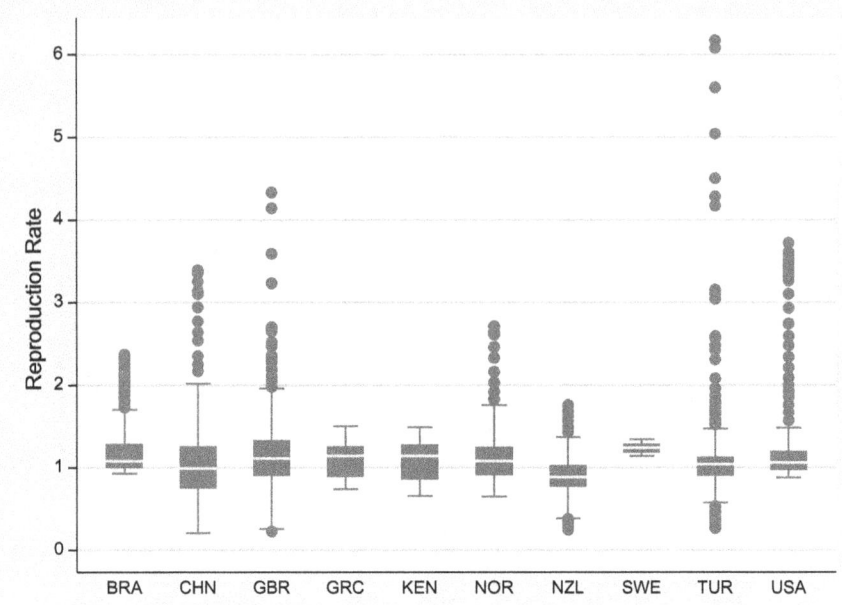

FIGURE 13.3 Reproduction Rate, 2020.

Summary of the Findings

The policy style in China is hierarchical and reactive, which is complemented by the Communist Party's support for policy experimentation (Qian 2019). Departing from this assessment, in Chapter 3, Stephen Ceccoli argues that the Chinese government's response to the pandemic demonstrated centralized leadership and hierarchical trust, but also that it took the government some time to adopt this approach. Ceccoli contends that during the first three weeks of the crisis, policymaking was disjoint and the implementation of the policies lax. The case study reveals that the highly centralized coordination of resources produced a situation in which bottlenecks emerged and resources were spent inefficiently. Only in the subsequent period, the approach became more efficient due to the decision to coordinate the resources both vertically and horizontally. By restructuring its policy style, China could leverage its policy capacity and 'crush' the infection curve rather swiftly. However, as suggested by Figure 13.3, the problem was severe in China, and when it was hit by the virus, the level of uncertainty was particularly high, which explains why it took the government some time to figure out the most effective approach and why there was considerable temporal variation in the reproduction rates.

The Turkish policy style has been characterized by imposition and reaction (Bolukbasi and Ertugal 2019). Did the country follow this general policy style when responding to the COVID-19 crisis or did it deviate from it? In Chapter 4, Lacin Idil Oztig contends that the Turkish imposition style was maintained through the crisis, but with one important modification. While usually reacting to policy issues when they had already become virulent, the Turkish government appeared as an anticipatory actor in this particular crisis. Despite comparatively low levels of political trust (see Figure 13.1) and policy capacity (see Figure 13.2), the government handled the pandemic effectively. It adopted stringent containment measures, facilitated their implementation by means of vertical and horizontal coordination, and instituted different types of sanctions for those who would not comply with these measures adopted.

In Chapter 5, Nikolaos Zahariadis and Vassilis Karokis-Mavrikos characterize the policy style in Greece as "administrative" and similar to that of China and Turkey. Interestingly, so far, Greece did not receive much attention in the emerging academic debate on policy styles, which makes the authors' systematic assessment of its policy style a welcome contribution to the broader literature on national policy styles. Zahariadis and Karokis-Mavrikos characterize the Greek policy style as reactive and impositional as well as allude to a low policy capacity and a low degree of inclusiveness. As shown in Figure 13.1, trust in politicians was relatively low in Greece in 2019. As anticipated by the theoretical framework in Chapter 1, this constellation resulted in the development of a highly centralized response plan to the crisis with the adoption of stringent measures and corresponding instruments for their proper implementation. The authors find that this approach became more centrifugal during the second wave of the pandemic, but still remained centralized in essence. They explain that the moderate deviations from the original policy approach resulted from the government realizing the costs incurred on the economy and its attempt to ease these.

In Chapter 6, Shadrack W. Nasong'o classifies the Kenyan policy style as 'administrative' and thus similar to that of China, Greece, and Turkey. In Kenya, policymaking remains exclusive and centralized despite attempts for decentralization. Public trust in political institutions is low (see Figure 13.1), and therefore citizens regarded the measures adopted as disproportionate given the degree to which the country was affected by the pandemic, which was relatively mild. As a result, people protested against the government's policy approach to containing the spread of COVID-19. Nasong'o compellingly demonstrates that Kenya's response to the pandemic was highly centralized and exclusive, mirroring the regular national policy style.

Overall, the four chapters on centralized policy responses provide a very coherent set of findings and demonstrate that a strong political will can compensate for lacking administrative capacity. In this regard, it is worth noting that, compared to China and Turkey, the Greek approach was more anticipatory and more consistent throughout the observation period. The case of Kenya aligns with the patterns observed for the first three countries.

The next two chapters on Norway and New Zealand are associated with the expectation of centripetal elements in the crisis mitigation approaches. In Chapter 6, Jörgen Sparf explains that the Norwegian policy style corresponds to that of the 'ministerial' model, which assigns individual ministers and ministries influence over the state capacity. Norway is characterized by high levels of trust in political institutions as indicated by Figure 13.1. Sparf contends that the autonomy of public agencies and local authorities as well as the inclusion of a great number of actors in the policymaking process resulted in an accommodative policy response to COVID-19. The case study reveals the tendency to curtail the autonomy of sub-national levels and centralize decision-making powers. The national response privileged health over economic concerns and a centralized national strategy over the flexibility of the local level. Thus, the politics of pandemic management did not resemble the regular patterns of policymaking. Instead, the Norwegian policy style oscillated between a managerial and an adversarial style, which is an intriguiging finding.

W. John Hopkins and Annick Masselot's assessment of the policy responses by the New Zealand government in Chapter 7 stresses the comparatively low level of administrative capacity but high level of trust in political leadership and the high degree of inclusiveness. The measures taken by the government were stringent but generally time-limited and based on the recommendation of scientific experts. The government's transparent and inclusive communication strategy has encouraged citizens to work collectively, fostering national unity and pride around a common goal of defeating the virus. This helped the government to achieve a COVID-free status and to become a role model for many other countries in how to respond to the crisis.

This set of chapters appears less coherent compared to the previous. The response plans by New Zealand and Norway indeed demonstrate the centripetal elements which were anticipated by the high levels of political trust in these two countries. However, the chapter authors associate New Zealand with an accommodative policy style and Norway with a blend of adversarial and managerial policy style, which does not align with the corresponding hypothesis. Thus, of the two countries, the policy response by the New Zealand government can be explained best by the theoretical framework.

Chapter 9 analyzes the British response to the COVID-19 pandemic. To this end, Theofanis Exadaktylos follows closely the classification of the United Kingdom in the literature, which has been characterized by two opposing views. One has regarded the British policy style as adversarial and impositional, and the other one as consensual (Richardson 2018b). While Jordan and Richardson (1983) stressed the consensual aspects of the British policy style, in more recent reflections, Richardson (2018a; 2018b) argues that the adversarial and impositional elements offer a more accurate description. This assessment aligns with the empirical picture Exadaktylos paints in his chapter since the initial response by the British government contained many centrifugal elements, arguably with the intension to diffuse responsibility and avoid direct criticisms on poor crisis management. However, subsequently, the British government adopted a centralized policy approach, while still attempting to diffuse responsibilities to the devolved administrations and local authorities. In this way, it could save its public image as a competent crisis manager.

In Chapter 10, Valesca Lima and José de Arimatéia da Cruz provide an in-depth analysis of the policy response to the pandemic by the Brazilian government.

The chapter reveals both the use of centrifugal elements and an overall inconsistent policy approach. The policy style of President Bolsonaro was marked by adversarialism and exclusiveness. Brazil's policy approach lacked the political will to propose proportionate and (horizontally and vertically) coordinated policy action. As a result, it became one of the countries hit most severely by the crisis in terms of death rates.

Kristin Taylor, Rob DeLeo, Deserai Crow, and Thomas Birkland studied the COVID-19 politics in the United States and alluded to the existence of centrifugal response plans in Chapter 11. Drawing from the instructive discussion by Peters (2019), the authors concentrate on the high level of administrative capacity and inclusivity of the US policy style, while acknowledging that the United States cannot be associated with one single policy style because of the federal organization of its political system. Most importantly, the authors contend that the existing administrative capacity, especially at the central level, went unused in the COVID-19 pandemic response. Consequently, the response to the crisis lacked coordination and was decentralized and fragmented.

The three chapters on the United Kingdom, Brazil, and the United States share their emphasis on the strategic dimension of the policy responses to COVID-19. In the beginning, the governments in the countries at hand lacked the political will to adopt appropriate measures. However, the British government changed its strategy and adopted stricter policy responses. The government of Brazil maintained its strategic consideration and minimal policy response to the pandemic. Similar to the case of Brazil, in the United States, there was no political will to leverage the state's administrative capacity and to institute a strict and coordinated policy approach.

Chapter 12 by Evangelia Petridou explores in-depth the Swedish response plans, which attracted considerable attention by publics and academics alike. Sweden is characterized by an inclusive, deliberative, consensual, problem-solving-oriented policymaking process, which Petridou in the chapter classified as "managerial". Both policy capacity and public trust are notability high in Sweden. These factors resulted in a depoliticized policy approach with a decentralized implementation of the national, mostly voluntary guidelines. The individual trusts the state to make collective decisions, and the state trusts that the individual will, in turn, trust the state and comply with these decisions. This "agreement" between Swedish people and the Swedish political system became very clear in the policy approach adopted.

The adoption of a lenient approach was a deliberate political decision based on government's trust in scientific advice. The outcome was a consistent, decentralized approach which makes Sweden a case apart from the rest.

Assessing the Hypotheses

The editors put forward four hypotheses in Chapter 1, which we can now assess in light of the empirical findings reported by the country chapters. The first hypothesis (H1) postulated that an administrative policy style and lower trust would prompt the adoption of more centralized response plans. The evidence on China, Greece, and Turkey reported by the corresponding chapters supports the logic on which this hypothesis rests. In addition to these three countries, the policy response by the Kenyan government aligns with this hypothesis. Among these four states, the response pattern was most consistent over time in Greece, Kenya, and Turkey. Being the first country that was hit by the novel virus and having no international benchmarks to rely on and to draw lessons from, it took the Chinese government some time to develop and consolidate its policy strategy, which explains why the country's policy response was volatile in the very beginning.

The second hypothesis (H2) postulated that an adversarial policy style and lower trust would prompt the adoption of more centrifugal response plans. The insights provided by the case studies on Brazil, the United Kingdom, and the United States confirmed H2. For the United Kingdom, the relationship postulated, however, only holds for the initial phase of the crisis. The British government subsequently adopted a more centralized response plan in response to pressure from the public and the high number of COVID-related deaths. The willingness of the British government to change its course of action indicates that the country's political institutions function well and that the government can adapt to dynamic public health challenges. The marked opposite could be observed for Brazil, where the centrifugal elements were maintained despite the massive adverse impact of the virus on the country's population. In the United States, the federal government also resisted pressure to adopt a centripetal policy approach, but there, some state governments had the willingness and capacity to fill in the gap (see, e.g., Rocco et al. 2020).

The third hypothesis (H3) postulated that an accommodative policy style and higher trust would prompt the construction of more centripetal response plans. This response pattern could only be observed for New Zealand. The other country that qualified for testing this hypothesis was Norway, but the country chapter indicated that its policy style was not accommodative but rather shifted between an adversarial and a managerial policy style. Despite this characterization of the Norwegian policy style, we can confirm that the country adopted a centripetal response plan. In other words, we could observe the expected outcome, but when following the conceptual model of this volume, we would argue that it was rather brought about by the high levels of trust in political institutions than the features of the national policy style. This interpretation of the Norwegian case is intriguing and important because it is one of the few cases that call into question the relevance of national policy styles for the design of the COVID-19 response plans.

The fourth hypothesis (H4) postulated that a managerial policy style and higher trust would prompt the construction of more decentralized response plans. Sweden has a managerial policy style, and the Swedish policymakers enjoy high levels of trust, and the policy approach to the pandemic was indeed decentralized. While Sweden fits perfectly with this hypothesis, it entails the question whether there exist other cases that would support the logic on which the hypothesis rests. In other words, does this hypothesis reflect the *sui generis* character of the Swedish response plan or could we potentially find support for H4 in other countries too? Interestingly, Norway, which would have been closest case to Sweden in terms of its national policy style and levels of political trust, adopted a different policy approach.

Of all the hypotheses guiding this collective analysis, the fourth appears to have received the most limited type of evidence largely because of the paucity of observations. The hypothesis that was supported by most case studies is the first predicting centralized response plans in countries with an administrative policy style and low levels of political trust.

Novel Insights

This volume produced several novel insights, which concern the study of national policy styles, the relevance of political trust for studying policy responses, and the role policy learning played in the evolution of the crisis response plans.

Importance of Policy Styles

Compared to the other recent attempts to assess the analytical value of policy styles (Howlett and Tosun 2019; 2021), this volume has one key advance: all chapters have analyzed the same policy problem and the governments' responses to it over the same observation period. Consequently, this volume created a methodologically sound design for a comparative assessment of how national policy styles matter in times of crisis. In this context, a striking finding is that we could identify distinguishable patterns in how governments responded to COVID-19. As already flagged above, the most coherent response pattern could be observed for those countries that have an administrative policy style. Nonetheless, we could also identify certain patterns for the other countries.

While this was not explicitly hypothesized, the findings revealed that the right-wing populist governments reacted in a particular way to the public health crisis as compared to the other governments. And in this context, what is perhaps the most important observation is that response patterns by the authoritarian regimes in China, Kenya, and Turkey took the pandemic seriously and adopted strict policy measures accordingly, whereas Brazil and the United States, as democratic regimes but ruled by right-wing populist leaders, behaved in the opposite manner. While it would certainly go beyond the scope of this chapter and even this volume to elaborate in detail on the relationship between the pandemic and democracy, the findings provided here confirm the observation by Croissant (2020) that the pandemic reveals the limited ability of populist governments to cope with the crisis effectively.

One could also argue that the chapters on China, Kenya, and Turkey showed that authoritarian regimes demonstrated a strong political will to be seen as governed by strong and effective leaders in order to prevent publics in their countries to question their ability of effective crisis management. The leaders in these three countries were willing to take whatever was needed to flatten the infection curve and to be perceived as successful pandemic managers. Evidently, in all three countries, compliance proved to be difficult, which then entailed additional and drastic responses to non-compliance by increasing the monitoring and sanctioning.

Overall, the volume has made a compelling case for the value of bringing the concept of national policy styles back in comparative public policy. At first glance, this is a remarkable finding since the policy responses to the pandemic could be regarded as the least likely case for arriving at this conclusion given that it constituted a crisis, and responses to crises follow their own rules and patterns (Boin et al. 2017; Boin and Lodge 2021; Boin, Lodge, and Luesink 2020; Lodge and Wegrich 2012). When reflecting on this further though, almost all chapters have shown that the policy responses to COVID-19 "normalized" after a certain period, which, in turn, increased the likelihood that they would correspond to a given policy style if such a style existed.

Importance of Political Trust

Another key achievement of this volume can be seen in the fact that it combines the concept of national policy styles with political trust. This approach is important for two reasons. First, it shows that national policy styles can be seminally integrated with other concepts in order to deliver more refined explanations for policy adopted in response to a crisis or non-crisis events or issues. Hitherto research did not attempt such an original approach to theorizing. When the notion of policy styles first emerged, the scholarly debate concentrated on whether policy styles comprise the entirety of national policies or whether there is intra-country variation in how sectoral policies are made (e.g., Freeman 1985). This question, despite its value (see also Cairney 2021), has dominated the research agenda and therefore arguably deviated attention away from the question whether policy responses are an outcome of the interaction between policy styles and political trust.

Second, by bringing together national policy styles and political trust, this volume succeeded in developing a compelling link between the stage of policy formulation and policy implementation. Several chapters alluded to the importance of political trust for the social acceptance of the COVID-19 measures adopted. New Zealand adopted a very strict approach and was successful in fighting the virus, which would not have been feasible without the trust of its population. The same holds true for Sweden, which adopted the exact opposite policy approach, but there, too, the population trusted the government, and that its policy approach was informed by scientific evidence. Otherwise, the Swedish people could have demanded the government to take a more rigorous policy approach.

The observation period of this volume ends in 2020 when COVID-19 vaccines were not already rolled out, and the vaccination campaigns had fully started in very few countries. When shifting the analytical focus to the people's willingness to get vaccinated, the question of political trust will become even more important as, for example, Debus and Tosun (2021) have shown. And the willingness of the population to get vaccinated voluntarily will then determine the design of the governments' vaccination policies. In this regard, one would expect that countries with high levels of political trust will not have to contemplate making vaccination mandatory whereas those with low trust levels will me more likely to do so.

In sum, this volume contributes to the literature on comparative public policy by elucidating in what ways and to what degree political trust matters for explaining both the adoption of policy responses and their implementation, which, in turn, produces feedback effects and can then again affect the formulation of policy responses. Political trust tends to play a limited role in comparative public policy, which, as this volume has demonstrated, is unfortunate since it provides a compelling concept for connecting the different stages of the policy phase and therefore facilitates more complete explanations of social phenomena.

Policy Learning

Several chapters highlighted the importance of policy learning when explaining policy responses to the COVID-19 pandemic. They alluded to two types of learning: learning from abroad and learning from their own experience. The chapters on Greece and the United Kingdom, for example, stressed the role of observing the predicament of Italy in spring 2020 for the governments' responses to the pandemic. The United Kingdom is also the country that was shown to have learned from errors made during the first wave. More broadly, several chapters contended that there was a certain period at the beginning of the pandemic when the governments were open to experimenting with a trial-and-error approach. In some countries, such as Germany and the Netherlands (both not covered here), the governments announced that they would make mistakes when formulating policy responses because of the distinct feature of the crisis (Engström, Luesink, and Boin 2021). In the beginning, the public in these two countries applauded them for doing that, but as the pandemic and the restrictions carried on, citizens became less accepting of such narratives.

Similar to the assessment that crises put the governments and their actions in the limelight, another crisis-related feature of COVID-19 politics refers to the link between policy change and policy learning. Several chapters showed either explicitly or implicitly that learning mattered for the evolution of the policy responses. In most cases, learning resulted in major policy change such as in the case of China or the United Kingdom. In the case of Sweden, in particular, the chapter author could identify that learning took place, but it resulted in minor policy change only. In this context, it is plausible to argue that Sweden with its deliberately mild response plan was the country that had to invest most in policy learning in order to justify a possible deviating approach to the Swedish people and the international community. Concerning the latter, the European countries, in particular, scrutinized the Swedish approach very closely, which also resulted from the interdependencies concerning some policy dimensions such as restrictions on intra- and extra-European travel.

Recently, the study of policy learning has entered into a new phase with a more systematic analysis of its types, triggers, and hindrances as well as its pathologies (Dunlop and Radaelli 2020). This volume contributes to this literature because it connects the policy learning with the politics of public health crises.

The Way Forward

Like every other scholarly endeavor, this study has limitations. Despite the valuable insights provided by the country studies, there exist several avenues for further improving our understanding of the politics of national responses to the COVID-19 pandemic. The paths for future research comprise conceptual, theoretical, and empirical aspects.

Conceptual Advances

The notion of policy styles has struggled with whether it applies to policymaking, policy implementation, or both. The original formulation has argued that it covers both (Richardson, Gustafsson, and Jordan 1982), but recent re-formulations and empirical applications have predominantly concentrated on policymaking (Howlett and Tosun 2019; 2021). There is good reason to interpret the notion of policy styles as one that holds a greater potential for explaining policymaking than for explaining policy implementation since the latter is less state-centered and involves actions by different actors, including most importantly compliance with the policies adopted by the policy addressees. For example, street-level implementation involves a wide range of actors. In this context, the special issue by Gofen and Lotta (2021) showed how differently different types of street-level bureaucrats and policy implementers were affected by the pandemic in terms of how they delivered public service. Health professionals and police officers had no choice but to offer direct interactions in policy delivery where teachers and providers of social services had to switch to online delivery.

Consequently, we can state that the features of the COVID-19 pandemic and the policy responses corroborate the need to distinguish between policymaking and policy implementation when studying national policy styles. As argued above, political trust as used in this volume provides an analytical tool for connecting these two stages of the policy cycle, but this still means that additional theorizing is needed to attain an integrated analysis.

A related suggestion concerns the distinction between policy delivery and compliance. In other words, if policy scholars continue to apply the notion of policy styles to policy implementation, it appears necessary to differentiate between the perspective of those who are in charge of delivering a policy, also by means of monitoring and enforcement, and the audience of the policies who must comply with their respective stipulations. The conceptual framework of this book indicates that it is rather compliance than policy delivery that has been studied in the context of the pandemic. This is indicated by the focus on political trust, which is likely to determine compliance rather than the delivery of COVID-related policies by implementing actors.

However, compliance entails a shift away from the state-centered perspective of policy styles to a more governance-oriented one (Richardson 2018b). Therefore, it would flow more naturally from the concept of policy styles to concentrate on how public actors delivered policies during the pandemic. However, this aspect, with the exception of the special issue on street-level bureaucracy by Gofen and Lotta (2021), has received comparatively scant attention. And yet, one could, for instance, see certain patterns when looking at the design and management of the vaccination campaigns. Countries like Israel and the United States adopted a pragmatic approach to vaccination, whereas Germany adopted a more centralized and bureaucratic approach to vaccination. To better capture aspects related to policy delivery, it is useful to integrate policy styles with administrative styles.

Theoretical Advances

The notion of policy styles has the advantage that it aligns with the basic reasoning of comparative policy and that it stresses the importance of politics for policymaking. However, what it does not pay attention to is to what extent governments respond to public demand (Hobolt and Klemmemsen 2005). Policy styles seem to be immune to public demand or at least seem to accommodate public demand in a manner that still corresponds to the standard operating procedures of a political system. However, the crisis character of COVID-19 also manifests itself in the salience of this issue and the need for governments to explain both action and non-action. This reasoning is supported by the fact that in almost all countries affected by moderate to high level of COVID-19, the heads of government or state appealed to the public by delivering speeches, in most cases for justifying the emergency measures and the instituting a lockdown. It is difficult to accommodate this particular feature of the pandemic with the existing notion of policy styles. Another important point in this regard is not only whether we could observe responsive government during the crisis but also responsible government (Mair 2009).

Along these lines, it appears that the public's perception of the COVID-19 measures adopted could have been affected by how the measures adopted by the other countries were depicted by the news media. In this regard, it is possible that either a performance perceived as very good or very bad of the mitigating measures adopted by other states affected the public's judgment of how its own government handled it. For example, we would expect that publics in European countries were more willing to accept or even to demand strict regulatory measures when observing the high number deaths in Italy (Capano 2020), which could have been associated with a poor performance in handling the crisis. In mid-2020, New Zealand was regarded as a country that performed very well and managed to crash the infection curve very effectively and was free of COVID for a certain period (Chapter 8 by Hopkins and Masselot). Likewise, in late 2020, when a fatigue with the (renewed) lockdown measures emerged, European publics could have been inclined to regard the Swedish approach as performing better with its lenient approach than what some other European governments had in place.

Empirical Advances

One important dimension of the policy styles approach concerns the degree to which governments anticipate policy problems and approach them proactively. In this context, it appears important to assess to what extent governments during the COVID-19 crisis based their policy strategies on the anticipation of testing possibilities, vaccination, and the achievement of herd immunity (Mazey and Richardson 2020). For example, it is possible that some governments may have abstained from instituting a second lockdown because they considered it realistic to have access to vaccination within a short period of time. In this regard, it would also be beneficial to pay enhanced attention to the scientific advice structure the individual governments had established. Did they follow one chief advisor? Did they have a whole group of advisors? What was the background of the advisors? These questions indicate that the COVID-19 pandemic offers a unique opportunity for advancing our understanding of evidence-based policymaking and clarifying the role of scientific evidence for policymaking (Yang 2020).

At the same time, the pandemic could represent a critical event that will make all countries become more anticipatory in their approaches to policymaking (Mazey and Richardson 2020), therefore representing a variable for characterizing or explaining policy styles rather than being the phenomenon to be explained. In this regard, a broader point was made by Howlett and Tosun (2020) in their reflection on policy styles and whether they should be conceived as independent or dependent variables. The authors contend that policy styles can be both and that policy scholars only need to make sure to state their stance on the analytical function of the notion accordingly. In this volume, policy styles were regarded as an independent variable, but it would also have been possible to ask whether the feedbacks from the pandemic outcomes produced a specific policy style or whether policy styles converged across countries in the particular case of COVID-19. The question of whether we could observe a cross-country similarity in responding to the crisis with respect to the degree of anticipation/reaction and cooperation/imposition with societal groups in the governments' reactions to the pandemic represents a very promising avenue for future research.

As suggested, the policy styles approach emphasizes the role of interest groups, and interestingly, this dimension has received even little attention in comparison to whether governments were anticipatory or reactive in policymaking during the COVID-19 crisis. Some research has alluded to the possibility that the post-pandemic measures could be 'captured' by interest groups to cater to their needs rather than the needs of other societal groups (Gawel and Lehmann 2020). However, this line of reasoning has not been explored systematically yet. It appears as if the pandemic created a policymaking situation in which interest groups did not exert the usual influence they do on public policy, which would be a very important insight if supported by empirical studies

Conclusion

The COVID-19 pandemic offers a unique opportunity for policy scholars to subject their established concept, theories, and methods to a 'stress test.' This volume corroborates the value of the concept of national policy styles, while it also identifies the need to study it in tandem with political trust. Considering that COVID-19 is a 'crisis' in conceptual terms, the contribution to this volume also had to account for this specific aspect of policymaking. The outcome is a remarkably coherent set of studies, which offers an instructive discussion of the analytical value of national policy styles. It also alludes to additional characteristics of policymaking that future research can address by further refining the concept of policy styles or by combining policy styles with other theoretical perspectives.

References

Ahammed, Tanvir, Aniqua Anjum, Mohammad M. Rahman, Najmul Haider, Richard Kock, and Md J. Uddin. 2021. "Estimation of novel coronavirus (COVID-19) reproduction number and case fatality rate: A systematic review and meta-analysis." *Health Science Reports* 4 (2): e274.

Boin, Arjen, Paul 't Hart, Erik Stern, and Bengt Sundelius. 2017. *The politics of crisis management: Public leadership under pressure* . Cambridge: Cambridge University Press.

Boin, Arjen, and Sanneke Kuipers. 2018. "The crisis approach." In *Handbook of disaster research*, eds. Havidán Rodríguez, William Donner, and Joseph E. Trainor. Cham: Springer, 23–38.

Boin, Arjen, and Martin Lodge. 2021. "Responding to the COVID-19 crisis: A principled or pragmatist approach?" *Journal of European Public Policy* 28 (8): 1131–1152.

Boin, Arjen, Martin Lodge, and Marte Luesink. 2020. "Learning from the COVID-19 crisis: An initial analysis of national responses." *Policy Design and Practice* 3 (3): 189–204.

Bolukbasi, H. Tolga, and Ebru Ertugal. 2019. "Napoleonic tradition, majoritarianism, and Turkey's statist policy style." In *Policy styles and policy-making: Exploring the linkages. Routledge textbooks in policy studies*, eds. Michael Howlett and Jale Tosun. London, New York, NY: Routledge, 351–74.

Cairney, Paul. 2019. "Policy styles in the United Kingdom: A majoritarian UK vs. devolved consensus democracies?" In *Policy styles and policy-making: Exploring the linkages. Routledge textbooks in policy studies*, eds. Michael Howlett and Jale Tosun. London, New York, NY: Routledge, 25–44.

———. 2021. "The concept of a sectoral policy style." In *The Routledge Handbook of Policy Styles*, eds. Michael Howlett and Jale Tosun. London, New York, NY: Routledge, 77–88.

Capano, Giliberto. 2020. "Policy design and state capacity in the COVID-19 emergency in Italy: if you are not prepared for the (un)expected, you can be only what you already are." *Policy and Society* 39 (3): 326–44.

Capano, Giliberto, Michael Howlett, Darryl S. L. Jarvis, M. Ramesh, and Nihit Goyal. 2020. "Mobilizing policy (In)Capacity to fight COVID-19: Understanding variations in state responses." *Policy and Society* 39 (3): 285–308.

Chakraborty, Chiranjib, Ashish R. Sharma, Manojit Bhattacharya, Govindasamy Agoramoorthy, and Sang-Soo Lee. 2021. "Asian-origin approved COVID-19 vaccines and current status of COVID-19 vaccination program in Asia: A critical analysis." *Vaccines* 9 (6): 1–27.

Croissant, Aurel. 2020. "Democracies with preexisting conditions and the coronavirus in the Indo-Pacific region." https://theasanforum.org/democracies-with-preexisting-conditions-and-the-coronavirus-in-the-indo-pacific/.

Debus, Marc, and Jale Tosun. 2021. "Political ideology and vaccination willingness: Implications for policy design." *Policy Sciences* 54 (3): 477–491.

Dunlop, Claire A., and Claudio M. Radaelli. 2020. "The lessons of policy learning: Types, triggers, hindrances and pathologies." In *A Modern Guide to Public Policy*, eds. Giliberto Capano and Michael Howlett. Cheltenham: Edward Elgar, 222–241.

Engström, Alina, Marte Luesink, and Arjen Boin. 2021. "From creeping to full-blown crisis: Lessons from the Dutch and Swedish response to COVID-19." In *Understanding the Creeping Crisis*, eds. Arjen Boin, Magnus Ekengren and Mark Rhinard. Cham: Springer Nature, 105–30.

Freeman, Gary P. 1985. "National styles and policy sectors: Explaining structured variation." *Journal of Public Policy* 5 (4): 467–96.

Gawel, Erik, and Paul Lehmann. 2020. "Killing two birds with one stone? Green dead ends and ways out of the COVID-19 crisis." *Environmental and Resource Economics* 1–5.

Gofen, Anat, and Gabriela Lotta. 2021. "Street-level bureaucrats at the forefront of pandemic response: A comparative perspective." *Journal of Comparative Policy Analysis: Research and Practice* 23 (1): 3–15.

Grin, Eduardo J., and Fernando L. Abrucio. 2019. "The co-evolutionary policy style of Brazil." In *Policy styles and policy-making: Exploring the linkages. Routledge textbooks in policy studies*, eds. Michael Howlett and Jale Tosun. London, New York, NY: Routledge, 115–36.

Hale, Thomas, Noam Angrist, Rafael Goldszmidt, Beatriz Kira, Anna Petherick, Toby Phillips, Samuel Webster, Emily Cameron-Blake, Laura Hallas, Saptarshi Majumdar, and Helen Tatlow. 2021. "A global panel database of pandemic policies (Oxford COVID-19 Government Response Tracker)." *Nature Human Behaviour* 5 (4): 529–538

Hobolt, Sara B., and Robert Klemmemsen. 2005. "Responsive government? Public opinion and government policy preferences in Britain and Denmark." *Political Studies* 53 (2): 379–402.

Howlett, Michael, and Jale Tosun, eds. 2019. *Policy styles and policy-making: Exploring the linkages*. Routledge.

———. 2021. *The Routledge handbook of policy styles*. London: Routledge.

Jordan, A. G., and Jeremy J. Richardson. 1982. "The British policy style or the logic of negotiation?, In Policy Styles in Western Europe, ed. Jeremy J. Richardson. London: Allen & Unwin, 80–110.

———. 1983. "Policy communities: The British and European policy style." *Policy Studies Journal* 11 (4): 603–15.

Jordan, Grant, and Paul Cairney. 2013. "What is the 'dominant model' of British policymaking? Comparing majoritarian and policy community ideas." *British Politics* 8 (3): 233–59.

Lodge, Martin, and Kai Wegrich. 2012. "Introduction: Executive politics in times of crisis." In *Executive Politics in Times of Crisis*, eds. Martin Lodge and Kai Wegreich. Cham: Springer, 1–15.

Mair, Peter. 2009. *Representative versus Responsible Government*. MPIfG - Max-Planck-Institut für Gesellschaftsforschung.

Mazey, Sonia, and Jeremy Richardson. 2020. "Lesson-drawing from New Zealand and Covid-19: The need for anticipatory policy making." *The Political Quarterly* 91 (3), 561–570.

McConnell, Allan, and Paul't Hart. 2019. "Inaction and public policy: Understanding why policymakers 'do nothing'." *Policy Sciences* 52 (4): 645–61.

Migone, Andrea R. 2020. "Trust, but customize: Federalism's impact on the Canadian COVID-19 response." *Policy and Society* 39 (3): 382–402.

Newton, Kenneth, Dietlind Stolle, and Sonja Zmerli. 2018. "Social and political trust." In *The Oxford handbook of social and political trust*, ed. Eric M. Uslaner. Oxford: Oxford University Press, 961–76.

Pamuk, Zeynep. 2021. "COVID-19 and the paradox of scientific advice." *Perspectives on Politics* 122: 1–15.

Peters, B. G. 2019. "The American policy style (s): Multiple institutions creating gridlock and opportunities." In *Policy styles and policy-making: Exploring the linkages. Routledge textbooks in policy studies*, eds. Michael Howlett and Jale Tosun. London, New York, NY: Routledge, 180–98.

Qian, Jiwei. 2019. "Policy styles in China: How to control and motivate bureaucracy." In *Policy styles and policy-making: Exploring the linkages. Routledge textbooks in policy studies*, eds. Michael Howlett and Jale Tosun. London, New York, NY: Routledge, 201–21.

Richardson, Jeremy, ed. 1982. *Policy styles in Western Europe*. London: Routledge.

———. 2018a. *British policy-making and the need for a post-brexit policy style*. Springer.

———. 2018b. "The changing British policy style: From governance to government?" *British Politics* 13 (2): 215–33.

Richardson, Jeremy, Gunnel Gustafsson, and Grant Jordan. 1982. *The concept of policy style*, In *Policy styles in Western Europe, ed. J. Richardson*. Allen & Unwin, London.

Rocco, Philip, Daniel Béland, and Alex Waddan. 2020. "Stuck in neutral? Federalism, policy instruments, and counter-cyclical responses to COVID-19 in the United States." *Policy and Society 39* (3): 458–477.

Roozenbeek, Jon, Claudia R. Schneider, Sarah Dryhurst, John Kerr, Alexandra L. J. Freeman, Gabriel Recchia, Anne M. van der Bles, and Sander van der Linden. 2020. "Susceptibility to misinformation about COVID-19 around the world." *Royal Society Open Science* 7 (10): 1–15.

Uslaner, Eric M., ed. 2018. *The Oxford handbook of social and political trust*. Oxford: Oxford University Press.

Yang, Kaifeng. 2020. "What can COVID-19 tell us about evidence-based management?" *The American Review of Public Administration* 50 (6–7): 706–12.

INDEX

Note: **Bold** page numbers refer to tables; *italic* page numbers refer to figures and page numbers followed by "n" denote endnotes.

Abrucio, F. L. 178
accommodative policy style 13, 238, 240
Act Relating to Control of Communicable Diseases 123
administrative: arrangements 10, 26, 60; capacity 4, 5, 11, 19, 20, 45, 52, 86, 89, 91, 92, 94, 129, 130, 136, 140, 145, 159, 192, 193, 197–200, 213, 224, 225, 237–9; policy capacity 4, 10, 11, 26–8, 32, 60–3, 70, 149, 159, 193–5; policy style 7, 13, 59, 71, 73, 74, 79–83, 239, 241
adversarial 11, 159; legalism 195; policy style 13, 41–3, 130, 157, 164, 166, 169, 170, 172, 240
agenda/agenda setting 65, 81, 86, 177, 178, 184, 195, 242
anticipatory approach 60, 66, 72, 74
anticipatory *vs.* reactive problem-solving 9, 10, 23–6, 42, 63, 71
anti-science 14
Ardern, J. 136, 141–4, 146, 149
aspirations 10, 27, 62, 159
AstraZeneca 169
Atkinson, M. M. 25
austerity 79, 81, 83, 94, 160, 161, 164
authoritarian regime 241
autonomy 10, 27, 62, 63, 71, 102, 103, 120–2, 129, 130, 158, 159, 176, 177, 213, 216, 224, 238; axiomatic trust 30, 32

Bakir, C. 19, 62
Barmé, G. 53
Bauer, P. C. 30
bi-constitutionality 162
Biden, J. 198, 200, 204, 205
BioNTech 69, 168
Bjørnå, H. 127
blame avoidance 12, 20, 51, 164, 204
Boin, Arjen 4, 5, 7, 47, 231, 242
Bolsonaro 175–87, 187n3, 239; approval ratings for *182*; federalism 175–8, 186, 187
Bouckaert, G. 18
"O Brasil Não Pode Parar" (Brazil Cannot Stop) 185
Brazil 174–6, 187, 197, 233, 234, 239–41; Federal administration 175, 177–9, 181, 184–7; federalism 176–9; government acts 179–81; normative acts 181–3; policy capacity 174, 234; policymaking 175–9, 187; policy style 176, 177, 179–87; public health advice **183,** 183–5; trust 185–7
Brazilian Bar Association (OAB) 186
Buck, M. 127
bureaucracy 10–12, 19, 27–9, 43, 59, 61, 129, 213
Bush, G. W. 194, 198

Calef, D. 192
Canterbury Earthquake Recovery Authority (CERA) 141

Capano, G. 18
cash transfer program 174
Ceccoli, S. 19
Center for Systems Science and Engineering 232
centralization 7, 8, 13, 14, 42, 61, 79, 80, 82–6, 93, 129, 130, 162, 176, 177, 197, 204, 211, 233
centralized leadership 42–4
centralized response 7, 8, 42, 47, 52, 54, 59, 60, 71, 88, 90, 92–4, 129, 164, 187, 237, 240, 241
central level 119, 120, 239
centrifugal response 9, 12–13, 42, 79, 80, 90–4, 157, 158, 160–4, 167–70, 175, 187, 204, 237–40
centripetal response 12, 13, 45, 149, 240
Chapple, S. 140
Chief Medical Officers (CMOs) 163, 165, 168
Chikungunya 174
China 7–8, 41–2, 101; command and coordination 47–9; communication and information management 49–52; People's Republic of China (PRC) 43; policy capacity 13, 41, 43, 45, 54, 236; policymaking 41, 42, 44, 54; policy style 13, 41–55, 236; resource management 52–3; and the US 6
Christensen, T. 123, 127
Civil Contingencies Committee 170n6
Civil Defence and Emergency Management Act 2002 (CDEM) 138–9
Civil Solidarity Platform 64
COBRA 162, 170n6
Coleman, W. D. 25
collaboration 22, 71, 73, 89, 105, 124, 129, 215, 216, 233
commissions of inquiry 119, 121, 126, 213
communication 5, 8, 9, 20, 42, 46, 49–52, 66, 71, 85, 89, 92, 107, 123, 128, 136, 140–3, 149, 160, 181, 183, 185, 192, 197, 200–2, 222, 238
Communist Party of China (CPC) 43
compliance 4, 6, 11, 28, 71, 72, 86–8, 94, 95, 128, 136, 140, 184, 197, 222, 242, 244, 245
consensual 23, 63, 162, 212, 238, 239
constitutional monarchy 120, 136
consultation 10, 23, 24, 26–8, 63, 81, 103, 121
cooperative federalism 175–7, 186, 187
coordination 5, 8, 9, 12, 20, 42, 43, 46–9, 54, 71, 83, 85–7, 93, 94, 101, 107, 123, 124, 130, 139, 140, 167, 175–7, 186, 198–200, 205, 215, 217, 224, 236, 237, 239

Corona Commission 126, 128, 130, 216, 224, 225
CoronaVac 69
Coronavirus Action Plan 163
coronavirus-denial 175
Coronavirus Leading Small Group (CLSG) 46–8
Corruption Perceptions Index (CPI) 62, 140
COVID-19 231–3, 235–47; in Brazil 174–87, *182,* **183**; in China 45–53; crisis 4–7; disease guide 67; in Greece 83–95, *85, 90, 93*; helpline 67; in Kenya 101, 105–13; law 218; national responses 18–20, 31–2; in New Zealand 134–7, 139–50; in Norway 123; survey characteristics and overall adherence **183**; in Sweden 211, 215–18, **219–21,** 222–5; in Turkey 59, 66–9, *70,* 71–4; in the United Kingdom 166; in the United States 192, 196–205, **203**
COVID-19 cases and deaths 7, 41, 67, 69, 70, 73, 85, 106, 135, 179, 197
COVID-19 Specialists Committee 84–6, 90, 91
Crawford, Sue, E. S. 9
crisis/crises 4–7, 10–13, 19, 20, 23, 26, 28, 30, 48, 51, 94, 124, 129, 141, 196, 201, 205, 231, 242, 247; communication 20, 49, 123, 200, 222; of democracy 21, 178; management cycle 7; and political power 6, 7; preparedness 215–16
Croissant, A. 241
Cummings, D. 163, 170n8
curfew 67–9, 88, 90, 102, 106–9, 113

Da, S. 50
Debus, M. 243
decentralization 74n1, 121, 129, 143, 164, 174, 177, 192, 193, 237
decentralized response 7, 9, 12, 13, 32, 92, 186, 200, 240
decision-making 8, 9, 12, 28, 42–4, 46, 53, 59, 64–6, 80, 85, 86, 107, 113, 119, 128–30, 136, 139, 141, 143, 149, 157–60, 162–4, 167, 176, 195, 201, 205, 212, 213, 225, 238
declaration of emergency 182
Defense Production Act 204
DeLeo, R. A. 74n2
democracy 8, 21, 30, 41, 45, 65, 80, 127–8, 137, 147, 178, 185, 187, 213, 241
democratic institutions 178, 187
Department of Health and Human Services (HHS) 198
Department of Health and Social Care (DHSC) 163, 164, 169

Department of Prime Minister and Cabinet (DPMC) 139
devolution 102, 104, 158, 175, 178, 205, 233
Disaster Risk Management (DRM) framework 138
District Health Boards (DHB) 142–3
Dotson, J. 48
dual federalism model 175, 176
dualism 19, 120, 178, 212

East Nordic administrative model 212, 224
East–West model 119–20, 212
'Eat Out to Help Out' 165
Emergency Response Law (2007) 48
end to austerity 160
enforcement 60, 72, 74, 92, 101, 108, 109, 140, 147, 218, 222, 242
England 31, 161–8
Epidemic Preparedness Act 2006 (EPA) 139
equivalency principle 124
Erdogan, R. T. 59, 64–6, 68, 69, 71
Ervasti, H. 82
Esaiasson, P. 214
Eurobarometer 65–6
European Union (EU) 18, 157, 197
Eurostat (2018) 66
exclusion 59, 61, 71, 102, 105, 107, 121, 158
expert(ise)/science/scientist 17, 22, 26, 27, 46, 50, 51, 59, 66, 71, 73, 79, 84, 86, 90, 135, 163, 168, 169, 196, 201

fatigue measure 246
federalism 8, 18, 175, 176; Bolsonaro's 175, 176, 178, 186, 187; cooperative 175–7, 186, 187; dual 175, 176; fragmented 199; and policymaking 176–9; in the United States 195
federative pact 175
fiduciary trust 30, 32
financial relief 123, 126, 215, 223
first wave 6, 79, 83–6, *85,* 88, 89, 91, 93, 94, 128, 233, 243
Flinders, M. 162
Four-Level COVID-19 Alert System 135, 141, 142, 145, 147, 150n1
fragmented authoritarianism (FA) 44
Freedom House Index (2020) 65
Freitag, M. 30
Fukuyama, F. 42

General Insurance Scheme 63
Ghersetti, M. 214
Gilson, L. 31
Goble, R. 192
Gofen, A. 244

Government Effectiveness Index 62
government-managed quarantine (MIQ) system 135, 147
Government offices 212–13, 216
Great Britain *see* UK
Greece 79–80, 94, 95, 237; administrative style and trust *93,* 93–4; COVID-19 cases population *90;* first wave 83–6, *85;* frustration and concern 87–91; national responses 20; policy capacity 79, 80, 237; policymaking 85, 87, 95; policy style 79, 80, 93, 94, 95, 237; second wave 91–3
Greek National Health System (GNHS) 82–4, 87, 91, 92
guerilla policy style 44

Hajer, M. 80
Hale, T. 202
Hardalias, N. 86
Health Act 1956 (HA) 139
Health and Medical Services Act 217
health care system 18, 24, 31, 62, 82–3, 130, 142, 175, 196–7, 216, 217
Health Emergency Regulations 47, 48, 52
health experts/advisors 59, 71, 82, 107, 112, 113, 184
Heclo, H. 21
Heilmann, S. 44
herd immunity 160–4, 169, 170n8, 179, 180, 246
Her Majesty's Revenue and Customs (HMRC) 165
HES code 68
hierarchical trust 45, 54, 236
HIV/AIDS 113, 194
H1N1 pandemic 86, 128–30, 198
Holmberg, S. 214
Hooghe, M. 32
Howlett, M. 9, 22, 26, 42, 233, 234, 246
Hubei Province Health Commission 47–8
Huntington, S. 21
Hwang, C. 19
hytte 125

IDEA approach 201
imposition style 10, 27, 59, 236
inclusion 13, 21, 27, 28, 41, 45, 120, 121, 129, 147, 159, 164, 174, 175, 177, 204, 238
inclusiveness 10–13, 27, 28, 32, 41–3, 45, 54, 59, 60, 70, 71, 73, 79, 81, 82, 85, 86, 92, 130, 136, 149, 159, 192, 195–6, 205, 224, 225, 237, 238
Independent Policing Oversight Authority (IPOA) 109
inequality 19–20, 66

infections prevention consumables
(IPCs) 112
Infectious Disease Law 48, 51, 52, 55n8
Influenza – Flu 66, 101, 107, 134, 139,
144, 194
institutional change, 80, 85, 94
intensive care unit (ICU) 62, 83, 84, 87, 91,
106, 134, 162, 183, 184
issue networks 21
institutional trust 45, 175
instrumental trust 30, 32
Italy 18, 19, 67, 83, 84, 86, 162, 179, 184,
243, 246

Jacobs, L. 52
Johansson, B. 214
Johnson, B. 160, 167, 168, 180
Jordan, G. 21, 158, 233, 234, 238
Justice and the Development Party (JDP)
59, 61–5, 70, 73

Karokis-Mavrikos, V. 237
Kenya 101–2, 106–8, 112–13; economic
relief and recovery measures 109–11;
healthcare system in **104,** 104–6;
opportunism 111–12; policy capacity
234; policymaking 101–3, 113; policy
style 101, 108, 111, 113, 237; stringent
enforcement 108–9
Kenya Medical Research Institute
(KEMRI) 107
Kenya Medical Supplies Agency (KEMSA)
109, 111, 112
Kenyatta, J. 102
Kenyatta, U. 103, 106, 107, 109–12
Kettl, D. F. 18
Khadiagala, G. M. 110
Kibaki, M. 102, 103
Knill, C. 24
Kristinsson, G. H. 129
Kristoff, N. 42

Lægreid, P. 120, 123, 127
Lampton, D. M. 55n4
Law Commission 138
Law on the Prevention and Treatment of
Infectious Diseases (1989) 48
leadership 6, 8, 20, 41–3, 45, 49, 94, 103,
111, 136, 141–5, 159, 160, 176, 187, 194,
200, 205, 238
Leading Small Groups (LSGs) 43
Lee, S. 19
legitimacy 6, 11, 32, 43, 71, 86, 119–21,
137, 147, 149

Levi, M. 31
Lieberthal, K. G. 55n4
Lijphart, A. 61
Li, L. 45, 54–5n2
Li Wenliang 52, 53
local authorities 44, 45, 89, 120, 122, 129,
164, 167, 170, 186, 216, 238
Local Government Act (1992) 121
local level 20, 59, 83, 89, 92, 119, 121, 123,
129, 160, 163, 167, 187, 216, 224, 225, 238
lockdown 6, 8, 9, 11, 12, 19, 32, 42, 48, 52,
69, 71, 83–95, 101, 106–9, 113, 125, 126,
128, 129, 135, 138, 139–42, 144–8, 157,
160–9, 175, 179–81, 202, 211, 218, 231,
245, 246
Lotta, G. 244

macro-relationships 31
Mahoney, J. 85, 94, 95
majoritarian model 61
managerial policy style 7, 13, 129–30, 213,
224, 238–40
Marien, S. 32
Matthíasson, P. B. 129
measures *see* stringency of measures
medical associations 63, 73
Mei, C. 19, 45–7
Meng Xin 50, 51
Mertha, A. 44
micro-relationships 31
Micro, Small, and Medium Enterprises
(MSMEs) 109, 110
ministerial model 119, 120, 212, 237
Ministry of Health (MoH) 59, 63, 66–8, 71,
74n1, 82, 105, 125, 142, 146
Ministry of Health and Care Services
122, 125
Ministry of Interior 59, 61, 71, 82, 107
mitigation strategy 144
Mitsotakis, K. 83
Möllering, G. 30
monitoring 20, 44, 52, 67, 82, 88–92, 169, 245
Moon, M. J. 19
multi level governance 123, 124
municipalities 53, 64, 88, 121, 125, 175–7,
181, 184, 186, 215, 216, 224, 225

National Board of Health and Welfare
(NBHW) 216, 222
National Coordination Committee on the
Response to the Coronavirus Pandemic
(NCCRCP) 101, 107
National Health Commission (NHC)
46–50, 53

National Health Preparedness Plan 123
National Health Service (NHS) 159, 162–4, 166–8
National Hospital Insurance Fund (NHIF) 105
National Institute for Economic Research (NIER) 223
National Public Health Organization (NPHO) 85, 86, 88, 89
national responses 5–14, 18–20, 29, 31–2, 46, 79, 80, 120, 123, 126, 128, 129, 136, 142–5, 211, 215, 224, 238, 244; Finland 128; Greece 20; Iceland 128; New Zealand 142; Norway 128; Sweden 215; Turkey 20; UK126
Newton, K. 30
New Zealand 134–6, 149–50, 150n1; communication 141–2; disaster management in 138–40; elimination strategy 135, 141, 144, 147, 148; human life, value of 144–5; legal context 136–8; lockdown 145; national responses 142; Parliamentary power 137; policy capacity 149, 235; policy style 136–49, 238; quarantine 146; recovery plans 147–9; robust test and contact-tracing system 145–6; "team of 5 million" 146–7; trust, high levels of 140–1
Nordic model 119–20
normalization process 68, 69
Norris, P. 30, 81
Northern Ireland 158, 162, 163, 165
Norway 128–30; contagion mitigation measures 125–6; Corona Commission 128; crisis management in 124; data and method 123; financial support 126–7; health sector 124; labor market policy 126; national responses 128; policy capacity 129, 235; policymaking in 119–22, 126, 129, 130; policy styles in 119–20, 129–30, 233, 237, 238, 240; preparedness 123–5, 124; trust 127–8
Norwegian Directorate of Health (NDH) 122, 125
Norwegian Institute of Public Health (NIPH) 125, 126, 129
Norwegian Labor and Welfare Administration (NAV) 127
Norwegian Ministry of Finance 129
Norwegian Ministry of Health 124
Norwegian Ministry of Justice and Public Security 125
Nyong'o, A. P. 102

Obama, B. 194, 198, 199
Officials Committee for Domestic and External Security Coordination (ODESC) 139
Olsen, J. P. 130
Ostrom, E. 9
Oxford COVID-19 Government Response Tracker 232
Ozbudun, E. 63

pandemic: 3–14, 18–20, 41, 42, 45, 54, 59–74, 79, 83, 85–8, 91, 93, 101, 102, 106, 107–13, 119–30, 134–6, 139, 141–6, 148, 149, 150, 157–62, 165–9, 174–87, 191–205, 211–25, 231–47; boards 67; as drama 5; response plan 85, 180, 200
Pandemic and All-Hazards Preparedness Act (PAHPA) 194
parity principle 215
parliament 21, 26, 61, 64, 65, 103, 111, 120, 121, 127, 159; New Zealand 137
Parsons, S. 170n9
Pei, M. 47
Perry, E. J. 44
personal protection equipments (PPEs) 6, 110–12, 182, 199, 216
Peters, B. G. 10, 27, 62, 102, 191–3, 195
Pew Research Center 196
Pew Research Survey 66
Pierson, P. 176
police 17, 53, 68, 69, 94, 108–9, 113, 147, 244
policy capacity 10–13, 26–8, 32, 41, 43, 45, 54, 60–3, 79, 80, 87, 88, 90, 94, 129, 149, 159, 174, 192–5, 204, 234–7, 239; Turkey 60–3, 73; United States (U.S.) 93–5
policy community 21, 22, 82, 158
policy feedback 93, 94, 121, 243
policy implementation 11, 17, 24, 28, 63, 121, 174, 177, 180, 242, 244
policy learning 19, 136, 241, 243–4
policymaking 4, 6, 7, 9, 10, 13, 231–3, 236–9, 244–7; in Brazil 175–9, 187; in China 41, 42, 44, 54; in Greece 85, 87, 95; in Kenya 101–3, 113; in Norway 119–22, 126, 129, 130; in Sweden 212–13, 224, 225; in Turkey 59–63, 70–3; in the United Kingdom 25, 157–60, 164, 166; in the United States 191–5, 204, 205
policy memories 45
policy style 4, 7, 9–14, 11, 17–32, 158, 169–70, 231, 233, 234, 241–2, 244–7; accommodative 10, 13, 120, 238, 240; administrative 7, 13, 59, 71, 73, 74,

79–83, 239, 241; adversarial 13, 41–3, 130, 157, 164, 166, 169, 170, 172, 240; in Brazil 176, 177, 179–87; China and 13, 41–55, 236; concept of 22–8; dimensions of 28; effects of 11, 13; Greek 79, 80, 93, 94, 95, 237; in Kenya 101, 108, 111, 113, 237; managerial 7, 13, 224, 238, 240; in New Zealand 136–49, 238; in Norway 119–20, 129–30, 233, 237, 238, 240; in Sweden 211–13, 224, 233; in Turkey 59, 60, 70, 71, 73, 74, 236–7; typology of *28*; United Kingdom 23, 157–62, 164–9, 233, 238; in the United States 191–7, 200, 201, 204, 205, 239

political leadership 20, 41, 94, 103, 113, 136, 141, 142, 144, 194, 238

political power 6, 7, 61, 63, 80, 233

political trust 3, 4, 7, 9–13, 29, 30–1, 32, 42, 44, 45, 54n2, 59, 60, 65, 93, 95, 127, 130, 136, 140–1, 174, 176, 184, 187, 196, 197, 204, 211, 213–14, 233, 237, 238, 241, 242–3, 244, 245, 247

polycentric governance 119

populism 175

power 8, 11, 19, 24, 29, 43, 44, 61, 62, 80, 102, 103, 129, 136–9

preparedness 5, 7, 14, 66, 87, 91, 107, 123, 126, 134, 139, 163, 193, 194, 198, 215, 216

presidential decree 67

presidentialism 61, 174

Prickett, K. 140

provincial health directorates 68, 71

proximity principle 215

public agencies 80, 120–2, 124, 128, 130, 212–14, 216, 222, 238

Public Health Agency of Sweden (PHAS) 211–18, 222–5

public policy 4, 9, 11, 14, 20, 21, 25, 26, 31, 65, 176, 178, 191, 194, 242, 243, 247

Public Readiness and Emergency Preparedness Act (PREPA) 194

Qian, J. 43

quarantine 46, 48, 49, 67, 69, 72, 124, 135, 146, 157, 181

Reagan, R. 194

referral process 213

representation/represent/representative 4, 5–8, 14, 21, 22, 23, 41, 64, 103, 105, 111, 124, 126, 134, 141, 137, 234

reproduction rate 235, 236, *236*

reproduction rate and COVID-19 235, 236

responsibility principle 124, 215

Richardson, J. 9, 21–4, 27, 74n2, 158, 212, 233, 234, 238

Rosenberg, C. E. 5, 14n1

Rothstein, B. 30, 214

Ruin, O. 212

Rule of Law Index 62, 140

SARS 46, 48, 49, 52

SARS-CoV-2 3

Schrad, M. L. 45

Schroeder, P. 44

Scientific Advisory Board (SAB) 59, 60, 67, 68, 71, 73

Scientific Advisory Group for Emergencies (SAGE) 163, 166

Scotland 158, 162, 165

second wave 7, 14, 41, 53, 79, 83, 87, 88, 90–4, 128, 165–7, 169, 170, 214, 223, 225, 233, 237

self-quarantine 101, 106, 146

Shapps, G. 165

Sistema Único de Saúde (SUS, Unified Health System) 175

social inequality 19–20

social trust 29, 45, 160

Sohlberg, J. 214

Solberg, E. 125

special jurisdiction 121, 122

staffing 10, 27, 62, 81, 94, 159

state-owned companies 120

state-society relations 9, 10, 23, 24, 26–8, 60, 63–5, 74, 80

"stay home campaign" 67

Stein, J. 127

Stoker, L. 31

Stolle, D. 30

storting 120

street-level bureaucrats 244, 245

stringency of measures 9, 11, 18, 92, 125, 145, 163, 202–3; daily cases *vs. 161*; daily recorded deaths *vs. 161*; face-covering requirements 203, **203**; lockdown 145; quarantine 146; recovery plans 147–9; robust test and contact-tracing system 145–6; "team of 5 million" 146–7

Sunak, Rishi 165

Supreme Election Council 64

Supreme Federal Court (STF) 175, 186

Sustainable Governance Indicators (SGI) 122

Sveriges Riksdag 218, 223, 224

Swaine, M. 48, 49

Sweden 211; contagion mitigation measures 217–18, **219–21**, 222; crisis communication 222; crisis preparedness 215–16; evaluation 224; financial relief

223; guidelines 224–5; health care sector 216–17; national responses 215; policy capacity 235, 239; policymaking 212–13, 224, 225; policy style 211–13, 224, 233; political trust in 213–14
Swedish Association of Local Authorities and Regions (SKR) 216
Swedish Civil Contingencies Agency (MSB) 215, 216, 222
Swedish Commission on Vulnerability and Security (2001) 215
Swedish Employment Service, The 223
synchronized messages 9
Sztompka, P. 30

Tang, W. 45
Tegnell, A. 222
Thatcher, M. 25, 158
Thelen, K. 85, 94, 95
Tosun, J. 9, 22, 26, 42, 233, 234, 243, 246
transboundary problems 5
travel corridors 165
Trump, D. 178, 198–202, 204, 205
trust 29–30; axiomatic 30, 32; and Brazil 185–7; China 42, 44–54; fiduciary 30, 32; and Greece 89, 90, *93*, 93–4; hierarchical 45, 54, 236; high 12–13, 32, 42, 45, 71, 86, 89–91, 128, 130, 149, 213, 214, 240; institutional 45, 175; instrumental 30, 32; interpersonal 31, 214; Kenya 106, 113; low 12, 13, 42, 60, 71, 72, 79, 84, 92–4, 162, 169, 170, 178, 185, 186, 239, 240, 243; and New Zealand 140–1; and Norway 127–8; political 4, 7, 11–14, 29–32, 42, 44–5, 54n2, 59, 60, 65, 82, 93, 95, 127, 130, 136, 140–1, 160, 174, 176, 184, 187, 196, 197, 204, 211, 213–14, 233, 237, 238, 241–5; in politicians 127, 214, 234, *234,* 237; social 29, 45, 160; and Sweden 213–14; and Turkey 65–6; and the United Kingdom 169–70; and the United States 196–7
Turkey 59–60, 70–4; administrative policy capacity 60–3, 73; to COVID-19 pandemic 66–9, *70;* health care system 62–3; hierarchical/imposition policymaking 72; majoritarianism 61; national responses 20; policy capacity 60–3, 70, 234; policymaking 59–63, 70–3; policy style 59, 60, 70, 71, 73, 74, 236–7; state-society relationship 63–5; trustworthy in 65–6
Turkish Medical Association 71, 73, 74
Tyce, M. 110, 111
"tyranny of the distance" 135

Unbridled Power 137
unemployment: benefits 126, 127; rate 69, 126, 148, 223
United Kingdom (UK) 157, 243; centrifugalism 160–4; first lockdown 164–6; national responses 126; policy capacity 159; policymaking 25, 157–60, 164, 166; policy style 23, 157–62, 164–9, 233, 238; second lockdown 166–7; third lockdown 167–9; trust and 169–70
United States (U.S.) 204–5; administrative policy capacity 193–5; centralization 204; communication 200–2; coordination structure 198–200; inclusiveness 195–6; policy capacity 192, 193–5, 204; policymaking 191–5, 204, 205; policy style 191–7, 200, 201, 204, 205, 239; stringency of measures 202–3, **203**; trust 196–7
University of São Paulo (USP) 181

vaccination/vaccine 66, 72, 82, 92, 157, 168, 180, 184, 186, 194, 197, 199, 200, 232, 242, 243, 245
Van der Schee, E. 31
Van Waarden, F. 24
Vetenskapsforum COVID-19 (VFC) 218

wales 31, 158, 162, 163, 165
Wallensten, A. 222
Wasike, A. 108
wealth 8, 121, 130
Weible, C. M. 17
welfare: state 90, 119, 120, 213, 214; system 121
Westminster model 157–60
West Nordic model 120, 122, 212
Wiggins, R.D. 170n9
Wilkes, R. 45, 54n2
Winter Energy Payment 148
World Health Organization (WHO) 6, 49, 51, 54, 73, 84, 87, 145, 163, 166, 174–6, 179, 180, 201, 216
World Press Freedom (2020) 65
Wu, C. 45, 54n2
Wuhan 46–53, 101, 135, 157
Wuhan Municipal Health Commission (WMHC) 48, 49

Xi Jinping 43, 46–8, 51, 53, 54

Yang, Q. 45

zero COVID vision 218
Zhong Nanshan 46
Zika 174

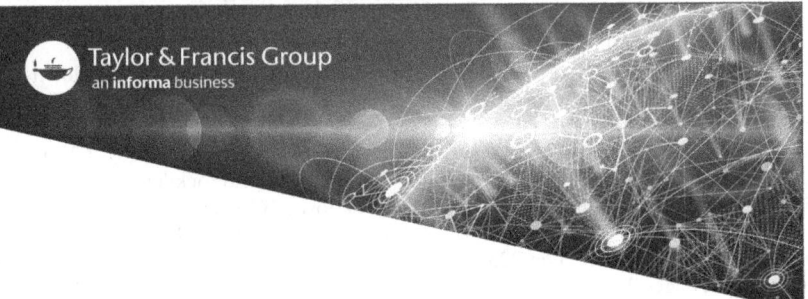
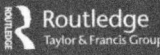
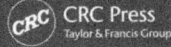